P9-DFJ-718

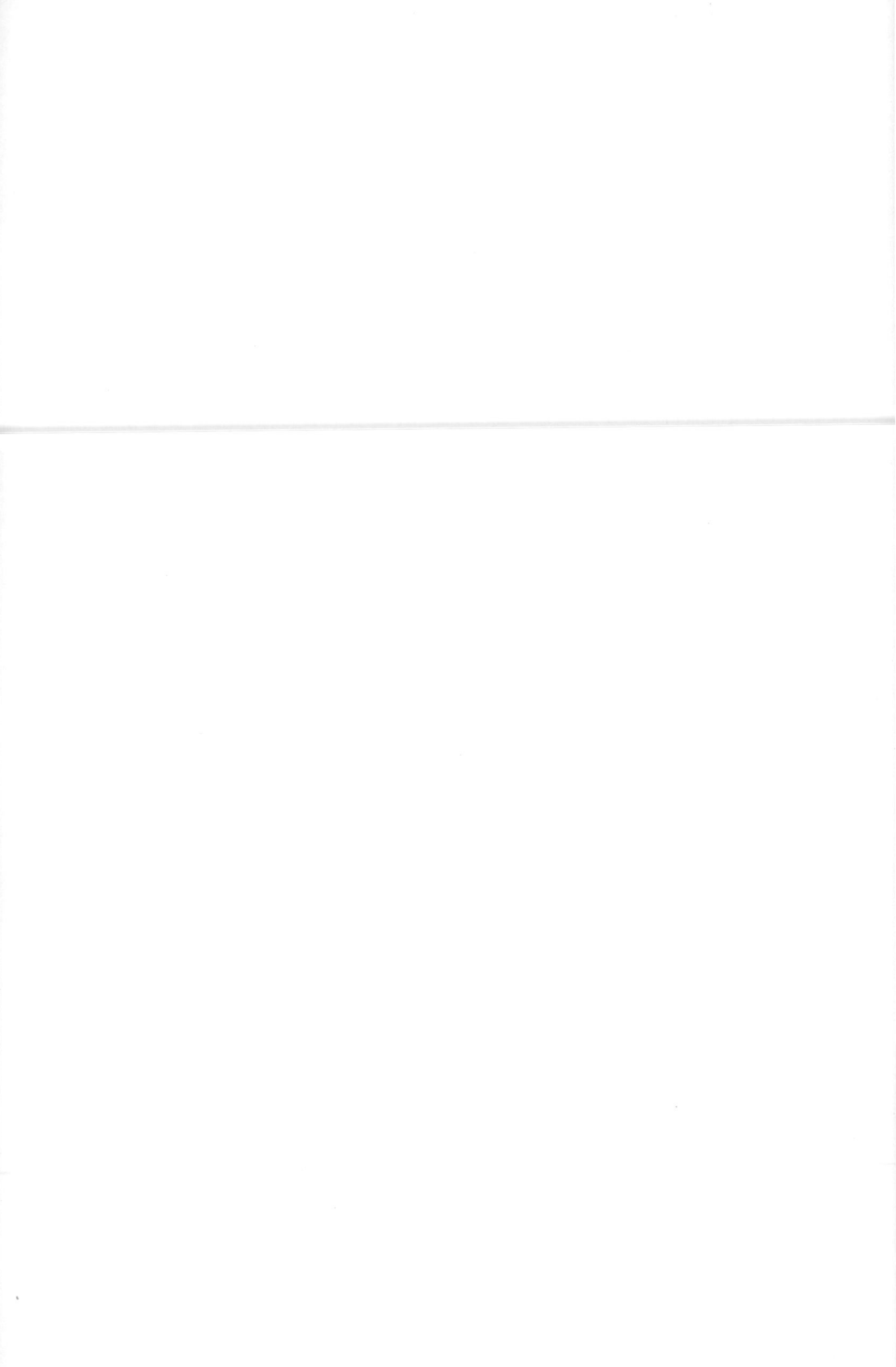

Borderline Personality Disorder

A Clinical Guide

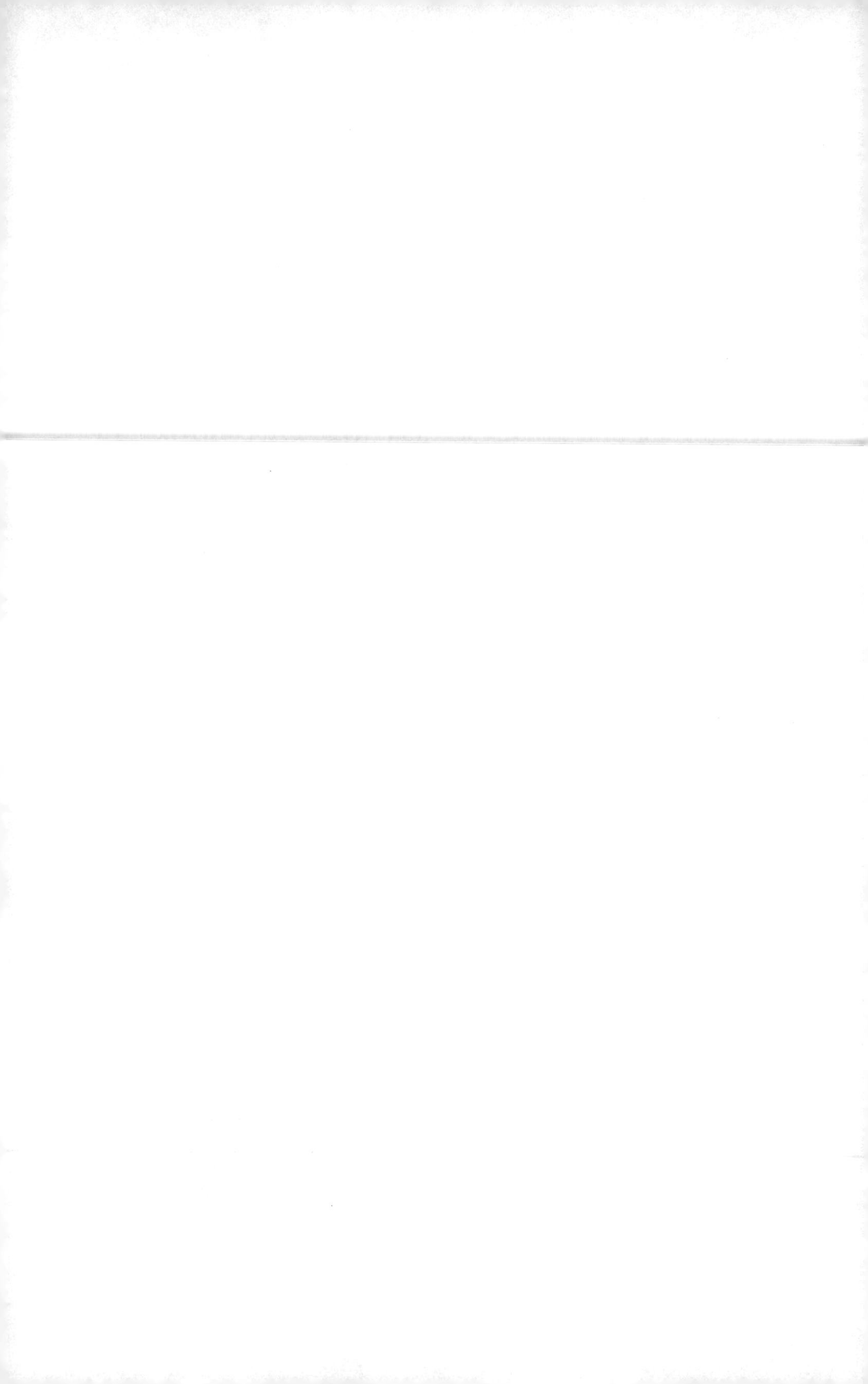

Borderline Personality Disorder

A Clinical Guide

John G. Gunderson, M.D.

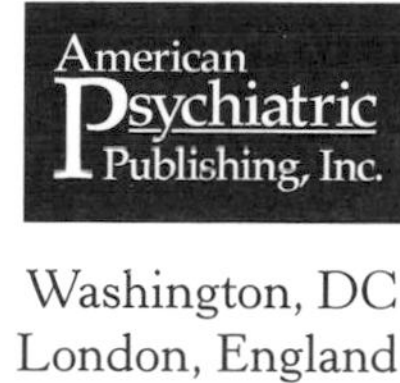

Washington, DC
London, England

Note: The authors have worked to ensure that all information in this book concerning drug dosages, schedules, and routes of administration is accurate as of the time of publication and consistent with standards set by the U.S. Food and Drug Administration and the general medical community. As medical research and practice advance, however, therapeutic standards may change. For this reason and because human and mechanical errors sometimes occur, we recommend that readers follow the advice of a physician who is directly involved in their care or the care of a member of their family.

Books published by American Psychiatric Publishing, Inc., represent the views and opinions of the individual authors and do not necessarily represent the policies and opinions of APPI or the American Psychiatric Association.

Manufactured in the United States of America on acid-free paper

04 03 02 01 4 3 2
First Edition

American Psychiatric Publishing, Inc.
1400 K Street, N.W.
Washington, DC20005
www.appi.org

Library of Congress Cataloging-in-Publication Data
Gunderson, John G., 1942-
Borderline personality disorder: a clinical guide / John G. Gunderson.— 1st ed.
p. ; cm.
Includes bibliographical references and index.
ISBN 1-58562-016-5
1. Borderline personality disorder. 1. Title.
[DNLM: 1. Borderline Personality Disorder. WM 190 G975ba 2000]
RC569.5.B67 G863 2000
616.85′852—dc21 00-056945

British Library Cataloguing in Publication Data
A CIP record is available from the British Library.

Contents

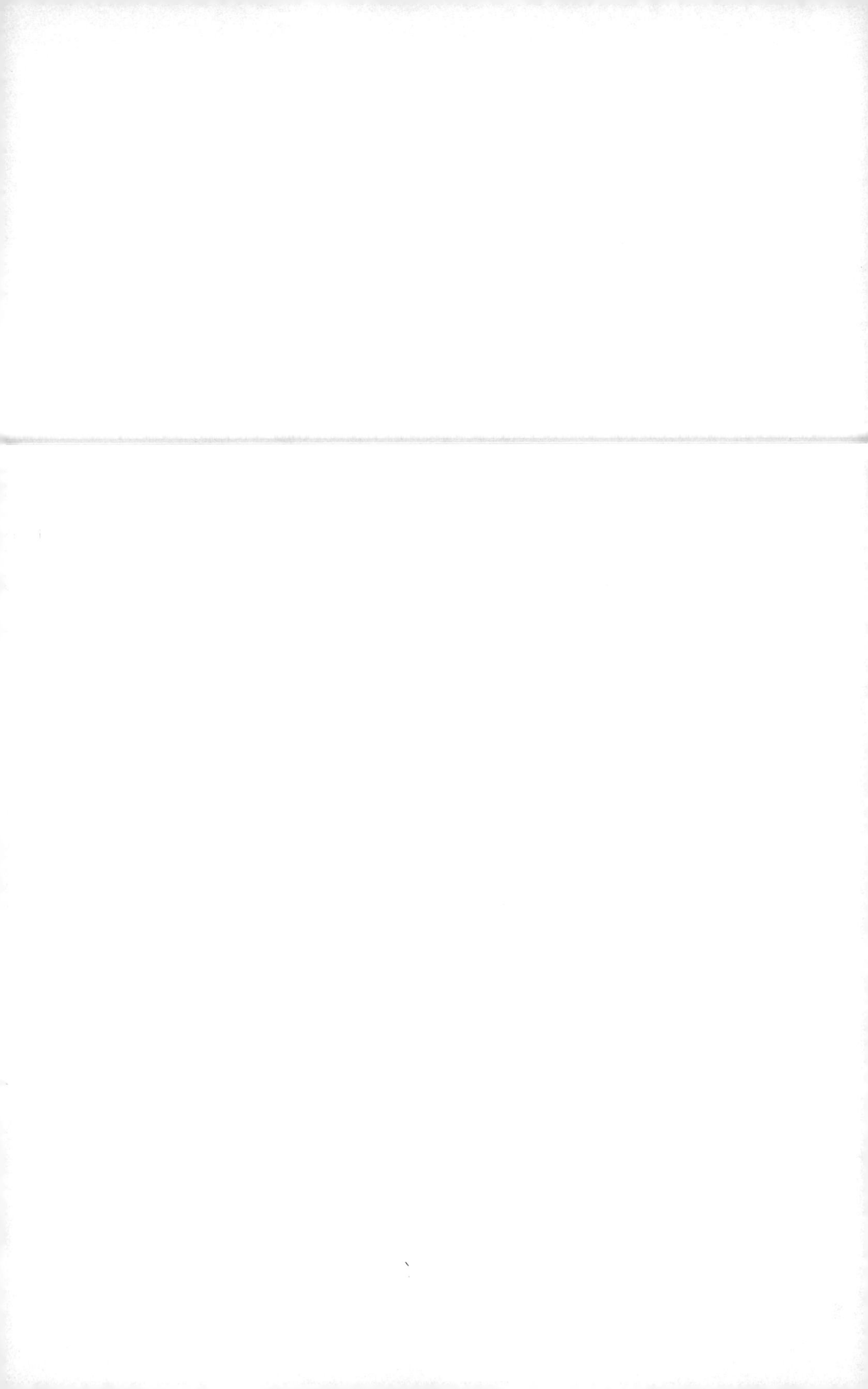

About the Author

John G. Gunderson, M.D., is Professor of Psychiatry at Harvard Medical School. At McLean Hospital in Belmont, Massachusetts, he serves as Director of Psychosocial and Personality Research and of the Outpatient Personality Disorder Service.

Dr. Gunderson has been integrally involved in the diagnosis and treatment of borderline patients since 1969. He has carried out important studies that have helped to define the diagnosis of borderline personality disorder and differentiate the condition from other disorders. He continues to work in advancing effective treatments for borderline patients.

PREFACE

IN 1995 I PROPOSED that the American Psychiatric Association (APA) develop official guidelines for the treatment of borderline personality disorder (BPD). The task force of the APA overseeing such developments weighed carefully the risks of establishing guidelines that would generally lack empirical support against the benefits of such guidelines for improving the standards of care (and diminishing the likelihood of liability to well-meaning but uninformed practitioners). Although the American Psychiatric Association did, happily, decide in 1997 to develop guidelines, I was already so sure that a new and better knowledge base was available that I continued to develop my initial proposal into what has become this book.

This book is a sequel to *Borderline Personality Disorder,* published in 1984. Both books summarize what is or was known—or believed—at the time of publication about treating borderline patients. This book differs from the earlier one in that treatment literature, clinical perspectives, and modalities are far more numerous, sophisticated, detailed, and empirically buttressed. The mushrooming of information, expertise, and specialization is the reason why the 1984 book, though it contains very little that needs retraction, can no longer serve as a sufficient guide for clinicians.

As noted in Chapter 1, my interest in this group of patients began when I was a resident in psychiatry at Massachusetts Mental Health Center. My academic contributions remained primarily descriptive during the 1970s, when my clinical experience was deepened by 7 years as an inpatient administrator. The twin credentials I'd earned from psychoanalytic training and from psychopathology research at NIMH sustained my involvement with what were experienced as very demanding and difficult patients. After the borderline personality disorder diagnosis became official in the 1980 DSM-III, my descriptive contributions had identified me as an "expert" and already assured my involvement with the treatment of borderline patients. Such involvement with these patients expanded throughout the 1980s and often seemed beyond my will to constrain. I was often asked to consult on troubled psychotherapies and at McLean Hospital's full array of clinical services. It involuntarily became my vocation—a career. By the early 1990s I could justifiably say, "Borderline personality disorder is what I do."

When McLean Hospital underwent fiscal crises occasioned by managed care in the early 1990s, I was shorn of my comfortable administrative role as director of its Psychosocial Program. My institutional role now depended even more directly on my clinical skills. It was a blessing of sorts. Since 1994, with colleagues, I've established an outpatient clinic at McLean Hospital for treating borderline patients.

The goal of that clinic, and that of this book, is to combine the advances from research with the practicalities of what is feasible in a managed care environment, given a wide range of borderline patients from diverse socioeconomic and intellectual backgrounds. This clinic experience complements that derived from my prior 7 years as an inpatient administrator, 15 years as a consultant to both cognitive-behavioral and psychodynamic partial-hospital programs, 20 years during which I've averaged more than three consultations a week on referred borderline outpatients, 30 years of supervisory experience, and 25 years and roughly 11,000 hours spent as a psychotherapist. The 6 years spent within my present outpatient clinic setting have concluded my education. What follows in this book is what I have learned.

I ended the 1984 book by referring to the appeal that borderline patients make to others to awaken, examine, and own the dark side of their own nature. This process has not lost its satisfaction for me. Still, my interest in treating borderline patients is no longer sustained by pride in having recognized expertise.I have been able to work capably with borderline patients for many years, but now I can often say, "I like working with them." It may be that aging without being close to so many suffering borderline patients would have taught me the same lessons, but I think my growth in tolerance and understanding of life's terrors and cruelties has been expedited by the companionship of these patients. Like Dr. Seuss's Grinch, my heart has grown a little bigger.

Acknowledgments

Because I was present for the birthing of this diagnosis, I have been in an ideal position to witness and appreciate the growing assembly of fellow clinicians and scientists whose perspectives have invigorated and rapidly increased our knowledge about these patients. So much has been learned that, in writing this book, I have been concerned that I might misunderstand or misrepresent an area of treatment or the contributions of colleagues. Notably, I experienced little concern about this in writing the 1984 predecessor, *Borderline Personality Disorder.*

To diminish the seriousness of my errors or oversights, I've taken advantage of the network of colleagues who have participated in the expansion of our knowledge about the treatments that this book reviews. Each chapter has had the advantage of reviews by two or more of these respected colleagues. Although these reviewers have not always admired the drafts I sent them (one suggested I "get a new author or omit the chapter"), their feedback has invariably enhanced the clarity and credibility of what I now pass on. They are listed below:

John Clarkin
Glen Gabbard
Marsha Linehan
Paul Links
Elsa Marziali
John Oldham
Joel Paris
Chris Perry
Bruce Pfohl
Lloyd Sederer
Larry Siever
Ken Silk
Paul Soloff
Michael Stone
Charles Swenson
Per Vaglum
Drew Westen
Mary Zanarini

Many of the colleagues who have contributed to advances in treatment have done so in so many different ways that I already assume that my citations will be incomplete and my selectivity will no doubt engender interpretation; that's fair, my slights of any colleagues are all unconscious.

In addition, and closer to home, have been the collaboration, instruction, shared experience, and support of the colleagues with whom I treat borderline patients. I refer particularly to Sara Bolton, Jay Bonner, Craig Boyajian, Len Glass, Trudi Kleinschmidt, Elizabeth Murphy, George Smith, and Joan Wheelis. Most have learned enough about me to take pleasure in telling me what I don't know. Each of these colleagues shares my passion for this work, and each brings a unique and complementary perspective to bear on our common interest. They too have each reviewed sections of this book and, even before that, have helped me shape its clinical message.

Finally, thanks to those who helped prepare the manuscript itself. Jason Fogler assisted immeasurably with the typing, the formatting, the organization, and even the substance during this book's preparation. After he departed to study for his Ph.D., this book was adrift until it was brought to shore by the virtuoso skills of Patti Brown. Thanks too for the editorial and technical help generously provided by the staff of American Psychiatric Publishing, Inc.

INTRODUCTION

THIS BOOK IS ABOUT clinical care of borderline patients. It is meant to be comprehensive, covering all the recognized therapies. It details long-term multimodal treatment, with an appreciation that no one modality is ever sufficient. It attempts to include the advances from empirical research and to synthesize them with what I've learned from clinical experience. Above all, it is meant to be useful and practical, primarily for clinicians, but also for patients' families and health care administrators. Although no treatment is excluded from consideration because of its cost, all treatments are considered with issues of cost effectiveness and feasibility in mind. My most ambitious goal for the book is that it improve the quality of care for borderline patients.

The first two chapters cover the issues of the diagnosis itself: what the diagnosis means, the biases that affect its usage, and its primary differential diagnosis considerations. Special attention is given to borderline patients' behavioral specialty: their self-destructiveness. Perhaps the most important message for clinicians is that we do these patients a favor by identifying the diagnosis and educating them (and their families) about it. This observation reflects why this book is written: there is now a great deal that is known about what to do, and what not to do, to treat borderline patients effectively. Patients and families welcome learning what is known, and, as often as not, the success of treatments rests upon their being included as responsible allies.

Although I believe it is essential for clinicians to be guided by a theory that gives them new ways to organize their knowledge about their patients or to understand them, this book does not attempt to provide such a theory. Of the three theories that guide most clinicians—biological, cognitive-behavioral, and psychodynamic—I've been most strongly influenced by and identified with the last. That viewpoint anchors much of this book and may unwittingly prejudice some of what I conclude. Still, as noted in the Acknowledgments, I've tried to avoid such prejudice by seeking critical reviews from experts immersed in other theories. In any event, the theory most central to this book's goals is a theory about therapies.

Chapter 3 offers an empirically and clinically anchored theory on the sequencing of goals (i.e., targets for intervention), on processes of change, and on the modalities that are best suited for a patient's changing needs. It superimposes a logic on treatment planning and, by design, it anticipates the sequence of the chapters that compose the rest of the book.

After Chapter 3, the book proceeds to chapters concerning the implementation of overall treatment plans (Chapters 4 and 5). These chapters emphasize the need for someone to develop the plan, establish an appropriate level of care, and include rehabilitative services that address the borderline patients' typically severe impairments in social functioning. Chapters 6 through 11 describe the specific modalities in a sequence consistent with the length of time needed to meet the primary goals of each modality.

Chapter 4 outlines the primary clinician's responsibilities. In an era when managed care hovers in the background of treatment authorization, and where care of borderline patients moves across multiple settings, it is easy to ignore the central requirement of having some one clinician be identified to all, including the patient, as being in charge—the *primary* clinician.

This chapter introduces a principle that emerges from the current multimodal, multi-treater environment: the *principle of split treatment.* What has been made necessary in this environment is here elevated into a virtue. This book repeatedly points out how a treatment having two or more components not only adds breadth to the treatment goals but also offers a structure that safeguards treatment against the borderline patients' usual intrapsychic splits—that is, it allows a borderline patient who is angry or frustrated by a treater or a therapy to use the second component to *hold,* or *contain,* the patient's angry or fearful elaborations on that experience. Thereby it prevents flight from treatment. This shift flies in the face of the traditional warnings against the dangers created by splits between treaters—splits ostensibly evoked by borderline patients.

Chapter 5 concerns four levels of care. Here empirical evidence is introduced about the potential value of the two most intensive levels: hospital care (level IV) and residential or partial hospital (level III). The four levels are not seen here as competitive but as having different goals, directions, structures, and staffing. Of most interest may be the endorsement given to a newer level of care, intensive outpatient programs (IOPs). IOPs represent a type of level II care that, although not widely available, may be more effective and certainly seems more cost beneficial than the type of partial hospital services to which IOPs offer an alternative.

Reflecting the fact that medications have quietly become the single most widely and uniformly used treatment for borderline patients, two chapters

(6 and 7) are devoted to psychopharmacology. Chapter 6 offers an extensive account of the seemingly irrational in vivo complexities surrounding prescribing medications and then evaluating their effectiveness. In contrast, Chapter 7 offers a rational algorithm to guide selection of medications that should usefully inform prescribing physicians.

Cognitive-behavioral (CB) therapies are on the rise; indeed, dialectical behavior therapy (DBT) has rapidly become the most BPD-specific and empirically substantiated treatment for borderline patients. Unquestionably it is the major advance in therapeutics of the 1990s. Chapter 8 tries both to acquaint the uninitiated with DBT and to place it in some perspective—that is, to see what it does and does not do and how it fits alongside other complementary modalities. Two other notable developments are cited in Chapter 8. One is the potential for short-term CB therapies to be effective for discrete goals. The second is that formal psychoeducation is often valued.

Chapter 9 encourages clinicians to involve families far more than has been customary. It describes how clinicians can use consumer-friendly psychoeducational interventions. Of note is that many interventions, albeit brief and not called therapies, may be very valuable. Of further note is that traditional dynamic family therapies are placed in a late stage of treatment. For most families, parental coaching and assisted problem solving is the primary treatment. Preliminary data that demonstrate the value of such coaching and problem solving are offered. A chapter appendix offers suggested psychoeducational publications, videos, films, and Web sites for families and others.

Chapter 10 underscores the role that interpersonal groups (IPGs) should play in the first year or so of most borderline patients' treatment. This type of treatment is readily exportable and nicely complements the functions served by individual therapies or psychopharmacology by addressing the interpersonal impairment that is central to most borderline patients' disorder. The available empirical evidence underscores the need for more use of and more research on IPGs.

Two chapters are devoted to psychoanalytic psychotherapy, the modality that for several decades was considered the treatment of choice for borderline patients. This modality has itself been the subject of at least 53 books. Chapter 11 argues that the modality should be used selectively, on account of the motivation and aptitude required by both patients and therapists. Otherwise skilled dynamically oriented therapists still need special training and experience, and perhaps special personality traits, to do such therapies well. Chapter 12 delineates the phases of psychotherapeutic progress and change over a period of 4 or more years. Both the corrective power of the relationship and the growth made possible by learning (i.e., insights) are described. The case is made that progress should be ongoing and its absence should be cause for review and consultation. This optimistic message is set against the need for a protracted multiyear process.

The book concludes with Chapter 13's comments about the future. Now that the borderline diagnosis has achieved a secure place in the consciousness of the mental health world, its recognition should be expanded and become established in the public consciousness. The dramatic advancements in treatment for borderline patients described and celebrated in this book can be expected to continue. Beyond some few basic standards for care, it is argued that the adoption of more formal or extensive standards would at this time be stultifying and potentially harmful. The present diversity of theory and research creates a healthy, vibrant vehicle for continued growth.

Borderline patients require an array of clinical services, any of which can be harmful or helpful. All the services can be helpful only if those providing them recognize the borderline diagnosis and if clinicians can capably deploy what is known to make their particular services effective for borderline patients. This book offers guidelines on how to make such services effective. Borderline patients are rarely untreatable, but to treat them effectively requires clinicians with specialized knowledge and training. When such conditions are present, beneficial changes occur that greatly reduce patients' dysphoric mental states and enhance social functioning. As side effects of skilled treatment, there is a concurrent reduction in the burden on borderline patients' significant others, the burden on treaters, and the otherwise enormous public health costs.

1

The Borderline Diagnosis

THE BORDERLINE PERSONALITY DISORDER (BPD) diagnosis entered the American Psychiatric Association's DSM-III in 1980 (American Psychiatric Association 1980) and 12 years later, in 1992, was adapted by the World Health Organization's *International Statistical Classification of Diseases and Related Health Problems,* Tenth Revision (ICD-10) (World Health Organization 1992). The growth in the recognition and use of this diagnosis during the period from 1975 to 1990 has been remarkable. It is easily the most widely and commonly used diagnosis for personality disorders in modern clinical practice (Loranger 1990, Loranger et al. 1997). Individuals with borderline personality disorder constitute about 2%–3% of the general population (Swartz et al. 1990; Zimmerman and Coryell 1989), about 25% of all inpatients, and about 15% of all outpatients (Koenigsberg et al. 1985; Widiger and Weissman 1991).

Origins of the Diagnosis

The origins of the borderline diagnosis, illustrated in Figure 1–1, are usually traced to the clinical observations of Adolph Stern (1938), a psychoanalyst in office practice, who recognized that a subgroup of his patients disregarded the usual boundaries of psychotherapy and did not fit into the existing classification system, a system concerned primarily with dividing psychoses from neuroses. A scholarly review of the work preceding Stern's can be found in Mack (1975). The patient group became somewhat more widely recognized in the early 1950s as a result of several influential papers by Robert Knight (1953, 1954). He expanded the descriptor *borderline* from relating only to the border with neurosis to be equally relevant to the border with psychosis. Like Stern, he began by decrying the "wastebasket" diagnostic status for such patients.

However, he added that failure to identify the unique needs of these patients was responsible for the troubling disagreements between staff members on inpatient units; he further stated that this failure led clinicians to ignore providing the structure such patients needed in order to avoid regressing. After Knight, the term *borderline* to denote troublesome patients who were neither psychotic nor neurotic retained some currency, but primarily within the community of psychoanalysts who worked in hospital settings. (See Sidebar 1–1.)

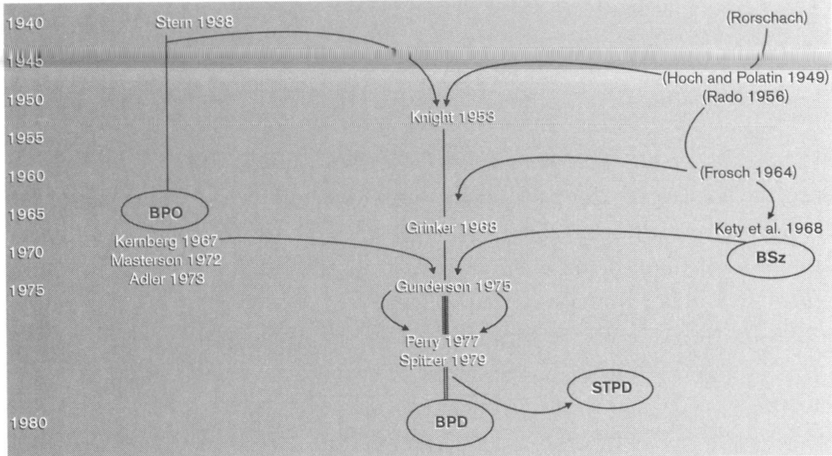

FIGURE 1–1. Development of the borderline construct, I.
BPO = borderline personality organization. BPD = borderline personality disorder. STPD = schizotypal personality disorder. BSz= borderline schizophrenia.

Sidebar 1–1: Where Were the Borderlines Before the Diagnosis?

A review of medical records from Danish and British psychiatric institutions before the diagnosis was used shows that such patients existed (Gunderson et al. 1983; Kroll et al. 1982). Although Freud himself used the term *borderline* only to differentiate delinquent acting-out adolescents from those with neuroses (Aichhorn 1925/1945, Introduction), years later Wolberg (1973) rediagnosed one of Freud's most famous cases, the "Wolf Man," as being borderline. Certainly before the diagnosis, clinicians (Aichhorn 1925/1945; Alexander 1930; Reich 1949) described impulse-driven disorders presaging what was to become the BPD diagnosis. Therefore there is every reason to believe that borderline patients were present in clinical settings long before the diagnosis.

Still, it is possible that what was formerly rare is now far more common. Grinker et al. (1968) suggested that borderline psychopathology is a by-product of social changes during the twentieth century. It is possible that the earlier burdens of manual labor and the earlier restrictions of travel, communication, and leisure time offered the structures, survival activities, and monitors that silently kept such psychopathology in check. Millon (1987) developed a thesis (subsequently elaborated by Paris 1992) about sociocultural causes for BPD that, if taken to its extreme, is consistent with the possibility that BPD would have been far less common in other eras. At present, this thesis can be tested only by epidemiological work showing whether the incidence and prevalence of BPD varies between cultures and their levels of modernity.

Use of the term *borderline* for atypical, clinically troubling cases staggered along in the periphery of psychiatric thinking without notable progress until developments in the late 1960s. At this point, the confluence of three independent investigations forced the questions about a borderline diagnosis into the mainstream of psychiatry's consciousness.

The first of these investigations came from Otto Kernberg (1967). Even as a relatively young man, Kernberg authoritatively added to the psychoanalytic perspective of the borderline construct. He defined *borderline personality organization* as one of three forms of personality organization, to be differentiated from sicker patients, who *had psychotic personality organization*, and healthier patients, who had *neurotic personality organization* (see Figure 1–2). Borderline personality organization was characterized by failed or weak identity formation, primitive defenses (namely, splitting and projective identification), and reality testing that transiently lapsed under stress. Kernberg's scheme was a conceptual advance within the psychoanalytic community by virtue of integrating object relations with ego psychology and the instincts and by virtue of giving a rationale and organization to a basic classification system. However, the impact of his scheme within the larger mental health community derived more from the optimistic therapeutic mandates that he derived from his way of understanding these patients than from the concept itself (see Kernberg 1968, 1975).

The second seminal contribution was provided by Roy Grinker et al. (1968), a senior and respected statesman within American psychiatry. Armored with a brief personal analysis by Freud himself, Grinker had become chairman of psychiatry at the University of Chicago and editor of the *Archives of General Psychiatry.* As one of the early champions of the need for empirical research, and having already made major contributions to studies of depression

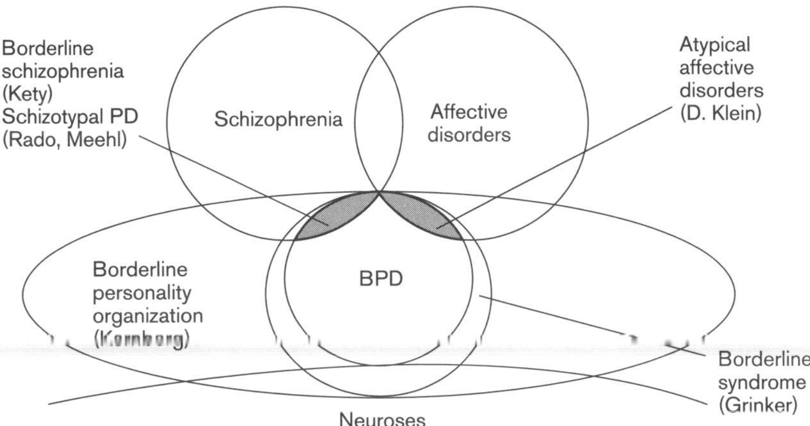

FIGURE 1–2. Concepts of borderline disorders.
Source. Reprinted from Gunderson JG: *Borderline Personality Disorder.* Washington, DC, American Psychiatric Press, 1984. Copyright 1984, John G. Gunderson. Used with permission.

and posttraumatic stress disorder (PTSD), Grinker undertook the first empirical study of borderline patients. With his publication of *The Borderline Syndrome* in 1968, Grinker established the accessibility of this patient group to clinical research methods and offered the first empirically based criterion set. The criteria were 1) failures of self-identity, 2) anaclitic relationships, 3) depression based on loneliness, and 4) the predominance of expressed anger.

The third major investigation to impel borderline patients into the consciousness of the mental health community was not intended to address these patients at all. In the Danish adoption studies that proved to be the cornerstone for establishing a biogenetic basis for schizophrenia, Kety and colleagues were forced to develop criteria by which to identify whether nonpsychotic relatives had schizophrenia-spectrum (i.e., "borderline schizophrenic") disorders (Kety et al. 1968). (Despite the power of adoptive designs to test heritability, the basic prevalence of schizophrenia is so small—about 1%—that it would have taken a nonfeasible number of adoptees to see statistically enhanced rates of schizophrenia per se in relatives.) Hence, the genetic transmission of schizophrenia was established by documenting the higher-than-expectable rates of relatives with "borderline" (meaning atypical) schizophrenia. Once genetic transmission was established, it became critically important to develop replicable ways to identify who these "borderline schizophrenics" were. Although these individuals were subsequently shown to have schizotypal, not borderline, personality disorder (Gunderson et al.

1983), the effect of this work was to stimulate further research interest in the borderline diagnosis and to move the theorizing about such patients into the realms of genetic transmission and biological therapies.

It was in the historical context of these independent investigations—analytic, descriptive, and genetic—that my own contribution began. At Massachusetts Mental Health Center in 1969, I conducted a small study characterizing the diagnostically "wastebasket" patients who most distressed my group of beginning residents. My interest subsequently intensified while at the National Institute of Mental Health (NIMH), where I became aware of the three investigations—and the three primary investigators—cited above. This interest prompted a collaboration with Carpenter and Strauss to disentangle borderline patients from those with a diagnosis of schizophrenia (Gunderson et al. 1975), more important, it prompted the review and synthesis of all the relevant literature in collaboration with M. Singer. That review, *Defining Borderline Patients: An Overview* (Gunderson and Singer 1975), received such surprising acclaim when it was published in 1975 that my involvement was greatly intensified. What followed was the development of a structured interview (Diagnostic Interview for Borderline Patients [DIB]; Gunderson et al. 1981), with which the diagnosis could be made reliably and with which we were able to identify a set of discriminating characteristics (Gunderson and Kolb 1978). These characteristics were used by Spitzer as overseer of the development of DSM-III in a survey of clinical practices and, with the addition of the criterion about identity diffusion that derived from Kernberg, the characteristics were all validated as being the most discriminating in clinical practice (Spitzer et al. 1979). The disorder defined by these criteria narrowed the syndrome from the definitions offered by Kernberg and Grinker (see Figure 1–2). In 1980, the BPD diagnosis, amid considerable controversy, entered the official classification system, DSM-III.

It was official, but what was it?

SHIFTS IN THE BORDERLINE CONSTRUCT: FROM ORGANIZATION TO SYNDROME TO DISORDER

The borderline construct has undergone several major shifts since the 1960s (Gunderson 1994). It was first a personality *organization,* then a *syndrome;* it is now a *disorder* (see Figure 1–2). These three versions of the construct reflect more general epochs within the field of psychiatry, as psychiatry itself has shifted from a psychoanalytic paradigm, to a remedicalization with empirical and pharmacological bases, to the ongoing search for psychiatric diagnoses to convey meaning in terms of specific etiology and specific treatment.

The identification of patients as borderline became very widespread in the United States and elsewhere during the 1970s. As is described in Chapter 3 of this book, this increase in usage was largely due to the optimistic endorsements of ambitious long-term psychoanalytic treatments by Kernberg (1968) and Masterson (1971). What was meant by calling a patient borderline was intellectually tied to borderline personality organization (BPO), an intrapsychic organization that aided psychodynamic clinicians in understanding these patients. In practice, *borderline* usually meant an angry, manipulative patient who was going to be a problem but who might be treated with long-term, psychoanalytically based hospitalizations or psychotherapies.

In the aftermath of DSM-III and the adoption of standardized criteria, the term *borderline* became used by a much wider segment of the mental health community. A study of first admission diagnoses in Denmark showed a dramatic increase in usage of this diagnosis between 1970 and 1985: the increase in Copenhagen was fivefold (Mors 1988). Within academic circles, the borderline diagnosis shifted from intrapsychic organization to descriptive syndrome—that is, a cluster of phenomena that co-occurred with greater-than-chance frequency and that could discriminate borderline patients from other types of patients. The value of the syndromal concept was that it incited researchers to establish the syndrome's meaning through studies of the syndrome's course, genetics, comorbidity, development, and treatment response, and, of course, by demonstrating its discrimination from other disorders in all these areas. It also opened the door to a new array of therapeutic modalities. Figure 1–3 identifies the sequence by which the borderline construct has been refined to include the domains of cognition, affect, impulse, and trauma. The figure also highlights the progression by which a group of enterprising empiricists have added validating evidence with respect to phenomenology, family history, course, treatment response, and development.

Figures 1–4 and 1–5 illustrate the remarkable explosion of publications and research that occurred between 1968 and the 1990s. Of particular note is the parallel rate of growth of published articles, both clinical and empirical, although the number of clinical reports remained nearly ten times as great as the number of empirical studies. The number of books on borderline personality disorder showed a similar logarithmic rise in number up to 1994 (Figure 1–5). Notably, the percentage of those books reflecting a psychoanalytic perspective has steadily declined, from 80% in 1974 to only 23% of those written between 1995 and 1999. Also notable is that the last 5 years has seen a dramatic decline

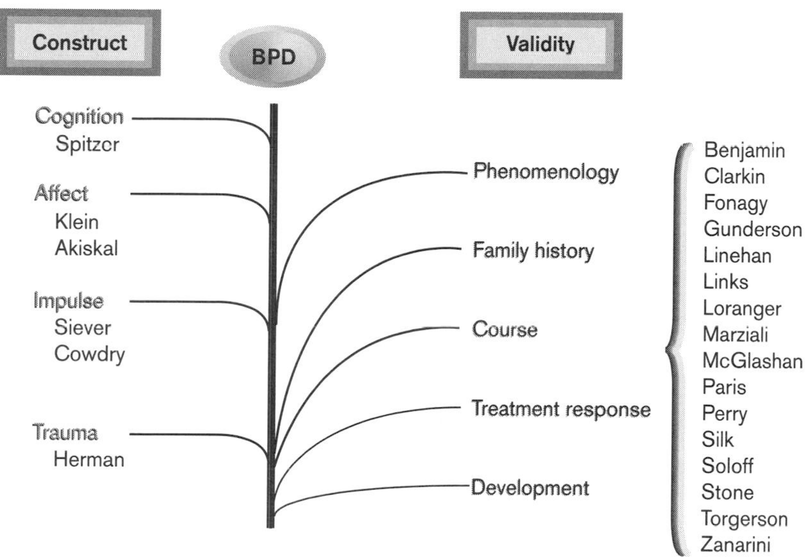

FIGURE 1–3. Development of the borderline construct, II.

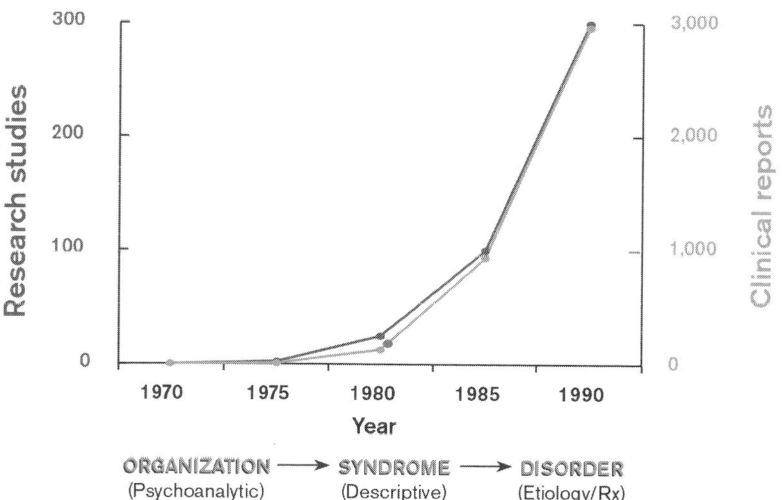

FIGURE 1–4. Number of research studies and clinical reports on borderline personality disorder, 1970–1990.

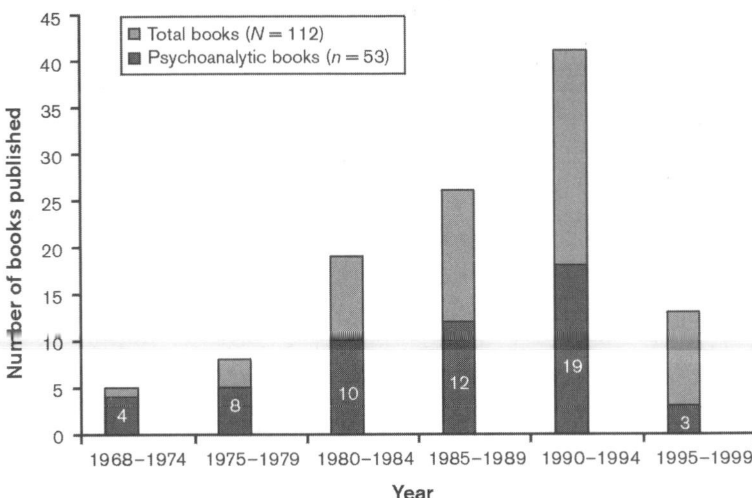

FIGURE 1–5. Number of books on borderline personality disorder, 1968–1999.
Source. Search of Library of Congress database, 1999.

in the number of new books. I think this is because psychoanalytic and other clinical observations have already said most of what they can say. The field awaits a synthesis and implementation of what has been learned, and, as described throughout this book, it awaits advances that are more empirically based.

Since DSM-III, the descriptive characteristics of BPD have been the subject of an enormous amount of research. These studies have demonstrated that 1) there is a high level of comorbidity with Axis I disorders and personality disorders (Chapter 2 of this book); 2) 29 longitudinal studies have shown considerable heterogeneity in course (Grilo et al. 1998); and 3) it is possible to identify subgroups based on defenses, medication response, neurobiological impairment, trauma, and factor analyses. Still, despite these evidences of heterogeneity, the overall results have tended to validate the integrity and clinical utility of the diagnosis. The latter is discussed in Chapter 2; but from a scientific point of view, the validating evidence derives from the following developments:

- Establishing a course that is distinctive from that of either psychotic or depressive disorders
- Demonstrating that few borderline patients resolve into a psychotic or a mood disorder

- Establishing a pathogenesis marked by low heritability (Torgersen et al., in press), family environment with high conflict and unpredictability (Gunderson and Zanarini 1989) and high frequencies of sexual abuse (Gunderson and Sabo 1993; Zanarini et al. 1997)
- Establishing that both modalities and techniques specific to this diagnosis have preferential benefits

Therefore, although boundaries remain blurred into a variety of other diagnostic types (see Chapter 2 of this book), the diagnosis has established itself as a viable disorder awaiting the more conclusive evidence of measurable neuropathology (see Chapter 13 of this book).

AN EXPLICATION OF THE DSM-IV CRITERIA

The DSM-IV criteria set for BPD is changed only modestly from the original in DSM-III. Changes were based on an extensive series of descriptive studies (see Gunderson et al. 1996).

Table 1–1 shows the nine criteria in DSM-IV (American Psychiatric Association 1994) for diagnosing borderline personality disorder, as well as changes in the criteria from DSM-III-R to DSM-IV. The criteria are listed in the table in rank order of their diagnostic value (differing from their order in DSM-IV), and only significant changes are shown. The text that follows is an amplification of each criterion to emphasize its clinical meaning.

1. *Unstable, intense relationships.* This criterion describes the interpersonal manifestations of intrapsychic splitting. A hallmark of borderline psychopathology is the inability to see significant others (i.e., potential sources of care or protection) as other than idealized, if gratifying, or devalued, if ungratifying. Kernberg (1967) is responsible for identifying the importance of the Kleinian construct of splitting for BPD. His theory traces splitting to unmitigated anger, initially intended toward still-needed caretakers. As such, this criterion is developmentally closely tied to the abandonment criterion.
2. *Impulsivity.* This criterion evolved out of the early literature describing the problems within psychotherapies of acting out as a resistance to, or flight from, feelings and conflicts. Empirical studies then found that the impulsivity of borderline individuals is to some extent different from that found in manic/hypomanic or antisocial patients by virtue of its being self-damaging. Thus, the person with BPD who is a substance abuser

TABLE 1–1. DSM-III-R and DSM-IV diagnostic criteria for borderline personality disorder (adapted)

1. A pattern of unstable and intense interpersonal relationships characterized by alternating between extremes of [over]idealization and devaluation
2. Impulsivity in at least two areas that are potentially self-damaging, e.g., spending, sex, substance abuse, reckless driving, binge eating. (do not include suicide or self-mutilating behavior covered in Criterion 5).
3. Affective instability [: marked shifts from baseline mood to depression, irritability, or anxiety] *due to a marked reactivity of mood, e.g., intense episodic dysphoria,* irritability, or anxiety, usually lasting a few hours and only rarely more than a few days)
4. Inappropriate, intense anger or lack of control of anger (e.g., frequent displays of temper, constant anger, recurrent physical fights)
5. Recurrent suicidal behavior, gestures, or threats, or self-mutilating behavior
6. Identity disturbance [uncertainty about at least two of the following: self-image, sexual orientation, goals or career choice, type of friends, values]; markedly and persistently unstable *self-image* and/or *sense of self*[a]
7. Chronic feelings of emptiness [or boredom]
8. Frantic efforts to avoid real or imagined abandonment (do not include suicidal or self-mutilating behavior covered in Criterion 5)
9. *Transient, stress-related paranoid ideation or severe dissociative symptoms*[b]

Note. Text in italics is significant text that was not in DSM-III-R (American Psychiatric Association 1987) but was introduced in DSM-IV (American Psychiatric Association 1994). Text in brackets is significant text that appears in DSM-III-R but does not appear in DSM-IV.
[a]E.g., he or she may feel that he or she does not exist or embodies evil [author's note].
[b]Or depersonalization, derealization, or hypnagogic illusions [author's note].
Source. Adapted from American Psychiatric Association: *Diagnostic and Statistical Manual of Mental Disorders,* 3rd Edition, Revised. Washington, DC, American Psychiatric Association 1994. Also adapted from American Psychiatric Association: *Diagnostic and Statistical Manual of Mental disorders, 4th Edition.* Washington, DC, American Psychiatric Association, 1994. Used with permission. Copyright 1987, 1994 American Psychiatric Association.

would be likely to relapse if angry at his or her AA sponsor or because of that sponsor's absence or unavailability. This one criterion, impulsivity, provides a way of incorporating as symptoms what are otherwise considered distinct disorders (e.g., bulimia and substance abuse). It is not uncommon for borderline patients to substitute one impulse pattern for another—for example, exchanging cutting for purging for abusing drugs. As noted elsewhere, the impulsivity of borderline patients has been considered a basic temperamental disposition and has linked BPD to antisocial personality disorder (see Chapter 2 of this book).

3. *Affective instability.* This criterion developed out of the work of early clinical observers (e.g., Grinker et al. 1968; Zetzel 1971) who were im-

pressed by the intensity, volatility, and range of the borderline patient's affects. As described earlier, such observations prompted D. Klein (1975, 1977), Akiskal (1981, 1985), and Stone (1979, 1980) to propose that the basic psychopathology of borderline individuals involved the same problems of affective regularity found in people with mood disorders—originally depression, now bipolar II disorder. Linehan and other cognitive-behavioral clinicians have adopted the concept of affective dysregulation as the borderline individual's core psychopathology, suggesting that intense emotions propel the behavioral problems (Chapter 7). Such theories have encouraged the testing and widespread use of mood-regulating medications (Chapter 6). Revisions of this criterion since DSM-III have tried to distinguish the affect shifts of borderlines as being more reactive (read "less autonomous") and less enduring than those in mood disorders.

4. *Anger.* As noted, Kernberg (1967) first suggested that the source of borderline psychopathology involved excessive aggression, due either to a temperamental excess or to the infant's response to excessive frustration. The result, whether genetic or environmental, was too much anger, which caused further problems, such as splitting (criterion 1) and self-destructive behaviors (criterion 5). Although the criterion about recurrent suicidality (see item 5 below) reads as if it is easy to observe, it is often not apparent in a borderline patient's presentation.

   The patient's anger can be discovered by the clinician's taking a history or actively inquiring about anger (many borderline patients are aware of feeling angry much of the time, even though they rarely express it); sometimes the anger becomes apparent only after a patient's acting-out behaviors (criteria 4 and 5), which have defended against this feeling, cease.

5. *Suicidal or self-mutilating behaviors.* Recurrent suicidal attempts, gestures, or threats or self-mutilating behaviors are the borderline patient's behavioral specialty. This criterion is so prototypical of persons with BPD that the diagnosis rightly comes to mind whenever recurrent self-destructive behaviors are encountered. The presence of this pattern helps signal concurrent BPD in patients whose presenting symptoms are depression or anxiety (Friedman et al. 1983, 1992). Clinicians must differentiate threats or acts that communicate a cry for help from those that have other motivations (see Sidebar 1–2). The clinical importance of this criterion is described in more detail later in this chapter (the section entitled "How to Explain the Diagnosis").

Sidebar 1–2: Borderline Personality as an Iatrogenic Disorder

Joe Triebwasser had only recently completed his psychiatry residency training at McLean when he wrote a paper bearing the title of this sidebar. Since I was his mentor, he was apprehensive about my reaction. The paper described instances where well-meaning therapists and staffs of inpatient services had unwittingly encouraged patients to get attention and care by raising the red flag of self-harm. As a psychiatrist responsible for administration for these patients, Triebwasser became impatient with the subsequent problems of trying to undo the effects of these naive interventions. He proposed that troubled adolescents or young adults were transformed into diagnosable borderlines by iatrogenic processes. To his relief, I thought the question of iatrogenicity was well founded and his examples compelling.

It is reassuring that the frequency with which mental health services now reinforce self-harm behaviors has greatly diminished as a result of better awareness about these dangers. What remains disturbing, however, is that borderline psychopathology exists without our help and for reasons that still remain difficult to reverse.

6. *Identity disturbance.* This criterion is derived from Kernberg's description of BPO (see the section in this chapter "Shifts in the Borderline Construct"). Since DSM-III, the criterion has undergone modifications intended to differentiate it from the generic identity issues that are normal parts of development, most notably adolescence. The identity disturbance criterion is meant to encompass the body image distortions seen in persons with anorexia or body dysmorphic disorder; more important, it is meant to recognize the pathological disorders of self that are more specific to borderline patients—that is, adults whose values, habits, and attitudes are dominated by whomever they are with to the extent that they feel they have no identity. Here too, the interpersonal context for these identity problems associates this criterion with early attachment failures.
7. *Emptiness.* Early analysts (Abraham 1927; Freud 1908/1959) conceived of an oral phase of development that, if unsuccessfully completed, created a disposition toward adult depression and dependent, object-hungry relatedness. This conceptualization was modified by object relations theorists (e.g., M. Klein 1932, 1946) who suggested that insufficiencies of early caretaking resulted in a failure to introject a soothing other (i.e., an internalized sense of oneself as being cared for), with a resultant in-

ability to self-soothe or to conjure up representations of soothing others. This internal absence leaves the child vulnerable and is theorized to be evident in the subjective experience of emptiness.

The early literature and the widespread use of the DIB (1981) brought this criterion to attention in partnership with boredom (Gunderson and Kolb 1978). Boredom was dropped in DSM-IV because it actually proved more characteristic of narcissistic personality disorder (Gunderson et al. 1996). Its linkage to emptiness in earlier accounts reflects the unclear clinical and theoretical discrimination between these two types of personality disorder (Singer 1977). Emptiness is a visceral feeling, usually in the abdomen or chest, not to be confused with fears of not existing or with existential anguish. Emptiness is an exemplary criterion—discriminating BPD from other types of depression (Westen et al. 1992) and linking the borderline individual's subjective experience to presumed developmental failures. Balint (1992) identified the feeling of "something missing" as the basic fault. Though emptiness is a valuable criterion, recent work has suggested that other aspects of the subjective experience of borderline patients may be equally or even more discriminating (see Sidebar 1–3).

Sidebar 1–3: The Subjective Experience of Being Borderline

Zanarini and Frankenburg (1994) identified the borderline patient's typical "hyperbolic" style, referring to his or her intense, insistent, and dramatic style of communicating feelings and wishes to others. As a sequel, Zanarini conducted a study documenting "the pain of being borderline" (Zanarini et al. 1998). Systematic enquiries of 50 dysphoric feelings and thoughts dramatically underscored her thesis: patients with BPD scored higher than patients without BPD on all 50! Patients with BPD spent far higher percentages of their time feeling overwhelmed (61.7%), worthless (59.5%), very angry (52.6%), lonely (63.5%), or misunderstood (51.8%). More revealing was that some borderline patients reported suffering for high percentages of the time for reasons and in ways that nonborderline patients rarely do: feeling abandoned (44.6%), betrayed (35.9%), evil (23.5%), out of control (33.5%), like a small child (39.1%), and like hurting or killing themselves (44%). The intensity of pain and the amount of time suffering pain reported by borderline patients proves, by itself, easily capable of discriminating patients with BPD from those without. Granted, the borderline sample was newly admitted inpatients, who can be counted on to maximize their reports of pain to garner support, but the results underscore that this disorder involves a terrible way to experience life.

8. *Abandonment fears.* This criterion reflects Masterson's seminal contribution to the borderline construct (Masterson 1972; Masterson and Rinsley 1975). The criterion needs to be differentiated from the more common, less pathological separation anxieties. Although borderline patients are quite aware of abandonment fears, some are so accustomed to acting out in response to such fears that they do not recognize the fears. This criterion was reframed as "intolerance of aloneness" by Gunderson and Singer (1975) and Adler and Buie (1979). Although Masterson attributed this trait to failure in the rapprochement subphase of development (ages 16–24 months), Mahler and Kaplan's (1977) empirical investigation indicated that children can develop these anxieties without noticeable problems in the rapprochement subphase or can fail to develop these fears despite very noticeable rapprochement failures. This criterion is now recognized as a symptom of early insecure attachment (Fonagy 1991; Gunderson 1996).
9. *Lapses in reality testing.* This criterion, added in DSM-IV, is a sharply demarcated derivative of the earlier clinical literature that spoke of psychotic transferences and the potential for psychotic regressing within unstructured treatment settings (see, for example, Hoch and Polatin 1949; Knight 1953). Indeed, speculation about the possible relationship of borderline psychopathology to schizophrenia was fueled by concerns about psychotic regression in unstructured settings as disparate as Rorschach testing and psychoanalysis (see Sidebar 1–4).

   John Frosch (1964) refined the description by distinguishing lapses in a *sense of reality* (not knowing whether one's experience is real) from a generally intact *ability to test reality* (being able to correct distortions of reality with feedback). The lapses in sense of reality that typify borderline patients involve depersonalization, derealization, and hallucinogenic phenomena (e.g., "I thought I heard my mother's voice, so I turned on the lights"). The ability to correct reality distortions would be exemplified by the fact that the patient can turn the lights on and be reassured by the fact that her mother isn't there. The addition of this criterion also ties the phenomenology of BPD to its possible pathogenesis insofar as such lapses in reality testing can be understood as sequelae of childhood neglect and abuse (Shearer 1994a; Silk et al. 1995).

Because the diagnostic system has traditionally set apart psychoses as major mental illnesses, there were reservations about introducing criteria suggesting transient lapses. If such lapses were present, they seemed when DSM-III was written to fit better with preconceptions that a reality-testing criterion was more consistent with the schizotypal personality disorder construct than with BPD. It took the accumulated data from many studies (Table 1–2) to document the presence of such phenomena in samples of patients with BPD.

TABLE 1–2. Prevalence of cognitive/perceptual symptoms in borderline personality disorder samples

Cognitive/perceptual problem	Study[a]	Range (%)
Depersonalization	1, 3, 5, 7, 8, 9	30–85
Derealization	1, 3, 4, 7, 8, 9	30–92
Paranoid experiences	3, 5, 6, 7, 8, 9	32–100
Visual illusions	3, 7, 8	77–88
Muddled thinking	4	52
Magical thinking	5, 6, 9	34–68
Ideas of reference	5, 6, 9	49–74
Odd speech	5, 6	30–59
Disturbed thoughts	2, 9	39–68

[a]Numbers in this column refer to the following studies: 1= Frances et al. 1984. 2 = Pope et al. 1985. 3 = Chopra and Beatson 1986. 4 = George and Soloff 1986. 5 = Jacobsberg et al. 1986. 6 = Widiger et al. 1987. 7 = Links et al. 1988. 8 = Silk et al. 1989. 9 = Zanarini et al. 1990.
Source. Reprinted from Gunderson JG, Zanarini MC, Kisiel C: "Borderline Personality Disorder," in *DSM-IV Sourcebook*, Vol 2. Edited by Widiger TA, Frances AJ, Pincus HA, et al. Washington, DC, American Psychiatric Association, 1996, p. 725. Used with permission. Copyright 1996 American Psychiatric Association.

A CLINICAL SYNTHESIS: INTOLERANCE OF ALONENESS

Aloneness is experienced as a terrifying loss of self (criterion 3) that the person with BPD may defend against by action (criterion 2) or by distorting reality (criterion 9). Aloneness can also be diminished either by the use of transitional objects (discussed in Chapter 12 of this book) or by another person's providing reassuring evidence that he or she cares for the person with BPD.

Identification of intolerance of being alone as one of the defining criteria for the diagnosis of BPD can be traced to the clinical and theoretical contributions of Modell (1963), Winnicott (1965), and Masterson (1972, 1976; Masterson and Rinsley 1975). Modell posited that borderline patients' basic developmental failure involved an inability to cope with the separateness of their caretakers—what Winnicott (1953) had defined as *transitional relatedness*. Masterson emphasized the abandonment fears of borderline patients and the origins of these fears in traumatic childhood separation experiences. The

DIB (Gunderson et al. 1981) operationalized this trait and established it as one of the more discriminating features of the disorder (Gunderson and Kolb 1978). The inability to conjure up representations of absent others (object inconstancy) was subsequently emphasized by Adler and Buie (1979). This intolerance of aloneness and this object inconstancy have been empirically confirmed (Richman and Sokolove 1992). The reason that the BPD diagnosis, so prevalent in clinical settings and now so much a part of the mental health world's consciousness, failed to be identified earlier is, I believe, due to the presenting phenomenology's being extremely dependent upon the interpersonal context. This formulation has been given empirical support in work by Perry and Cooper (1986) and more extensively by Benjamin (1993).

Whereas it was these clinical and conceptual characterizations of adult borderline patients that led to the development of the diagnostic criteria, there have been a sequence of British child analysts who have continued to explicate the childhood experiences that illuminate the pathogenesis of BPD (see Sidebar 1–4).

Sidebar 1-4: British Developmentalists–From Winnicott to Bowlby to Fonagy

Three British child analysts have lent their clinical and theoretical contributions to the understanding of the development of borderline psychopathology. D. W. Winnicott, originally a pediatrician, distinguished himself in the 1950s by his keen clinical observations, by his personal charisma, and by his creative conceptualization of key concepts such as the *holding environment* and *transitional objects.* The concept of the analyst's role as holding–that is, serving as a container for–the borderline patient's aggression has been widely used to understand the functions served by hospitals as well as to understand the need for the clinician's accepting the patient's hostilities without withdrawing. The concept of transitional objects has been picked up within object relations theory and developmental psychology. Modell (1963) used this concept to describe the function that borderline patients need their therapists to serve–that is, as if the therapists were extensions of their patients who lacked separate identities or feelings. This contribution later generated a round of empirical investigations (see Sidebar 11–2).

Bowlby's (1969, 1973, 1980, 1988) primary contributions started to gain influence in the 1970s. He was a child psychiatrist, analytically trained, who systematized his observations of children and thereby established an empirically based and observer-friendly scheme for child development organized around the acquisition of secure attachments. He proposed that all infants possess a basic instinct toward attachment to caretakers. Darwinian adaptations for survival impel infants to evolve interpersonal behaviors that function to maintain their proximity (availability and responsiveness) to a caregiver. Caretaker proximity is required for the development of internal feelings (i.e., by introjection or internalization) of security and lovability. Children whose early attachments were insecure become adults whose interpersonal behavioral adaptations are developed in response to inconsistent, absent, or frustrating caregivers. Ainsworth et al. (1978) later developed the Strange Situation experiment assessing toddlers' response to separation from their caregivers. She operationalized subtypes of insecure attachment. One pattern called *anxious/ambivalent* includes the need to check for caretaker proximity, signaling the need to establish contact by pleading or other calls for attention or help, and clinging behaviors. This pattern can alternate unpredictably with a different subtype of attachment pattern called *disorganized/disoriented* (Main and Solomon 1990), consisting of the denial of dependent needs, the apparent absence of separation anxiety, and a reluctance or fearfulness about becoming attached. Such behaviors, intermittently present in many patients with BPD, develop in response to primary caregivers who are depressed, disturbed, or abusive (Crittendon 1988; Main and Hesse 1990)–qualities that unfortunately are common in the childhood caretakers of many borderline patients (Gunderson and Zanarini 1989; Links 1990). This alternating attachment pattern is believed to be the core psychopathology for borderline patients by me (Gunderson 1996) and other clinician-scientists (Adler and Buie 1979; Benjamin 1993; Fonagy 1991; Perry and Cooper 1986).

Fonagy's influence is only beginning to be felt, and, although it is premature to place him alongside Winnicott and Bowlby, his work extends their contributions in creative and significant ways (Fonagy 1991; Fonagy et al. 1995a, 1995b, in press). Fonagy has added specificity and detail to the parent-child interactions that beget those anxious/ambivalent or disorganized/disoriented forms of insecure attachment typical of borderline patients. Specifically, Fonagy et al. (1991) used the Strange Situation experiment to identify parental misunderstandings (i.e., misattributions) of the child's internal states. Thus a caregiver who misperceives a frightened child and labels his or her feelings as angry, or who misconceives a child's normal attention seeking as being demanding, will respond in ways that impair the child's capability to develop stable and realistic concepts of himself or herself–that is, to capably "mentalize" their own and others' intentions, desires, or feelings. Fonagy has shown that this capability to reflect or mentalize is reliably measurable (Fonagy and Target 1987) and that it corresponds in a predictable way with a child's attachment status. He proposes that BPD develops in children who acquire only a limited capacity to depict feelings and thoughts in themselves and in others (Fonagy 1991, 1995a). His work essentially begins to chart the mental consequences of disturbed early attachments; it promises to clarify the mechanism of intergenerational transmission, to build bridges between cognitive and dynamic theories, and to identify improved therapeutic strategies for borderline patients (see Chapters 8 and 12).

Table 1–3 shows how borderline patients' feelings of being securely held, threatened by separation, or alone in relation to their primary object (i.e., their needed other) account for changes in their clinical phenomenology.

When the person with BPD feels cared for, "held," he or she appears like a depressed waif—easy to sympathize with, grateful for signs of care, and, like a healthier neurotic patient, receptive to therapeutic interpretations. Symptoms like depression, eating disorders, substance abuse, or PTSD often become the focus of therapy.

TABLE 1–3. How BPD patients' perceived attachment relates to borderline personality disorder phenomenology

Interpersonal context	Phenomenology	Others' responses	Clinical implication
Held/idealizing	Empty, dysfunctional, symptomatic	Sympathetic	Collaborative; interpretations; patient needs expressive, involving therapies
Threatened/devaluing	Angry, self-destructive pleas for help	Scared, guilty, angry	Confrontations; patient needs social supports, behavioral change
Alone	Terrified, dissociated, paranoid, substance-abusing, promiscuous	Rescue, avoid	Words unimportant; patient needs containment, medications

Source. Adapted from Gunderson 1984.

When the person with BPD is confronted with the potential loss of the caring, holding other, a different set of clinical phenomena becomes evident—phenomena that link the theme of intolerance of aloneness to the DSM-IV criteria for BPD. Now, prompted by fears of abandonment, the angry devaluation or the self-injurious behaviors become apparent, often with unexpected suddenness and intensity. The self-injurious behaviors may be potentially lethal, indicating a readiness to die unless the person whose absence is threatened, or someone new, establishes that he or she wants the person with BPD to live. Often, this involves not leaving the person with BPD or otherwise rescuing him or her. This sets in motion a characteristic dilemma in the other: the other feels guilty about any impending separation from the person with BPD but finds the prospect of staying very distasteful.

When the person with BPD feels that he or she is without a caring other, without a holding environment, a third set of clinically significant phenomena becomes evident. The experience of aloneness leads to a loss of a sense of reality (dissociative or hallucinogenic symptoms) or to paranoid ideation (which conjures up a malevolent other, a situation preferable to being alone). Alternatively, the experience of aloneness is obviated by desperate object-seeking behaviors (e.g., promiscuity), often made possible by the disinhibiting influence of alcohol or other drugs.

This formulation of intolerance of aloneness as the central or core psychopathology of borderline patients contrasts with dynamic formulations that give equal emphasis to borderline patients' fears of too much closeness—that is, fear of "fusion" (Lewin and Schulz 1992). In my view, when fear of fusion is equal to or greater than fears of aloneness, the patient is more likely to have predominantly schizoid or narcissistic psychopathology. The formulation offered here is consistent with Fairbairn's (1963) thesis (and subsequently Bowlby's) that humans have an innate drive for attachment; they are biologically object seeking.

It is only by longitudinal and interpersonally focused observations that these changing phenomena become evidence of a single underlying pathological process. Descriptive psychiatry has been too cross-sectional and too distant to see the interpersonal patterns. Psychoanalytic psychiatry has been too single-case–based and interpersonally intimate to identify the phenomenological pattern.

Misuses of the Borderline Diagnosis

Controversies persist within the mental health community about the borderline diagnosis. It is easy and not uncommon to misuse this diagnosis, and this possibility remains in large measure a result of the emotional responses such patients engender.

There are reasons for the overuse of the diagnosis, starting with the breadth of Kernberg's construct of borderline personality organization (BPO) and the value that his conceptualization retains for psychodynamic therapists. Notwithstanding the merits of his contribution, there is also a deep skepticism within the psychoanalytic community about defining diagnoses by external, observable (read "superficial") phenomena. Mental health professionals, whether analysts or not, whose primary identity lies in doing dynamic therapy may still use the borderline diagnosis for all "primitive characters" who show immature defenses like projection and acting out.

Occasionally, overuse can even come from the managed care environment. Little time is afforded for extended evaluations, and clinicians must identify diagnoses early on to justify their costs. From this perspective, it is convenient—as well as usually correct—to identify anyone who has carried out repeated self-destructive acts or who is an inappropriately angry young woman as "301.83" (the DSM-IV diagnostic code number for BPD).

One reason for underuse parallels the first source of overuse noted above. Some psychiatrists believe that the foundations of our diagnostic system should be more biologically based than is the borderline diagnosis. They believe that dynamic considerations are superficial and that the major therapeutic importance of diagnosis is to guide pharmacotherapies. This perspective can be inferred from the proliferating studies of bipolar II disorder, where "comorbid" (or overlap with) BPD has not, to my knowledge, yet been assessed. Offsetting this tendency, the borderline diagnosis remains useful for most biological psychiatrists because of its role in explaining patients with mood disorders who prove resistant to medications.

A second source of underuse is more subtle. Distinguished mental health professionals have suggested that the borderline diagnosis is pejorative (Vaillant 1992; Jordan et al. 1991). They argue that the diagnosis is primarily used by clinicians to label patients they don't like. After that, the critics split in their reasoning. Vaillant argues that just because you dislike a patient, you should not label him or her borderline (see Sidebar 1–5). Stiver (1991) and others from the Stone Center argue that the label misleadingly conveys that the patients are angry and manipulative and that it therefore interferes with a clinician's empathic availability for patients who are often better conceptualized as trauma victims. They are joined by Heller (1991), who argues that because the borderline label "implies a character problem," it causes doctors and therapists to shun patients with BPD rather than provide proper—meaning in Heller's view pharmacological—therapies. Both the Stone Center and Heller agree that the BPD label assigns too much accountability for socially undesirable behaviors.

Sidebar 1-5: "Wisdom Is Never Calling a Patient Borderline"

Beginning in 1974, George Vaillant entertained audiences with a talk by this name that eventually found its way to publication (Vaillant 1992). His thesis that the label *borderline* is used by clinicians for patients they don't like captures an unhappy truth–most clinicians don't like borderline patients. More to the point, most clinicians don't like patients who are angry, critical, rejecting, mocking, or even contemptuous toward them. Vaillant is right. Such attitudes don't warrant being diagnosed as borderline. Disliking a patient–that is, a hostile countertransference–isn't a reason to make the borderline diagnosis; it's a reason to understand one's reaction. Such reactions may, of course, occur because your narcissism is hurt. It may also be that you're a participant in a complicated process in which mutual hostilities are being provoked, a process that may signal the activities of someone with borderline personality disorder. Ironically, Vaillant couldn't give this talk, or even write his paper, without making ongoing reference to "his" borderline patients–thereby offering testimonial to the many positive ways the label guides his clinical work. Vaillant's wit, this time, surpassed his usual wisdom.

There is an alarming tendency for clinicians who are working within institutional settings—for example, hospitals and outpatient clinics—to underuse the borderline diagnosis. Zimmerman and Mattia (1999) showed that clinicians in a private practice group at the Rhode Island Hospital outpatient psychiatry clinic diagnosed BPD in only 0.4% of the patients, whereas, when a similar sample of patients was given structured interviews, the frequency rose to 14.4%—36 times as great! The authors argue that clinicians typically give priority to Axis I diagnoses and treatment, leaving insufficient time for Axis II assessments. Consistent with this conclusion is the much lower use of the BPD diagnosis in state mental health facilities than in nonstate facilities (Oldham and Skodol 1991). I believe this conclusion is true but that the underuse may have even more to do with a strong bias toward diagnosing and offering treatments for only what managed care payers and biological psychiatrists deem treatable.

THE BEHAVIORAL SPECIALTY: SELF-INJURIOUS BEHAVIOR

When John Mack (1975) called for a "behavioral specialty" to establish the borderline diagnosis, self-injurious behaviors offered a vivid and distinctive exemplar. Such behaviors are found in about 75% of borderline patients (Clarkin et al. 1983; Gardner and Cowdry 1985; Gunderson 1984; Zisook et al. 1994). In a sample of inpatients, 33% reported current actual plans to kill themselves (Zisook et al. 1994). The frequency with which self-*destructive* behaviors occur (e.g., unprotected sex with strangers, drinking while taking Antabuse) would increase this rate into the 90% range. Self-*injurious* behaviors, most often cutting (80%), but also frequently bruising (24%), burning (20%), head banging (15%), and biting (7%) (Shearer 1994b), are the most common symptoms by which people with borderline personality disorder come to clinical attention. For most people, and certainly for school counselors, clergy, friends, and family, the evidence of willful self-harm is an alarming indication of suicidal intentions. Indeed, such self-injurious acts often occur in people who have histories of suicide attempts (62%), with an average frequency of about three attempts. Moreover, the presence of a history of self-injurious behaviors doubles the likelihood of suicide (Stone et al. 1987). Of note is that a growing body of empirical evidence suggests that the likelihood of suicidal behaviors is not related to comorbid depression (Soloff 1994; Zanarini, personal communication, May 2000); is related (Brodsky et al. 1997; Shearer et al. 1990; Stone 1990) or is not related (Zweig-Frank et al. 1994) to childhood abuse; and may be related (Stone 1990) or may not be related (Fyer et al. 1988; Soloff et al. 1994) to comorbid substance abuse.

Judgments about the potential lethality of behavior(s) and the decisions about how best to respond are by no means simple matters. Indeed, the reasons for self-injurious behaviors are variable (see Table 1–4). A patient struggling with her impulse to cut wrote:

> I want to cut. I want to see pain, for it is the most physical thing to show. You can not show pain inside. I want to cut, cut, show, show. Get it out. What out? Just pain.

It is clearly here an expression of pain intended to be responded to. In recent years, this wish to communicate one's pain by self-mutilative behaviors has occasionally rendered this symptom socially contagious (see Sidebar 1–6). Yet it is unsafe ever to assume that self-mutilative behaviors are merely attention-getting. Chapter 4 of this book resumes a discussion of clinical management issues surrounding these behaviors. Chapter 7 of this book describes a behavioral therapy specifically targeted at diminishing such behaviors. Chapter 8 of this book offers suggestions to families and other nonprofessionals about how they can respond helpfully.

TABLE 1–4. Functions of self-injurious behavior

Function	% of patients
To feel physical pain—to overcome psychic pain	59
To punish self for being "bad"	49
To control feelings	39
To exert control	22
To express anger	22
To feel—to overcome numbness	20

Source. Adapted from Shearer 1994b. Used with permission.

Sidebar 1–6: Cutting: Social Contagion or Serious Disorder

In an article entitled "Cutting," published in the July 27, 1998, *New York Times Magazine,* Jennifer Egan (1998) suggested that cutting is an extreme expression of the same impulses that are making tattoos and piercing contagions among modern adolescents. Indeed, she noted that several communities have witnessed an epidemic of cutting among adolescent girls. This sociological perspective is an extension of Favazza's scholarly examination of the social and historical context for self-mutilation (Favazza 1996). He introduces his book by speculating that the remarkable lack of attention given to this widespread and long-standing aspect of human behavior reflects the horror and shameful fascination such behaviors hold. He notes that cutting was identified as the work of evil spirits by Jesus, who performed an exorcism, and that ritualistic cutting has been documented in various religions or other subcultural practices since the 13th century. He estimates that about 2 million Americans self-mutilate (about 750 per 100,000). Favazza develops a thesis that whether self-mutilative acts are culturally sanctioned or are the products of personal anguish, they often help relieve pain and that their adaptive, life-enhancing qualities deserve recognition. The danger of this sociological perspective is that it minimizes the personal and clinical significance usually attached to cutting. In modern cultures, it is far more common that self-mutilative behavior begins as a private act of desperation, reflecting either an inability to communicate in words or a failure of words calling for help to evoke the needed response. Not all those who self-mutilate have borderline personality disorder, but many do, and all need to be taken seriously. Because the diagnosis of BPD underscores a serious, long-standing mental health problem, the diagnosis should not be offered too readily to anyone who cuts or otherwise self-mutilates. However, the diagnosis should never be excluded because "we didn't want to believe it was serious." The latter response is likely to evoke further alienation and more serious acts of self-destruction.

Repeated self-destructive acts by any patient should alert clinicians to the fact that the acts may *not* be suicidally intended. Such self-destructive acts are usually done for self-punitive reasons (Shearer 1994) and are sometimes associated with an experience of relief from painful or intolerable affective states (Soloff et al. 1994), but these acts are also performed with progressively greater awareness of the controlling effects that such acts have on significant others. Indeed, the power that self mutilative behaviors have on others is probably the reason that it can become contagious in adolescents. Follow-up studies show that, in fact, about 8%–9% of borderline patients commit suicide (Perry 1993) and that the suicide rate is particularly high among those with comorbid substance abuse (Stone 1990). This rate is about 400 times the suicide rate in the general population (about 0.01%) and more than 800 times the rate (0.005%) found in young females (ages 15–34) (U.S. Department of Commerce 1995). Despite the high frequency with which borderline patients perform multiple self-destructive acts, the comparative frequency of acts that result in actual suicide is low (Soloff et al. 1994; Stone 1990).

Borderline patients do commit suicide, often under circumstances that may have begun as a gesture but in which they have miscalculated the response of those from whom a saving response was expected. Borderline patients will recount after serious overdoses that they were fully aware that they could die and that they were knowingly placing their fate in the hands of chance. Moreover, having once, or ever, made an actual suicide attempt greatly increases the likelihood of later suicide.

How to Explain the Diagnosis

When asked whether someone has borderline personality disorder, it is useful to be able to describe it in a way that is relatively jargon free, allowing patients, their families, or other laypersons to reach their own conclusions about whether the diagnosis fits. I say this to laypersons:

"People with a borderline personality disorder have grown up feeling that they were unfairly treated, that they didn't get the attention or care they needed. They are angry about that, and as young adults, they set out in search of someone who can make up to them for what they feel is missing. When they think they've found such a person, they set in motion intense, exclusive relationships, which then fail because they place unrealistic expectations on the other person. Upon failing, they feel rejected or abandoned, and either their rage about being treated unfairly gets reawakened or they feel they've been bad and caused the rejection, in which case they become suicidal or self-destructive. Sometimes, their descriptions of having been mistreated cause others to feel guilty and try to make it up to them. Sometimes their self-destructiveness evokes protective feelings in others, who then try to be rescuers. Such guilty or rescuing responses from others validate the borderline person's unrealistically high expectations of having their needs met, and the cycle is apt to repeat itself."

SUMMARY

The existence of patients fulfilling criteria for the borderline syndrome is well established, and the use of the diagnosis has become more uniform and universal. The meaning of the diagnosis is still undergoing revision as greater specificity is added to our understanding of the etiology and pathogenesis of this disorder (Gunderson and Zanarini 1989; see Paris 1994 for extended reviews). A basic thesis of this book is that the diagnosis already carries great specificity in terms of treatment, but that it requires a great deal of expertise to provide such treatment well, whereas it is very easy to do it harmfully. With the emergence of this diagnosis as a valid and widely recognized entity, it is important that clinicians begin using the diagnosis openly with patients and families. A way to do that has been presented. This chapter's larger message is that it is highly useful to be explicit and unapologetic in making this diagnosis and that to do otherwise is often a product of our countertransference feelings about such patients.

REFERENCES

Abraham K: Selected Papers. London, Hogarth Press, 1927

Adler G, Buie D: The psychotherapeutic approach to aloneness in borderline patients, in Advances in Psychotherapy of the Borderline Patient. Edited by LeBoit J. New York, Jason Aronson, 1979, pp 433–448

Aichhorn A: Wayward Youth (1925). New York, Viking, 1945

Ainsworth MDS, Blehar MC, Waters E, et al: Patterns of Attachment: A Psychological Study of the Strange Situation. Hillsdale, NJ, Erlbaum, 1978

Akiskal HS: Subaffective disorders: dysthymic, cyclothymic and bipolar II disorders in the "borderline" realm. Psychiatr Clin North Am 4(1):25–46, 1981

Alexander F: The neurotic character. Int J Psychoanal 11:292311, 1930

Akiskal HS: The nosologic status of borderline personality: clinical and polysomnographic study. Am J Psychiatry 142(2):192–198, 1985

American Psychiatric Association: Diagnostic and Statistical Manual of Mental Disorders, 3rd Edition. Washington, DC, American Psychiatric Association, 1980

American Psychiatric Association: Diagnostic and Statistical Manual of Mental Disorders, 4th Edition. Washington, DC, American Psychiatric Association, 1994

Balint M: The Basic Fault: Therapeutic Aspects of Regression, Evanston, IL, Northwestern University Press, 1992

Benjamin LS: Interpersonal Diagnosis and Treatment of Personality Disorders. New York, Guilford, 1993

Bowlby J: Attachment and Loss, Vol 1: Attachment. New York, Basic Books, 1969

Bowlby J: Attachment and Loss, Vol 2: Separation: Anxiety and Anger. New York, Basic Books, 1973

Bowlby J: Attachment and Loss, Vol 3: Loss. New York, Basic Books, 1980

Bowlby J: A Secure Base: Parent-Child Attachment and Healthy Human Development. New York, Basic Books, 1988

Brodsky BS, Malone KM, Ellis SP, et al: Characteristics of borderline personality disorder associated with suicidal behavior. Am J Psychiatry 154(12):1715–1719, 1997

Chopra HD, Beatson JA: Psychotic symptoms in borderline personality disorder. Am J Psychiatry 143:1605–1607, 1986

Clarkin JF, Widiger TA, Frances A, et al: Prototypic typology and the borderline personality disorder. J Abnorm Psychol 93(3):263–275, 1983

Crittendon PM: Relationships at risk, in Clinical Implications of Attachment. Edited by Belsky J, Nezworski T. Hillsdale, NJ, Erlbaum, 1988, pp 136–174

Egan J: Cutting: the thin read line. The New York Times Magazine, July 27, 1998, pp 21–25, 39–44, 48

Fairbairn WRD: Synopsis of an object-relations theory of the personality. Int J Psychoanal 44:224–225, 1963

Favazza M: Bodies Under Siege, 2nd Edition. Baltimore, MD, Johns Hopkins University Press, 1996

Fonagy P: Thinking about thinking: some clinical and theoretical considerations in the treatment of a borderline patient. Int J Psychoanal 72(Pt 4):639–656, 1991

Fonagy P, Target M: Attachment and reflective function: their role in self-organization. Development and Psychopathology 9(4):679–700, 1987

Fonagy P, Steele H, Moran G, et al: The capacity for understanding mental states: the reflective self in parent and child and its significance for security of attachment. Infant Mental Health Journal 13:200–217, 1991

Fonagy P, Leigh T, Kennedy R, et al: Attachment, borderline states and the representation of emotions and cognitions in self and other, in Emotion, Cognition, and Representation (Rochester Symposium on Developmental Psychopathology, Vol.

6). Edited by Cicchetti D, Toth SL, et al. Rochester, NY, University of Rochester Press, 1995a, pp 371–414

Fonagy P, Steele M, Steele H, et al: Attachment, the reflective self, and borderline states: the predictive specificity of the Adult Attachment Interview and pathological emotional development, in Attachment Theory: Social, Developmental, and Clinical Perspective. Edited by Goldberg S, Muir R, et al. Hillsdale, NJ, Analytic Press, 1995b, pp 223–278

Fonagy P, Target M, Gergely G: Attachment and borderline personality disorder: a theory and some evidence. Psychiatr Clin North Am 23:vii–viii, 103–122, 2000

Frances A, Clarkin J, Gilmore M, et al: Reliability of criteria for borderline personality disorder: a comparison of DSM-III and the Diagnostic Interview for Borderline Personality Disorder. Am J Psychiatry 141:1080–1084, 1984

Freud S: Character and erotism (1908), in Standard Edition of the Complete Psychological Works of Sigmund Freud, Vol 9. Translated and edited by Strachey J. London, Hogarth Press, 1959, pp 169–175

Friedman RC, Aronoff MS, Clarkin JF, et al: History of suicidal behavior in depressed borderline inpatients. Am J Psychiatry 140(8):1023–1026, 1983

Friedman S, Jones JC, Chernen L, et al: Suicidal ideation and suicide attempts among patients with panic disorder: a survey of two outpatient clinics. Am J Psychiatry 149(5):680–685, 1992

Frosch J: The psychotic character: clincal psychiatric considerations. Psychiatr Q 38:1–16, 1964

Fyer MR, Frances AJ, Sullivan T, et al: Comorbidity of borderline personality disorder. Arch Gen Psychiatry 45:348–352, 1988

Gardner DL, Cowdry RW: Suicidal and parasuicidal behavior in borderline personality disorder. Psychiatr Clin North Am 8(2):389–403, 1985

George A, Soloff P: Schizotypal symptoms in patients with borderline personality disorders. Am J Psychiatry 143:212–215, 1986

Grilo CM, McGlashan TH, Oldham JM: Course and stability of personality disorders. Journal of Practical Psychiatry and Behavioral Health 1(4):61–75, 1998

Grinker R, Werble B, Drye R: The Borderline Syndrome: A Behavioral Study of Ego Functions. New York, Basic Books, 1968

Gunderson JG: Borderline Personality Disorder. Washington, DC, American Psychiatric Press, 1984

Gunderson JG: Building structure for the borderline construct. Acta Psychiatr Scand 379 (suppl):12–18, 1994

Gunderson JG: The borderline patient's intolerance of aloneness: insecure attachments and therapist availability. Am J Psychiatry 153(6):752–758, 1996

Gunderson JG, Kolb JE: Discriminating features of borderline patients. Am J Psychiatry 135(7):792–796, 1978

Gunderson JG, Sabo AN: The phenomenological and conceptual interface between borderline personality disorder and PTSD. Am J Psychiatry 150(1):19–27, 1993

Gunderson JG, Singer M: Defining borderline patients: an overview. Am J Psychiatry 132:1–10, 1975

Gunderson JG, Zanarini MC: Pathogenesis of borderline personality disorder, in American Psychiatric Press Review of Psychiatry, Vol 8. Edited by Tasman A, Hales RE, Frances AJ. Washington, DC, American Psychiatric Press, 1989, pp 25–48

Gunderson JG, Carpenter WT, Strauss J: Borderline and schizophrenic patients: a comparative study. Am J Psychiatry 132:1257–1264, 1975

Gunderson JG, Kolb JF, Austin V: The Diagnostic Interview for Borderline Patients. Am J Psychiatry 138(7):896–903, 1981

Gunderson JG, Siever LJ, Spaulding E: The search for a schizotype: crossing the border again. Arch Gen Psychiatry 41(1):15–22, 1983

Gunderson JG, Zanarini MC, Kisiel CL: Borderline personality disorder, in DSM-IV Sourcebook, Vol. 2. Edited by Widiger TA, Frances AJ, Pincus HA, et al. Washington, DC, American Psychiatric Association, 1996, pp 717–731

Heller LM: Life at the Border. Okeechobee, FL, Dyslimbia Press, 1991

Hoch P, Polatin P: Pseudoneurotic forms of schizophrenia. Psychiatr Q 23:248–276, 1949

Jacobsberg I, Hymowitz P, Barasch A, et al: Symptoms of schizotypal personality disorder. Am J Psychiatry 143:1222–1227, 1986

Jordan J, Kaplan A, Miller J, et al (eds): Women's Growth in Connection: Writings from the Stone Center. New York, Guilford, 1991

Kernberg O: Borderline personality organization. J Am Psychoanal Assoc 15:641–685, 1967

Kernberg O: The treatment of patients with borderline personality organization. Int J Psychoanal 49:600–619, 1968

Kernberg O: Borderline Conditions and Pathological Narcissism. New York, Jason Aronson, 1975

Kety S, Rosenthal D, Wender P, et al: The types and prevalence of mental illness in the biological and adoptive families of adopted schizophrenics, in The Transmission of Schizophrenia. Edited by Rosenthal D, Kety S. New York, Pergamon, 1968, pp 345–362

Klein D: Psychopharmacology and the borderline patients, in Borderline States in Psychiatry. Edited by Mack I. New York, Grune & Stratton, 1975, pp 75–92

Klein D: Psychopharmacological treatment and delineation of borderline disorders, in Borderline Personality Disorders: The concept, the Syndrome, the Patient. Edited by Hartocollis P. New York, International Universities Press, 1977, pp 365–384

Klein M: The Psychoanalysis of Children. London, Hogarth Press, 1932

Klein M: Notes on some schizoid mechanisms. Int J Psychoanal 27:99–110, 1946

Knight R: Borderline states. Bull Menninger Clin 17:1–12, 1953

Knight R: Management and psychotherapy of the borderline schizophrenic patient, in Psychoanalytic Psychiatry and Psychology. Edited by Knight R, Friedman C. New York, International Universities Press, 1954

Knight R: Management and psychotherapy of the borderline schizophrenic patient, in Psychoanalytic Psychiatry and Psychology. Edited by Knight R, Friedman C. New York, International Universities Press,1954

Koenigsberg HW, Kaplan RD, Gilmore MM, et al: The relationship between syndrome and personality disorder in DSM-III: experience with 2,464 patients. Am J Psychiatry 142(2):207–212, 1985

Kroll J, Carey K, Sines L, et al: Are there borderlines in Britain? a cross-validation of US findings. Arch Gen Psychiatry 39(1):60–63, 1982

Lewin RA, Schulz C: Losing and Fusing: Borderline Transitional Object and Self Relations. New York, Jason Aronson, 1992

Links PS (ed): Family Environment and Borderline Personality Disorder. Washington, DC, American Psychiatric Press, 1990

Links PS, Steiner M, Offord D, et al: Characteristics of borderline personality disorder: a Canadian study. Can J Psychiatry 33:336–340, 1988

Loranger AW: The impact of DSM-III on diagnostic practice in a university hospital. Arch Gen Psychiatry 47:672–675, 1990

Loranger AW, Oldham JM, Tulis EH: Familial transmission of DSM-III borderline personality disorder. Arch Gen Psychiatry 39(7):795–799, 1982

Loranger AW, Janca A, Sartorius N (eds): Assessment and Diagnosis of Personality Disorders: The ICD-10 International Personality Disorder Examination. Cambridge, England, Cambridge University Press, 1997

Mack J (ed): Borderline States in Psychiatry. New York, Grune & Stratton, 1975

Mahler M, Kaplan L: Developmental aspects in the assessment of narcissistic and so-called borderline personalities, in Borderline Personality Disorders: The Concept, the Syndrome, the Patient. Edited by Hartocollis P. New York, International Universities Press, 1977, pp 71–86

Main T: The ailment. Br J Med Psychol 30:129–145, 1957

Main M, Hesse E: Parents' unresolved traumatic experiences are related to infant disorganization status: is frightened and/or frightening parental behavior the linking mechanism? in Attachment in the Preschool Years. Edited by Greenberg MT, Cicchetti D, Cummings EM. Chicago, University of Chicago Press, 1990, pp 161–184

Main M, Solomon J: Procedures for identifying infants as disorganized/disoriented during the Ainsworth Strange Situation, in Attachment in the Preschool Years. Edited by Greenberg MT, Cicchetti D, Cummings EM. Chicago, University of Chicago Press, 1990, pp 121–160

Masterson J: Treatment of the adolescent with borderline syndrome (a problem in separation-individuation). Bull Menninger Clin 35:5–18, 1971

Masterson J: Treatment of the Borderline Adolescent: A Developmental Approach. New York, Wiley, 1972

Masterson J: Psychotherapy of the Borderline Adult. New York, Brunner/Mazel, 1976

Masterson J, Costello JL: From Borderline Adolescent to Functioning Adult: The Test of Time. New York, Brunner/Mazel, 1980

Masterson JF, Rinsley DB: The borderline syndrome: the role of the mother in the genesis and psychic structure of the borderline personality. Int J Psychoanal 56(2):163–177, 1975

Meehl P: Schizotaxia, schizotypy, schizophrenia. Am Psychol 17:827–838, 1962

Millon T: On the genesis and prevalence of the borderline personality disorder: a social learning thesis. J Personal Disord 1(4):354–372, 1987

Modell A: Primitive object relationships and the predisposition to schizophrenia. Int J Psychoanal 44:282–291, 1963

Mors O: Increasing incidence of borderline states in Denmark from 1970–1985. Acta Psychiatr Scand 77(5):575–583, 1988

Oldham JM, Skodol AE: Personality disorders in the public sector. Hospital and Community Psychiatry 42(5):481–487, 1991

Paris J: Social risk factors for borderline personality disorder: a review and hypothesis. Can J Psychiatry 37(7):510–515, 1992

Paris J: Antisocial and borderline personality disorders: two separate diagnoses or two aspects of the same psychopathology? Compr Psychiatry 38(4):237–242, 1997

Perry JC: Longitudinal studies of personality disorders. J Personal Disord 7:65–85, 1993

Perry JC, Cooper SH: A preliminary report on defenses and conflicts associated with borderline personality disorder. J Am Psychoanal Assoc 34:863–893, 1986

Pope HG Jr, Jonas JM, Hudson JI, et al: An empirical study of psychosis in borderline personality disorder. Am J Psychiatry 142:1285–1290, 1985

Rado S: Psychoanalysis of Behavior: Collected Papers. New York, Grune & Stratton, 1956

Rado S (ed): Psychoanalysis of Behavior, Vol 2. New York, Grune & Stratton, 1962

Reich W: Character Analysis, 3rd Edition. New York, Orgone Institute Press, 1949

Richman NE, Sokolove RL: The experience of aloneness, object representation, and evocative memory in borderline and neurotic patients. Psychoanalytic Psychology 9(1):77–91, 1992

Roig E, Roig C, Soth N: The use of transitional objects in emotionally-disturbed adolescent inpatients. International Journal of Adolescence and Youth 1(1):45–58, 1987

Rorschach H: Psychodiagnostics, 5th Edition. Bern, Hans Huber, 1942

Shearer SL: Dissociative phenomena in women with borderline personality disorder. Am J Psychiatry 151(9):1324–1328, 1994a

Shearer SL: Phenomenology of self-injury among inpatient women with borderline personality disorder. J Nerv Ment Dis 182(9):524–526, 1994b

Shearer SL, Peters CP, Quaytman MS, et al: Intent and lethality of suicide attempts among female borderline inpatients. Am J Psychiatry 145(11):1424–1427, 1988

Shearer SL, Peters CP, Quaytman MS, et al: Frequency and correlates of childhood sexual and physical abuse histories in adult female borderline patients. Am J Psychiatry 147:214–216, 1990

Siever LJ, Gunderson JG: Genetic determinants of borderline conditions. Schizophr Bull 5:59–86, 1979

Siever LJ, Gunderson JG: The search for a schizotypal personality: historical origins and current status. Compr Psychiatry 24(3):199–212, 1983

Silk K, Lohr N, Westen D, et al: Psychosis in borderline patients with depression. J Personal Disord 3:92–100, 1989

Silk KR, Lee S, Hill EM, et al: Borderline personality disorder symptoms and severity of sexual abuse. Am J Psychiatry 152(7):1059–1064, 1995

Singer M: The experience of emptiness in narcissistic and borderline states, II: the struggle for a sense of self and the potential for suicide. International Review of Psycho-Analysis 4(4):471–479, 1977

Soloff PH: Is there any drug treatment of choice for the borderline patient? Acta Psychiatr Scand 379 (suppl):50–55, 1994

Soloff PH, Lis JA, Kelly T, et al: Self-mutilation and suicidal behavior in borderline personality disorder. J Pers Disord 8(4):257–267, 1994

Spitzer RL, Endicott J, Gibbon M: Crossing the border into borderline personality and borderline schizophrenia: the development of criteria. Arch Gen Psychiatry 36(1):17–24, 1979

Stern A: Psychoanalytic investigation and therapy in the borderline group of neuroses. Psychoanal Q 7:467–489, 1938

Stiver IP: The meaning of care: reframing treatment models, in Women's Growth in Connection: Writings from the Stone Center. Edited by Jordan J, Kaplan A, Miller J, et al. New York, Guilford, 1991, pp 250–267

Stone M: Contemporary shift of the borderline concept from a sub-schizophrenic disorder to a subaffective disorder. Psychiatr Clin North Am 2:577–594, 1979

Stone M: The Borderline Syndromes. New York, McGraw-Hill, 1980

Stone MH: The Fate of Borderline Patients. New York, Guilford, 1990

Stone MH, Hurt SW, Stone DK: The P.I. 500: long term follow up of borderline inpatients meeting DSM-III criteria, I: global outcome. J Personal Disord 1:291–298, 1987

Swartz M, Blazer D, George L, et al: Estimating the prevalence of borderline personality disorder in the community. J Personal Disord 4:257–272, 1990

Torgersen S, Lygren S, Oien PA, et al: A twin study of personality disorders. Compr Psychiatry (in press)

U.S. Department of Commerce: Statistical Abstracts of the United States. U.S. Department of Commerce, Economic Statistics Administration, Bureau of the Census, 1995

Vaillant GE: The beginning of wisdom in never calling a patient borderline. Journal of Psychotherapy Practice and Research 1(2):117–134, 1992

Westen D, Moses MJ, Silk KR, et al: Quality of depressive experience in borderline personality disorder and major depression: when depression is not just depression. J Personal Disord 6(4):382–393, 1992

Widiger TA, Weissman MM: Epidemiology of borderline personality disorder. Hospital & Community Psychiatry 42(10):1015–1021, 1991

Widiger TA, Trull T, Hurt S, et al: A multidimensional scaling of the DSM-III personality disorders. Arch Gen Psychiatry 44:557–563, 1987

Widiger TA, Frances AJ, Harris M, et al: Comorbidity among Axis II disorders, in Personality Disorders: New Perspectives on Diagnostic Validity. Edited by Oldham JM, et al. Washington, DC, American Psychiatric Press, 1991, 165–194

Winnicott DW: Transitional objects and transitional phenomena. Int J Psychoanal 34:89–97, 1953

Winnicott DW: The Maturational Process and the Facilitating Environment. London, Hogarth Press, 1965

Wolberg AR: The Borderline Patient. New York, Intercontinental Medical Book Corporation, 1973

World Health Organization: The ICD-10 Classification of Mental and Behavioural Disorders: Clinical Descriptions and Diagnostic Guidelines. Geneva, World Health Organization, 1992

Zanarini MC, Frankenburg FR: Emotional hypochondriasis, hyperbole, and the borderline patient. J Psychother Pract Res 3(1):25–36, 1994

Zanarini MC, Gunderson JG, Frankenburg FR: Cognitive features of borderline personality disorder. Am J Psychiatry 147(1):57–63, 1990

Zanarini MC, Williams AA, Lewis RE, et al: Reported pathological childhood experiences associated with the development of borderline personality disorder. Am J Psychiatry 54(8):1101–1106, 1997

Zanarini MC, Frankenburg FR, DeLuca CJ, et al: The pain of being borderline: dysphoric states specific to borderline personality disorder. Harvard Review of Psychiatry 6(4):201–207, 1998

Zetzel ER: A developmental approach to the borderline patient. Am J Psychiatry 127:867–871, 1971

Zimmerman M, Coryell W: DSM-III personality disorder diagnoses in a nonpatient sample. Demographic correlates and comorbidity. Arch Gen Psychiatry 46(8):262–269, 1989

Zimmerman M, Mattia JI: Differences between clinical and research practices in diagnosing borderline personality disorder. Am J Psychiatry 156:1570–1574, 1999

Zisook S, Goff A, Sledge P, et al: Reported suicidal behavior and current suicidal ideation in a psychiatric outpatient clinic. Ann Clin Psychiatry 6(1):27–31, 1994

Zweig-Frank H, Paris J, Guzder J: Psychological risk factors for dissociation and self-mutilation in female patients with borderline personality disorder. Can J Psychiatry 39(5):259–264, 1994

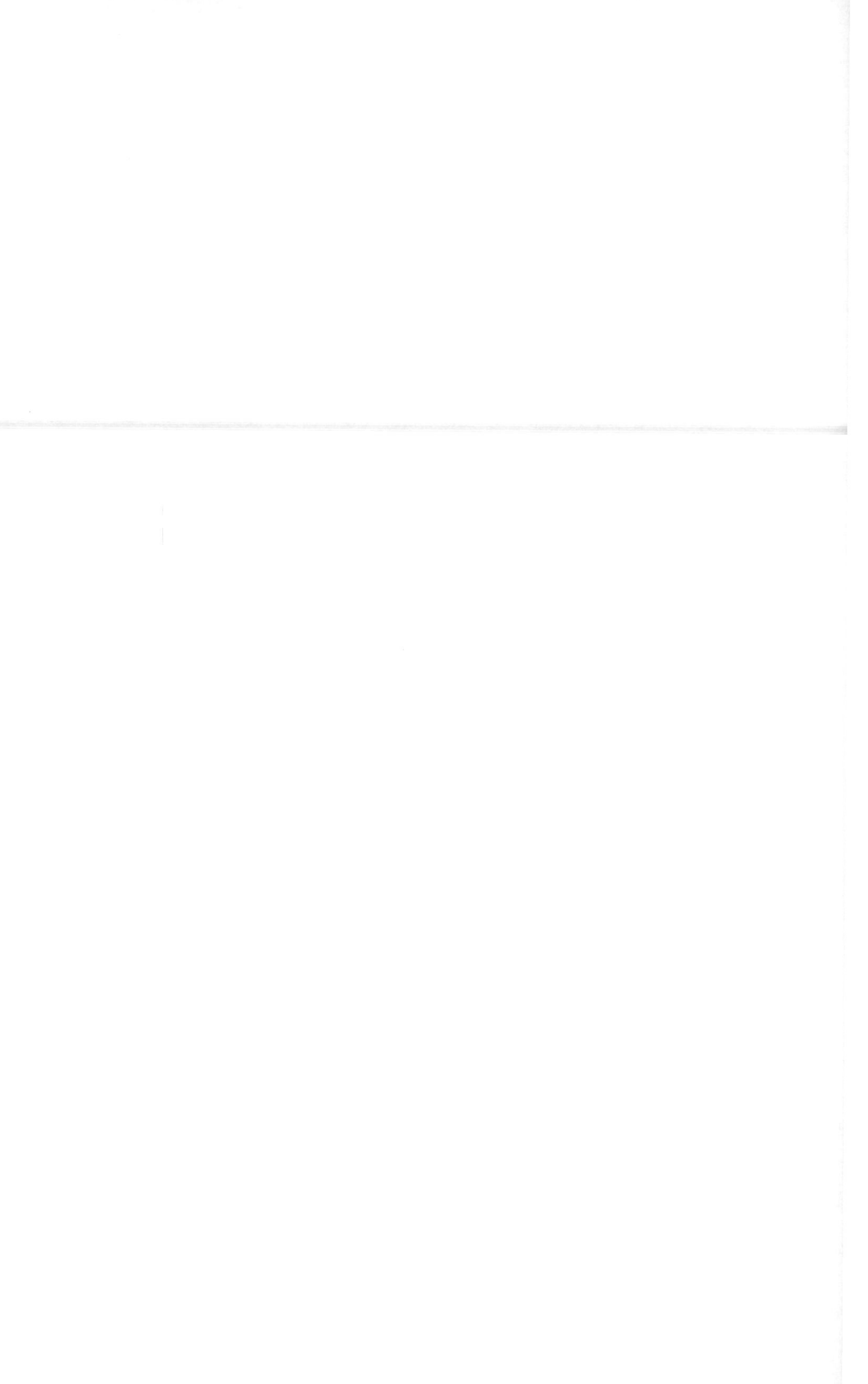

2

Differential Diagnosis

Overlaps, Subtleties, and Treatment Implications

Overall Function

Medical diagnoses are meant to reflect etiology and pathophysiology; they are also used by clinicians to develop appropriate treatment plans. This usage is most dramatically illustrated when a diagnosis indicates a specific and very effective therapy. Unfortunately, psychiatric diagnoses rarely provide such specificity; the causes are often unclear and usually multiple, and the treatment effects are almost always gradual and incomplete. Borderline personality disorder (BPD) exemplifies this; and, given its fuzzy borders with many other psychiatric diagnoses, the importance of making this particular diagnosis can easily be underestimated. However, recognizing the diagnosis is often of great importance, since ignoring it will always create clinical problems.

There are several specific reasons why identifying BPD is important.

First, it anchors the patient's and the clinician's expectations about course. Even when priority may be given to symptoms, behaviors, or situational crises, the perspective of a long-term seriously handicapped person sets realistic boundaries to what can be expected. Because BPD patients almost always present with depression, eating disorders, or substance abuse, it is only when the BPD diagnosis is identified that realistic prognostications can occur.

Second, the borderline diagnosis establishes a basis for developing a treatment alliance. It does this by offering patients a developmental and therapeutic context that they will experience as meaningful and appropriate. As described in this chapter, it often starts by the initial reassurance that borderline patients feel upon learning that their problems are shared by others and that their clinicians have a body of relevant knowledge to draw from.

Third, it prepares clinicians for what's ahead—including the option of referring the patient to those who may be better able to provide what is needed. Most specifically, it helps therapists focus on the characteristic defensive adaptations that these patients have made (e.g., regressing, idealizing, blaming) lest they unwittingly enact the roles that these patients commonly project (i.e., caretaker, controller, or abuser). Indeed, it is because of such countertransference enactments that astute clinicians began to appreciate that a particular type of personality psychopathology that lay behind the fluctuating phenomenology could help explain why clinicians had these problems. Fear of aloneness, for example, is a stable underlying trait that gives coherence to the descriptive characteristics of BPD (see Chapter 1 of this book) and conveys added meaning in terms of both etiology and treatment. Such a characteristic helps clinicians discriminate borderline personality disorder from posttraumatic stress disorder (Gunderson and Sabo 1993), narcissistic personality disorder (Plakun 1987; Ronningstam and Gunderson 1991), and depressive disorders (Westen et al. 1992).

The Changing Construct: From Schizophrenia to Depression to Posttraumatic Stress Disorder

Figure 2–1 begins to divide the population of individuals with personality disorders into subtypes created by temperaments, level of impairment, biogenetics, and phenomenological features. A hierarchy is present, such that—as in clinical practice (Herkov and Blashfield 1995; Westen 1997)—the presence of a more severe personality disorder makes fulfilling criteria for lesser types superfluous. In this respect the figure differs from DSM-IV (American Psychiatric Association 1994), in which the lesser types are considered comorbid. In this scheme—similar to one recognized by Kernberg (1986) and buttressed in large measure by empirical support from Livesley et al. (1992, 1998) and Skodol et al. (A. E. Skodol, T. H. McGlashan, C. M. Grilo, R. L. Stout, and J. G. Gunderson, unpublished manuscript, July 2000)—BPD remains one of the major forms of disorders of the self, alongside schizoid and antisocial personality disorders. Each of these disorders of self constitutes so severe an impairment that extended social rehabilitative treatments are required. The presence of these disorders must assume priority in treatment planning: their presence will greatly complicate, or override, the usual treatments of concurrent Axis I or even medical problems. As such they deserve categorical status or equal weight with Axis I. To mental health clinicians, BPD is by far the most important type of personality disorder. Socially isolated people with schizoid personality disorder or socially exploitative people with antisocial personality disorder are not self-destructive careseekers like those with borderline personality disorder. Although good epidemiological data are not available, borderline patients are estimated to constitute about 15%–20% of inpatients and 10%–20% of outpatients (see Table 2–1). They are in addition high consumers of emergency room services, crisis lines, and psychiatric consultative liaisons to other medical services (Ellison et al. 1989; Reich et al. 1989).

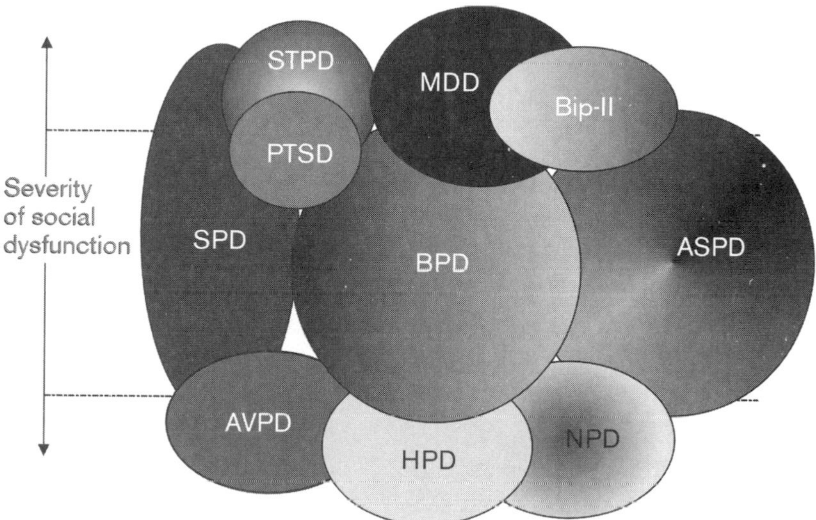

FIGURE 2–1. How borderline personality disorder (BPD) fits in with neighboring diagnoses.
AVPD = avoidant personality disorder. HPD = histrionic personality disorder. NPD = narcissistic personality disorder. ASPD = antisocial personality disorder. BPD = borderline personality disorder. SPD = schizoid personality disorder. PTSD = posttraumatic stress disorder. STPD = schizotypal personality disorder. MDD = major depressive disorder. Bip-II = bipolar II disorder.

TABLE 2–1. Demographics

Age at onset[a]	
Age group	**Percentage**
Adolescence (ages 13–17)	15
Early adulthood (ages 18–25)	50
Young adulthood (ages 26–30	25
Adulthood (ages 31–48)	10
Prevalence	
Population	**Percentage**
General population	0.4–3[b]
Inpatient populations	15–18[c]
Outpatient populations	15 25[d]
Socioeconomic status (SES)	Possible increase in low SES, otherwise evenly distributed
Gender	75% female
Race	No known variations

[a] The percentages estimated to have onset in each age group are based on the author's experience; no epidemiologic data are available.
[b] Coryell and Zimmerman 1989; Reich et al. 1989; Swartz et al. 1990; S. Torgersen, E. Kringlen, and V. Cramer, "The Prevalence and Demographic Associations of Personality Disorders in the Community," unpublished manuscript, June 2000.
[c] Dahl 1986; Loranger 1990; Widiger and Weissman 1991.
[d] Koenigsberg et al. 1985; Widiger and Weissman 1991.

Comorbidity and Differential Diagnosis

Table 2–2 offers a summation of the literature studying the concurrence between BPD and other diagnoses because of which differential diagnosis can be difficult. Although these estimates are from the sources cited in the table, readers should understand that the estimates are not based on epidemiologically generalizable samples. It is very clear from this extensive, albeit seriously flawed, literature that rates of overlap increase with higher levels of care (e.g., hospitalized samples will have much higher rates of overlap than outpatient samples). It is notable that, with the possible exception of the eating disorders, the concurrence rate for the other diagnoses is higher in the BPD samples than is the rate of the presence of BPD in samples with the other diagnosis (e.g., the rate of depression in BPD samples is roughly three times as high as the rate of BPD in depression samples). This phenomenon in concurrence rates has fueled the persistent idea that BPD represents an atypical form of Axis I disorder (to be discussed further in Chapter 12 of this book).

BPD and Depression

As shown in Table 2–2, most BPD patients meet criteria for depressive disorders—at least half with major depressive disorder (MDD), dysthymia, or both. Yet the descriptive characteristics of patients with these conditions seem so disparate—for example, gloomy, constricted depression patients versus angry, impulsive borderline patients—that it is not obvious why the differentiation of them should pose problems. A series of studies has established that the quality of the depressive experience of borderline patients is unique and quite distinct from that of depressed or other patient types (Kurtz and Morey 1998; Rogers et al. 1995; Westen et al. 1992) (see Figure 2–2 for distinctions between BPD and MDD). These studies have highlighted the emptiness, the primitive guilt, and the negative, devaluative attitudes of BPD depressions.

TABLE 2–2. Estimated co-occurrence of BPD and other diagnoses

Diagnosis	% of BPD with other diagnosis	% of other diagnosis with BPD
Depression	50	15
Dysthymia	70	10
Bipolar II disorder	10	20
Bipolar I disorder	5	15
Eating disorder	25	
Bulimia	20	20
Anorexia	5	20
Obesity	5	10
Posttraumatic stress disorder	30	No estimate
Substance abuse	35	10
Alcohol only	25	5
Somatization	5	10
Narcissistic personality disorder	25	~15
Antisocial personality disorder	25	~25

Source. Estimates based on the following review articles: Dolan et al., in press; Fyer et al. 1988; Gunderson and Sabo 1993; Gunderson et al. 1991, 1993, 1999; Herzog et al. 1992; Hudziak et al. 1996; McGlashan et al., in press: Stern et al. 1993; Tyrer et al. 1997; Zanarini et al. 1998a, 1998b.

Still, and despite the fact that BPD and MDD often co-occur, deciding which diagnosis should assume priority can be difficult (Gunderson and Phillips 1991; Rogers et al. 1995; Westen et al. 1992). This difficulty occurs when a patient meets criteria for MDD in the context of a troubled relationship,

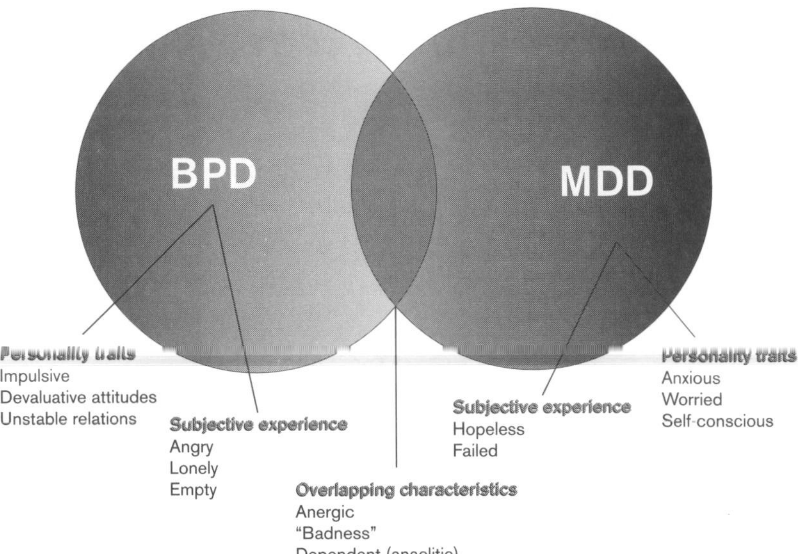

FIGURE 2–2. Distinctions and overlapping characteristics between borderline personality disorder (BPD) and major depressive disorder (MDD).

with a threat of separation, and with the onset of suicidal impulses or actions. The clinician must then make a judgment about whether the patient's suicidality is a communication motivated by the wish to gain a sympathetic and binding response (a borderline dynamic), or motivated by despair and hopelessness (a depressive mental state). Did the suicide "attempt" fail because of design or ineptitude? Even after a clinician knows a patient very well, it may be impossible to disentangle both sources of a patient's suicidality.

A complicating issue is that patients may appear to qualify for either diagnosis when they present, only to reveal later that the less phenomenologically evident diagnosis is primary. This occurs most dramatically for depressed patients who meet all criteria for MDD and have very modest responses to antidepressants, then have a very rapid remission when put in a hospital. The clinician may only then learn, for example, that the "depressed" patient had held her husband hostage by her dysfunction for several months—ever since he'd begun amicable discussions with her estranged mother. The borderline diagnosis is primary, in this instance, but the opposite can occur, as seen in this case example:

Vignette

A patient in whom BPD was diagnosed on the basis of self-mutilative behaviors was referred for psychotherapy, where it became clear that she was chronically isolated and had a developmental history marked by gloomy, introverted parents and adherence to rigid religious values. She reported, "I did not know I'd been depressed much of my life. I thought it was normal, just the way life is." Her acts of cutting were the outgrowth of long-standing moral preoccupations and offered her temporary relief from them. Here a depressive diagnosis was primary.

The clinical significance of this differentiation involves the optimism that clinicians communicate about pharmacological therapies (not about whether an antidepressant is desirable, since BPD also profits from them—see Chapter 6 of this book) and the importance that clinicians assign to the patient's engagement in psychosocial therapies. Although many MDD patients benefit from psychotherapies, they are often unnecessary, whereas BPD almost always involves sustained use of several somewhat specialized psychosocial modalities (see Chapter 3 of this book).

BPD AND BIPOLAR II DISORDER/CYCLOTHYMIC PERSONALITY

The similarity of the BP (bipolar disorder) and BPD acronyms is deserved. BPD and bipolar II disorder are in fact so similar, phenomenologically (see Figure 2–3) and otherwise (i.e., predominantly diagnosed in females with unstable relationships and heightened risk of suicide), that it is sometimes best not to think that these are two independent disorders (Kopacz and Janicak 1996; Gunderson et al. 1999). BPD is considered one of the bipolar disorders' most indistinct boundaries (Blacker and Tsuang 1992).

The overlap in phenomenology—mood lability and impulsivity—probably relates to a common underlying temperament—that is, a genetically derived disposition (Akiskal 1981; Gunderson et al. 1999; Silverman et al. 1991). This may account for the fact that mood stabilizers are often used for BPD patients. Yet in a more controlled trial, borderline patients failed to respond as dramatically to lithium as would be expected for patients with a variant of bipolar disorder (Links et al. 1990).

Table 2–3 offers some ways to distinguish BPD from bipolar II. Especial-

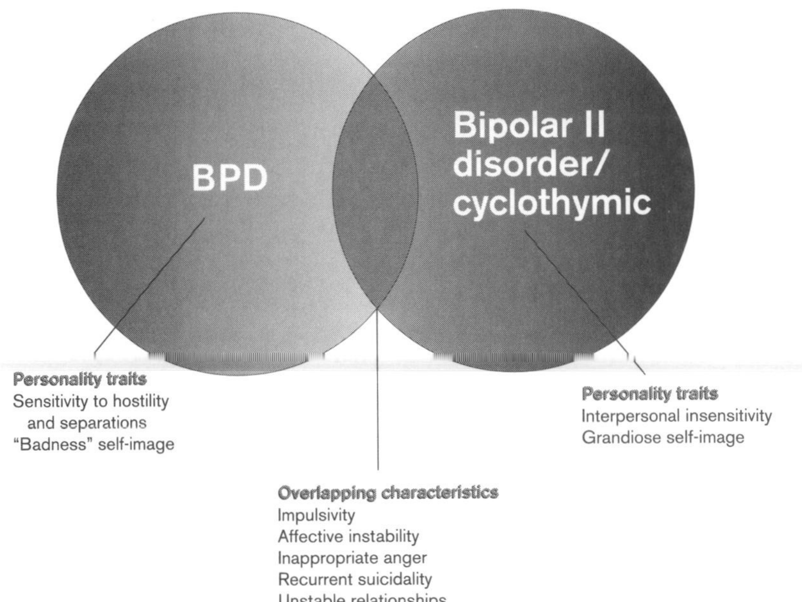

FIGURE 2–3. Distinctions and overlapping characteristics between borderline personality disorder (BPD) and bipolar II disorder.

ly telling can be the differential responsiveness of BPD and bipolar II patients to confrontation or interpretation (Bolton and Gunderson 1996). Borderline patients will react, sometimes constructively and sometimes not. Bipolar II patients are not fazed: they are likely to go on as if the intervention had not occurred—either by not responding at all, by changing the topic, or by glibly rationalizing. Both bipolar II and BPD patients may respond to external controls by rage or flight, but the borderline patients' responses will always and clearly be emotional. They will believe that much is at stake, either about their self-esteem or about the clinician's trustworthiness. A related finding by Benjamin and Wonderlich (1994) was that hospitalized borderline patients perceived more hostility and autonomy in others than did bipolar depressed inpatients.

Vignette

A 34-year-old man who had undergone a female-to-male sex change operation was flirtatious and had many affairs with members of both sexes. After being hospitalized for suicidal impulses, he quickly became the "life of the unit" and wondered aloud why his therapist

TABLE 2–3. Comparison of BPD and bipolar II disorder

Trait	BPD	Bipolar II
Mood lability/ impulsivity	Due to interpersonal sensitivity	Autonomous and persistent (person acts out)
Affects	Deep, intense; evoke strong empathic response	Lack depth, pain; hard to empathize with
Prototypical behavior pattern	Care seeking: seeks exclusivity, is sensitive to rejection	Begins energetic self-initiated activities that are left incomplete; requiring others to clean up
Defense	Splitting: polarizes realities and, if challenged, becomes angry at challenger or changes to opposite view	Denial: ignores undesirable realities and, if confronted with a reality, denies its emotional significance

would have thought he was suicidal. When the patient was confronted with the facts that his recent vocational and relational failures were doubtless related to these impulses, he angrily stood up and declared, "How dare you talk to me like that. You have no right to call me a 'loser'! Do you want me to kill myself?" He then promptly filed a formal complaint about his treatment.

The subtleties that differentiated this patient's diagnosis were the indiscriminate thrill-seeking or attention-seeking aspects of his behavior, his confidence that authorities would help him punish the transgressors (the confrontational staff), and the patient's interest in keeping all relationships transient (as opposed to exclusive and binding). Particularly important, in my experience, was the glibness of his feelings—it was hard to take them seriously or to empathize with them. These characteristics tilted the diagnostic balance toward bipolar II.

Unfortunately, there are relatively few studies examining the overlap in these diagnoses. About 10% of hospitalized borderline patients have bipolar II (Zanarini et al. 1998a). I suspect that many of the reports on bipolar II include large numbers of patients who meet criteria for BPD, yet this possibility, to my knowledge, has not been assessed. I think this is largely because the investigators of bipolar II are primarily interested in responsiveness to mood stabilizers. As the evidence accumulates that bipolar II patients respond to the same diversity of medications with the same lack of impressive effectiveness as is shown with borderline patients, attention to this overlap will increase.

The complexity of the interface between these disorders now offers a

Rorschach-test-like opportunity for clinicians to project their biases. The diagnoses of schizophrenia and depression in years past (and posttraumatic stress disorder [PTSD] most recently) offered a preferred haven for clinicians whose countertransference led them to want to reduce the level of accountability and hostility they assigned to BPD patients; a similar diagnostic process takes place in the case of the bipolar II label—but by a different mechanism. Many clinicians, perhaps especially biological psychiatrists, prefer Axis I diagnoses, because they offer a rationale for a pharmacological approach that will keep managed-care overseers at bay and will keep the level of involvement with such patients at a feasibly limited level (sometimes actually the clinician's preferred level). The diagnosis of BPD means that emotional involvement will be an essential aspect of meaningful treatment. Clinicians whose interest and skills are primarily psychotherapeutic will be prone to see the same patients as having BPD and may err by overlooking bipolar or cyclothymic phenomena that could respond to mood stabilizers. Borderline patients for whom the relationship to bipolar disorder should be honored are those with histories of early onset of depression, positive family histories, and tricyclic-induced hypomania.

BPD AND PTSD

The issue of differential diagnosis between BPD and PTSD involved the same basic question in 1990 as did depression in 1980 and as does bipolar II at present: are these really separable disorders? The question of the border with PTSD is usually raised when a depressed, self-mutilative, and impulsive patient has a developmental history marked by significant childhood trauma. The clinician then considers whether that reaction to trauma was sufficient to account for the presenting adult's emotional and behavioral problems (i.e., PTSD) or whether the trauma was itself emblematic of sustained developmental problems that formed the patient's disturbed personality (i.e., BPD). This vignette illustrates such a problem:

Vignette

A 44-year-old woman patient presented with flashbacks that disrupted her sleep and concentration. Her childhood included 8 hospitalizations between the ages of 13 and 18 for treatment of a congenital disease. Twenty-six years later she could still access the

> feeling of being "helpless and alone." In response, she would become agitated, with bursts of accusatory, offensive anger towards her husband and children, which she would then deeply regret as unfair. This remorse then prompted self-destructive or suicidal impulses.

The diagnosis of complex PTSD (Herman 1992) is warranted when such patients have flashbacks or sustained dissociative experiences and an interpersonal style marked by wariness and fears of attachment—such that in adulthood, social isolation is usual and only intermittently interrupted by brief, often alcohol-related, social forays. If the patient is very hungry for attention and protection and is expressive of angry feelings when hurt, the impact of trauma is less likely to have been dominant, and the patient is better conceptualized as having BPD. Westen (1990) points out that when patients are organized around their abuse experiences (i.e., when they have complex PTSD), they are more likely to respond with paranoid accusations of malevolence within the context of an ongoing relationship, whereas borderline patients are more likely to become accusatory when threatened by the loss of their other (see Chapter 1 of this book).

The interface between the disorders is complex (Gunderson and Sabo 1993; Herman et al. 1989). Abusive experiences predispose children to a variety of serious psychiatric illnesses, including BPD. For the roughly 70% of BPD patients who have childhood histories of physical or sexual traumas, it is the sexual abuse that most distinguishes them from traumas associated with antisocial personality disorder (ASPD). Adult BPD patients are vulnerable to developing PTSD by virtue of their recklessness and emotional hyperreactivity. Indeed, PTSD co-occurs in about 30% (lifetime 40%) of BPD patients (Swartz et al. 1990; Zanarini et al. 1998a). The social conditions needed for BPD to develop require emotional estrangement from parents. This estrangement gives abusive experiences during childhood an impact that is far more traumatic in warping character development than is the impact of similar events on children who have the opportunity to find support, talk about the events, and react with their families.

The presence of childhood trauma has clinical significance—as much for the attitudes of treaters as for the nature of the treatments required (Gunderson and Chu 1994). Many clinicians, influenced by their instinctive sympathy for victims of violence, may prefer the PTSD diagnosis for anyone with childhood traumas, because it encourages a deep involvement while sidestepping these patients' hostility (see Chapter 10 of this book).

Vignette

A 34-year-old unmarried woman sought psychotherapy because she "needs support." She related this to a series of recent events.

She loved her job but, after becoming convinced that she was underpaid, demanded more pay from her employer. She consequently lost her job. She also had a fight with her landlord, insisting on her rights. This too resulted in her being kicked out. In both instances, she perceived injustices in the situations correctly, but she experienced the injustice too personally and her anger was disproportionate. Depressed about the consequences of her fights and about the prospects of having no husband and no children, she moved back to live with her mother and with her 40-year-old brother. This brother had been sexually abusive to her when she was between the ages of 6 and 10. Her mother knew but had coped by alternating between helplessness and denial.

The patient presented as very sensitive, wary, vigilant to rejection and criticism, with a defensive response to interpretations. She acknowledged fears of intimacy and attachments. Her defensiveness made exploratory therapy unlikely. Even when a supportive therapist attempted to work with her, she resisted getting attached.

This patient might have been diagnosed as having BPD by virtue of her anger and need for support, but in my opinion she would better be identified as having complex PTSD, as proposed by Herman (1992). The bleakness of her interpersonal life and her resistance to any attachment set the effects of trauma apart from what is seen in BPD. Although the PTSD diagnosis is sometimes overused by clinicians sympathetic to victims, its clinical significance often means that a less intensive, exploratory, or close therapeutic relationship is possible than for BPD.

BPD and Eating Disorders

Eating disorders constitute one of the three most common presenting complaints of patients with BPD. Bulimia is the most common type of co-occurring eating disorder (Table 2–2). Individuals with bulemia are more impulsive than those with anorexia; the latter group are more perfectionistic and conscientious as people and are more purposeful and persistent in their personal deprivations than are those with bulemia. Even more significant is the way in which bingeing and purging offer outward expression of internal splits. Starving oneself, the ascetic ethic of denying one's appetites/needs, is "dutiful and good." Eating is "bad," associated with being too uncontrolled and too aggressive.

Sustained deprivation accompanied by persistent body image distortions or illusions of purity and perfection usually signifies the prototypic individual with anorexia nervosa. Insuch individuals, BPD is unlikely or, if present, less relevant.

Those with bulemia, however, alternate this state of "good" deprivation with angry and entitled feeling states based on feeling that they have suffered more than their share. Under these circumstances—rebelling against their self-imposed restrictions—they binge. No sooner does this occur than they conclude that they have been self-indulgent, feel deeply ashamed, and need to be punished. The punishment often takes the form of renewed anorexia or the more impulsive recurrence of self-destructive behaviors. Thus their purging, their impulsivity, and the volatility of their self-image are indicators of underlying BPD.

Other complications involve appearance. The starving borderline individual is making both a private statement of goodness and a public statement of neediness. Being underfed evokes solicitous responses. It also evidences an inability to take care of oneself—without having to acknowledge unrecognized or humiliating dependency needs. Finally, undereating can be a particularly effective way to torture mothers who see their provision of food as extensions of their love and who therefore make great efforts to accommodate the child's increasingly special food requirements. In this way, undereating is like most other self-punishing behaviors by borderline patients: it contains both intrapsychic and interpersonal meanings. Eating disorder behaviors leave responsibility for the patients' safety and welfare in the hands of others. Indeed, it is central to having BPD that eating (i.e., living) can be justified only if there is reassuring and concrete evidence that others want you to eat (i.e., want you to live) and that they will take responsibility for keeping you alive.

Borderline patients who are obese are likely to have a history of sexual abuse (Sansone et al. 1995) and, in my experience, often have a conscious desire to deflect sexual interests. Complex PTSD (see section above titled "BPD and PTSD") needs to be considered. In addition, in an era of multiple medications (see Chapter 7 of this book), secondary obesity in borderline patients is dramatically increasing. This can be a particularly unfortunate side effect in young women who already feel alienated. Education and treatment recommendations may be welcomed.

The distinction between patients with eating disorders and BPD from those with eating disorders but without BPD can usually be found in their developmental history. Borderline patients will typically evidence impulsivity and dysfunction related to markedly unstable family situations. Many patients with eating disorders and without BPD have histories in which family problems are not easily recognizable. These patients have developmental histories that typically reflect the narcissistic issues of counterdependence and expectations of high achievement. Such patients have more sensitivity to inferiority and fewer concerns about rejection than are evidenced by borderline patients.

BPD and Substance Abuse

When a patient has a history of heavy substance use and, along with it, a history of desperate, impulsive, self-endangering relationships, the clinician must determine whether these typically "borderline-like" relationships are really evidence of BPD or are simply behavioral by-products of the drugs—that is, outgrowths of a primary substance abuse disorder. If the substance abuse is primary, the behaviors and relationships are caused by drug-seeking or drug-related disinhibition. The patient is the victim of his or her drug needs and feels regretful about the relationships. Alternately, the drug use can be a behavioral by-product of the cravings of the person with BPD to soothe himself or herself (i.e., to self-medicate dysphoric feeling states). This drug use, described in Khantzian's "self-medication hypothesis" (Khantzian 1985), also has a desirable disinhibiting effect that permits otherwise unacceptably active efforts to seek relationships that offer the illusion of being cared for by others. From this perspective, the substance abuse would be a secondary symptom of the primary borderline personality disorder.

As with the general population, the most common type of substance abused by borderline patients is alcohol, but what is most specific to these patients is that the type of substance is not very important—that is, they are polysubstance abusers (Nace 1989). Their abuse tends to be—but is not always—episodic and impulsive, and they use whatever drug is available. Even if hard-core addicts have BPD, the treatment of their substance abuse needs to take priority. For such people, the structures, supports, and ideology of substance abuse programs are ideal and are essential for gaining control over their drug habit. Even for borderline patients whose substance abuse is episodic and clearly secondary, the treatment options used for substance abusers still have value—especially for patients who can accept the diagnosis of substance abuse but resist the idea of having more sustained problems with relationships and impulsivity. The ubiquitous and daily access to Alcoholics Anonymous or Narcotics Anonymous self-help services meets borderline patients' needs for support, crisis management, and networking in ways that the mental health system can rarely replicate.

Vignette

A 24-year-old woman with diagnoses of BPD and polysubstance abuse was transferred to a hospital after being kicked out of her third substance abuse program. In each case, she had violated every restriction by resuming her pain-drug habit. While failing several placements in residential programs, she became attached to a therapist, and gradually a new precipitant for her substance abuse relapse became apparent: relapse occurred when her mother (though geographically distant from the patient) traveled to see the patient's brother or was visited by him. At this point, the psychodynamic BPD issues took precedence over the substance abuse issues in the therapist's mind. Concretely, this idea surfaced when, in response to the patient's expressed wish to relocate home, her substance abuse counselor said, "When you have remained sober for 3 months," and the therapist reframed the criterion as "When you can manage visits between your mother and brother without relapsing."

Although this vignette illustrates how, with the understanding that comes from psychotherapy, priority can shift from a substance abuse diagnosis to a BPD diagnosis, such cases do not often work out so well. The presence of comorbid substance abuse appreciably increases the likelihood of suicide and diminishes the overall prognosis for the BPD patient (Stone 1990a). On the other hand, borderline patients who recover from substance abuse habits may have very good outcomes (Stone 1990b).

Still, few borderline patients can change or grow without therapies that are directed at their problems with close relationships and at the management of their angry and anguished feelings. It is therefore important for substance abuse programs to be sensitive to these ongoing issues for these patients—whose success in living, despite their appearing committed to sobriety, depends on other, more borderline-specific therapies.

BPD and Somatoform/Somatization Disorders

Borderline patients are care seekers. So are people with somatoform disorders, except that these people go to medical doctors, surgeons, and emergency rooms with physical complaints as a way to get care. Indeed, Zanarini and Frankenburg (1994) termed the borderline patient's use of emotional displays to elicit care "emotional hypochondriasis." This form of care seeking can be carried out with any significant other, but within medicine it usually involves the mental health disciplines. Some borderline patients are insistent on seeing psychiatrists (rather than psychologists or social workers) because they insist that their mental problems are somatic diseases (a very complex issue, discussed in Chapter 13 of this book). Patients who have multiple somatic complaints without obvious or well-documented physical pathology, i.e., somatizers, raise questions of malingering or hypochondriasis. The difference being that malingerers sometimes consciously but guiltlessly manufacture symptoms (sometimes called Munchausen syndrome), whereas the hypochondriac, having no more of a physical basis for their symptoms, consciously believe that medical care can relieve their symptoms. Borderline patients may use physical complaints in either way (Nadelson 1985). Though Cluster C personality disorders are even more likely to have somatoform disorders than BPD (Fink 1995; Stern et al. 1993), the risks associated with having BPD make it particularly important for medical services to be aware of. Some borderline patients may wish to be injured (i.e., they may consciously or unconsciously seek mistreatment) and thence liability issues can haunt unsuspecting doctors. Indeed, somatoform patients exemplify a striking example of why making the borderline diagnosis can be of critical importance. Knowing about BPD in a somatizing patient increases doctors' awareness about potential misuse and placebo effects from medications. It helps redirect the search for care into more explicit and less dangerous communications. It also encourages clinicians to emphasize basic healthcare messages about diet, sleep, and exercise that many borderline patients otherwise neglect. These messages are standard aspects of how cognitive-behavioral therapists assist chronic pain patients. Finally, it will be a help to such patients for other doctors to refer them for psychiatric care.

BPD and Narcissistic Personality Disorder

The differential diagnosis issue between BPD and narcissistic personality disorder (NPD) is usually triggered by the concurrence of inappropriate anger, feelings of entitlement, and suicidality (see Figure 2–4). People with either of these personality disorders are likely to use such defenses as devaluation, projection, and counterdependence (Perry and Perry, in press). This diagnostic question is more common in males because they are more typically unaware of dependency needs and thus more apt to seem narcissistic, i.e., they are more likely to present as distant and haughty. People with either type of personality disorder can become either angry or self-destructive in response to rejections or even criticisms. These apparent areas of overlap often yield discrimination upon closer scrutiny (see Sidebar 2-1).

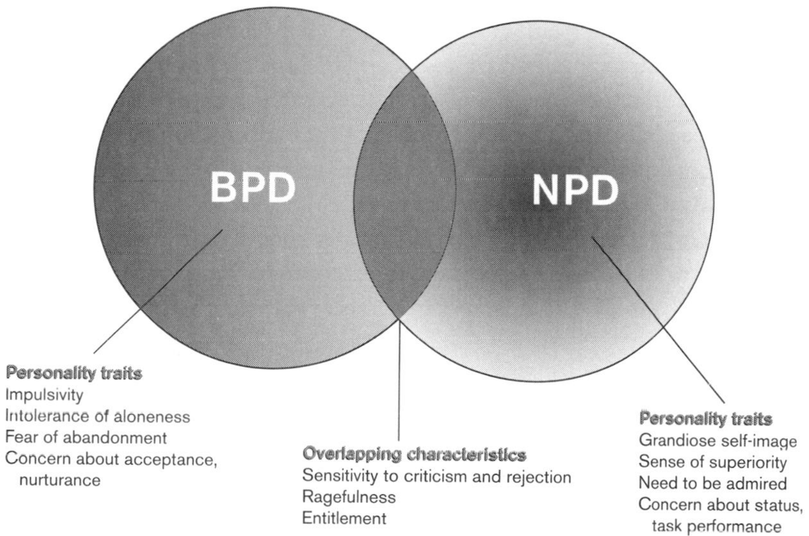

FIGURE 2–4. Distinctions and overlapping characteristics between borderline personality disorder (BPD) and narcissistic personality disorder (NPD).

Sidebar 2-1: Is Martha Stewart Borderline? I Think Not.

Yet in the biography other impressions that cast doubt on this diagnosis become evident. The behaviors, fears, and rages are not sustained patterns. They take place against a life patterned on high achievement in challenging and competitive fields of endeavor. The behaviors are reactive to events in which the issues do not involve feeling deprived and alone, but rather injured pride. Martha Stewart's self-esteem is tied to her public image of beauty, productivity, and perfectionism. That she is demanding of others is not in the service of nurturance, it is in the service of completing tasks according to her lofty standards. Although she is surely capable of rages, they ensue when she feels frustrated, criticized, or defeated, not when she feels neglected. Her self-esteem is precariously perched on standards of superiority, not precariously sustained by evidence of lovability.

On September 2, 1997, The *National Enquirer* headlined the story "Martha Stewart: Mentally Ill" and went on to report experts who judged her to have borderline personality disorder. Their conclusions were based on reading the unauthorized biography of her written by Jerry Oppenheimer, titled *Martha Stewart: Just Desserts.* The supposed experts cited the book's documentation of abandonment fears, demandingness, rages, self-destructive acts, threats, shifts from idealizing to devalued views of others, and impulsive acts. Using DSM criteria, they argued that she would appear to fulfill the current diagnostic standard for BPD.

The primary reason for consideration of the borderline diagnosis involves Martha Stewart's alleged response to her husband's leaving her. She became enraged with feelings like "How could he do this to me?" and "He has no right to do this." It is the functions he served for her that she felt abandoned by, not the man per se. His departure seemed an insulting and humiliating betrayal of her. There is little evidence that she felt she needed his love or support. For her, those needs would be admissions of weakness. More at stake seemed to be her belief in her ability to control him. These are narcissistic, not borderline, issues.

Reading her unauthorized biography could justify speculation about narcissistic personality disorder, but the twin dangers of such speculation are twofold: the potential for mistakes from such a data source and the potential for being the target of a response like Martha Stewart's response to the *National Enquirer.* Her response to the *Enquirer* is similar to her reaction to her husband: vindictive rage. She has brought suit against the newspaper for libel: defamation of character. Defamation is what hurt.

Vignette

Matthew, an 18-year-old man who used what seemed to be his girlfriend's idealization of him to sustain his fantasies of becoming a great poet, became very agitated and had suicidal ideas when he learned of his girlfriend's plans to relocate to another school—despite her assurances of ongoing love. In therapy, he talked about being enraged by the disparity between what she meant to him and what he meant to her—"otherwise, she would never leave." He hated himself for "being so stupid" as to let her mean so much.

There is no question that Matthew is narcissistically injured, but the differential diagnosis of NPD or BPD cannot be clarified without knowing 1) whether the injury revolves around the prototypically borderline fear of abandonment or around the prototypically narcissistic reaction to perceived threats to a grandiose self-image, 2) whether his relationship was sustained by his girlfriend's idealization (NPD) or by her caretaking (BPD), and 3) whether he has had a pattern of intense relationships that ended because of his becoming too needy (BPD).

Beyond the similarities noted above, however, these disorders diverge (Ronningstam and Gunderson 1991). Persons with BPD experience rejections as abandonments that trigger their fears of stark aloneness. For them, criticisms may be intolerable, because what is intended as discrete becomes generalized into an indictment of their whole person (i.e., their overall badness). Persons with NPD experience either rejection or criticisms as shameful humiliations that trigger feelings of defeat or inferiority, but, as Rinsley (1984) pointed out, do not involve issues of survival of self or others. Akhtar and Thomson (1982) believe that the grandiosity or feelings of omnipotence that characterize NPD patients mask (i.e., compensate for) covert convictions of inferiority. The self-destructive response of a borderline patient is likely to be impulsive, consistent with other impulsive behaviors; or, if it is a calculated response, it will be designed to regain caring attention. The self-destructive response of a person with NPD is less likely to be part of a pattern, and it is more likely to have lethal intentions.

People with either NPD or BPD feel entitled to special privilege, attention, or care. People with NPD believe they deserve it because they are unique and exceptional and have "earned" it. Persons with BPD feel entitled to special privilege, attention, or care because they have suffered and because they *need* more. Persons with NPD would be reluctant to recognize or acknowledge being needy; for them, it would be humiliating.

This differentiation has both theoretical and psychotherapeutic implications (Ronningstam and Gunderson 1991). The theoretical implications (discussed further in Chapter 12 of this book) involve the question of whether aggression—along with its symptoms, rage, hostility, and anger—is 1) a primary drive whose misdirection and dyscontrol create the psychopathology (i.e., is part of BPD) or is 2) reactive to environmental insults, so that its misdirection or dyscontrol is a symptom of an overly fragile self (i.e., is part of NPD). This question has therapeutic significance. The treatment of choice for NPD involves a long-term corrective attachment whose effectiveness depends on the therapist's empathy and sensitivity to not bruising the patient's self-esteem so much as to precipitate flight. A role for medications has not been established. Although long-term corrective attachment experiences are also important in the treatment of borderline patients, they, in contrast to patients with NPD, typically require pharmacological (Chapters 6 and 7 of this book) and social-rehabilitative (Chapters 8–10 of this book) modalities. As described in this book, initial treatments should be directed at behavioral and affect controls. Within their individual psychodynamic psychotherapies, borderline patients require that more attention be paid to boundaries, regressions, and negative transference issues (Chapter 12 of this book).

BPD and Antisocial Personality Disorder (ASPD)

Roughly 75% of BPD patients are female, roughly 75% of ASPD patients are male, and roughly 25% of patients with either diagnosis will meet criteria for the other (Zanarini and Gunderson 1997). Hatzitaskos et al. (1997) found that persons with BPD had more introverted hostility and that those with ASPD had more extroverted hostility. Antisocial personality is usually marked by action-oriented defenses and, as emphasized by Livesley et al. (1989), a cold, interpersonally exploitative way of relating to others (see Figure 2–5). The diagnostic dilemma often occurs when a female patient, otherwise prototypically borderline, has a pattern of calculated (conscious) deceitfulness (including malingering) and/or episodic violence. The diagnostic dilemma also occurs when a male patient with a clear pattern of violence or interpersonal irresponsibility has recurrent suicidality and deep-seated feelings of badness about himself that he struggles to keep out of his awareness.

The issue is often made no easier after a developmental history is obtained, since patients with either of these diagnoses often report neglect, abuse, and alienation (Robins 1966; Widom 1997; Zanarini et al. 1989). Their family experience often includes marital discord, abandonment, violence, and substance abuse. Kernberg's (1967, 1986) placement of these disorders together within the overarching construct of a borderline personality organization marked by broken identities, primitive defenses, and transient failures in reality testing seems incontrovertible. So disturbed is the development of many BPD or ASPD individuals that it seems unnecessary to invoke genetic causality. Yet it seems likely that the aggressivity and impulsivity shared by these patients has its roots in a temperamental predisposition (Paris 1997; Siever and Davis 1991; Zanarini and Gunderson 1997). Both disorders score similarly on the personality dimensions of high neuroticism and low agree-

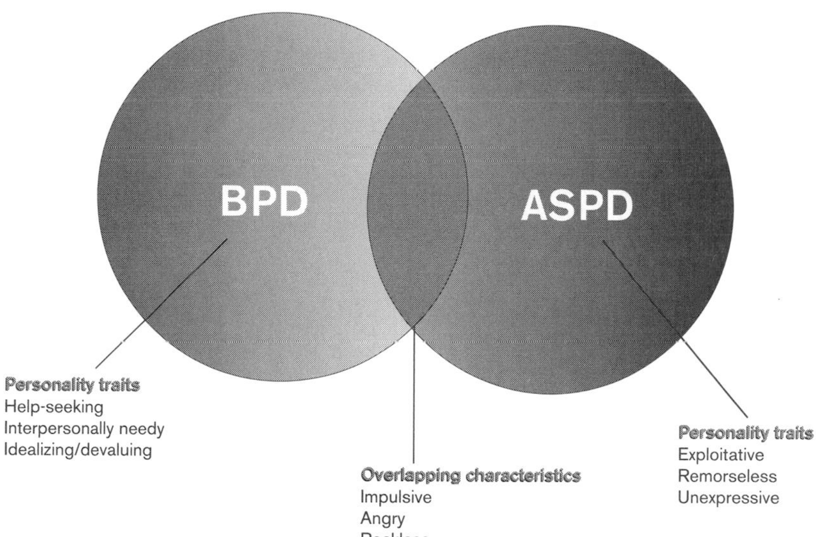

FIGURE 2–5. Distinctions and overlapping characteristics between borderline personality disorder (BPD) and antisocial personality disorder (ASPD).

ableness and conscientiousness (Widiger et al. 1994).

These similarities in phenomenology and development suggest that these two diagnoses may be highly related forms of psychopathology. Indeed, I think they are and that the distinctions are probably gender related, from both a genetic and an environmental perspective. (As a parallel observance, even infant boys can be differentiated from infant girls: the boys are more instrumental, the girls more affiliative [Gilligan 1982; Jordan et al. 1991]. This presumably genetic difference may be supported by environmental experiences that support girls' socialization and boys' task competence.) Relevant to this is the finding that adult borderline patients report a high frequency of use of transitional objects in their childhoods (Morris et al. 1986). Transitional objects, as observed by Winnicott (1953), are a normal way in which children attempt to diminish anxieties normally associated with separation from a caretaker. With borderline patients, transitional-object use often extends past its usual spontaneous ending by age 4 or 5 (Arkema 1981; Lobel 1981; Morris et al. 1986). The nursing staff on inpatient units confidently predict, when a newly admitted patient insists on his or her stuffed animal, blanket, or other inanimate source of comfort, that the person is borderline (Cardasis et al. 1997; Labbate and Benedek 1996). In contrast, Horton et al. (1974) reported, with conflicting replications (Cooper et al. 1985; Morris et al. 1986), that adult patients with ASPD report no use of transitional objects. This finding is consistent with both genetic and environmental pressure for boys to manage their needs, or drives, in ways that are less interpersonal than girls'.

Vignette

> Mr. A was a 23-year-old man with divorced parents who developed an intense, idealized relationship with his very supportive but inexperienced substance abuse counselor. Because of Mr. A's continuing to steal from his family and from stores and to drive too fast despite repeated encounters with the law, his mother sought consultation. When a change to a more confrontational and intensive therapy was recommended, he became very abusive and threatened his mother and stepfather with a knife. When his counselor, frightened by the patient's desperate calls and by his threats to kill himself, joined the mother in support of a change in treatment, Mr. A ran away. The next contact from him was a phone call apologizing for his flight and requesting that his mother send him money to pay a debt and transport him home.

Had Mr. A been 16 years old, I would have felt strongly that a borderline diagnosis should guide his treatment. Treatment would have probably required sustained care on level III (partial hospital). When I consulted and advocated a change in therapist, I still believed that his borderline issues (i.e., need for caring attention) were dominant, but it was unclear to what extent his past drug use, his potential violence, and his dishonesty (i.e., ASPD issues) made treatment unlikely to succeed. His phone call for help does nothing to resolve the question of whether his motives were exploitative or were guided by a real wish for rapprochement. By now, however, I felt that his request would be better responded to as if he primarily had ASPD.

The differentiation of these disorders has major significance to clinicians. To mistakenly diagnose a borderline patient as having ASPD often consigns a potentially treatable patient to minimal treatment. To mistakenly diagnose a patient with ASPD as being borderline is to initiate the ineffective use of valuable clinical resources and to expose other patients, even the treaters, to potential exploitation and, at worse, physical harm. Having said this, the case can be made that, when the diagnosis is in doubt, it is best to honor evidence of the patient's interest in treatment and to make a serious effort (Zanarini and Gunderson 1997). Tipping the balance toward treatment are 1) evidence of a hunger to be attached, 2) a capacity to bear negative feelings (e.g., shame, envy) or self-critical attitudes, 3) any history of sustained role functioning, 4) whether significant supports for the treatment can be called on from people the patient needs or respects, and 5) adequate monitoring of the patient's use of a therapy. Keeping an eye on these guidelines will allow clinicians to stop a therapy before harmful consequences occur. Unfortunately, for borderline patients who also fulfill criteria for ASPD, their responsiveness to treatment will usually be reduced (Clarkin et al. 1994).

SUMMARY

This discussion of the most common and difficult differential diagnosis issues has demonstrated that the boundaries separating BPD from neighboring disorders are often inherently unclear. The decision about making the diagnosis of BPD versus that of its overlapping neighbor should be guided by whether the treatment implications will benefit the patient. In most instances, making treatment plans that overlook the borderline diagnosis when it is present sets the stage for therapeutic impasses or worse (splits, regressions, countertransference enactments). Clearly woven into these diagnostic considerations are countertransference issues. There is an inevitable inclination to diagnose borderline personality disorder by those who believe they can treat it, to ignore it when clinicians feel that they cannot treat it, and to invoke it as a retrospective explanation for patients who prove noncompliant or unresponsive. Above all, this discussion intends to convey why thoughtful consideration of whether the borderline diagnosis is suitable—and informed recognition of its significance when it is present—can usefully inform clinical decisions.

REFERENCES

Akhtar S, Thomson JA Jr: Overview: narcissistic personality disorder. Am J Psychiatry 139:12–20, 1982

Akiskal HS: Subaffective disorders: dysthymic, cyclothymic and bipolar II disorders in the "borderline" realm. Psychiatr Clin North Am 4(1):25–46, 1981

American Psychiatric Association: Diagnostic and Statistical Manual of Mental Disorders, 4th Edition. Washington, DC, American Psychiatric Association, 1994

Arkema PH: The borderline personality and transitional relatedness. Am J Psychiatry 138(2):172–177, 1981

Benjamin LS, Wonderlich SA: Social perceptions and borderline personality disorder: the relation to mood disorders. J Abnorm Psychol 103(4):610–624, 1994

Blacker D, Tsuang MT: Contested boundaries of bipolar disorder and the limits of categorical diagnosis in psychiatry. Am J Psychiatry 149(11):1473–1483, 1992

Bolton S, Gunderson JG: Distinguishing borderline personality disorder from bipolar disorder: differential diagnosis and implications. Am J Psychiatry 153(9):1202–1207, 1996

Cardasis W, Hochman JA, Silk KR: Transitional objects and borderline personality disorder. Am J Psychiatry 154(2):250–255, 1997

Clarkin JF, Hull JW, Yeomans F, et al: Antisocial traits as modifiers of treatment response in borderline inpatients. J Psychother Pract Res 3(4):307–312, 1994

Cooper SH, Perry JC, Hoke L, et al: Transitional relatedness and borderline personality disorder. Psychoanalytic Psychology 2(2):115–128, 1985

Coryell WH, Zimmerman M: Personality disorder in the families of depressed, schizophrenic, and never-ill probands. Am J Psychiatry 146(4):496–502, 1989

Dahl AA: Some aspects of the DSM-III personality disorders illustrated by a consecutive sample of hospitalized patients. Acta Psychiatr Scand 328 (suppl):61–67, 1986

Dolan RT, Kreuger RF, Shea MT: Co-occurrence of Axis I and Axis II disorders, in Handbook of Personality Disorders. Edited by Livesley J. New York, Guilford (in press)

Ellison J, Barsky A, Blum NR: Frequent repeaters to an emergency service. Hospital and Community Psychiatry 40:958–960, 1989

Fink P: Psychiatric illness in patients with persistent somatization. Br J Psychiatry 166:93–99, 1995

Fyer MR, Frances AJ, Sullivan T, et al: Comorbidity of borderline personality disorder. Arch Gen Psychiatry 45(4):348–352, 1988

Gilligan C: In a Different Voice: Psychological Theory and Women's Development. Cambridge, MA, Harvard University Press, 1982

Gunderson JG, Chu JA: Treatment implications of past trauma in borderline personality disorder. Harv Rev Psychiatry 1(2):75–81, 1994

Gunderson JG, Phillips KA: A current view of the interface between borderline personality disorder and depression. Am J Psychiatry 148(8):967–975, 1991

Gunderson JG, Sabo AN: The phenomenological and conceptual interface between borderline personality disorder and PTSD. Am J Psychiatry 150(1):19–27, 1993

Gunderson J, Zanarini M, Kisiel C: Borderline personality disorder: a review of data on DSM-III-R descriptions. J Personal Disord 5:340–352, 1991

Gunderson JG, Triebwasser J, Phillips KA, et al: Personality and vulnerability to affective disorders, in Personality and Psychopathology. Edited by C. R. Cloninger. Washington, DC, American Psychiatric Press, 1999, pp 3–32

Hatzitaskos PK, Soldatos CR, Sakkas PN, et al: Discriminating borderline from antisocial personality disorder in male patients based on psychopathology patterns and type of hostility. J Nerv Ment Dis 185(7):442–446, 1997

Herkov MJ, Blashfield RK: Clinician diagnoses of personality disorders: evidence of a hierarchical structure. J Pers Assess 65:313–321, 1995

Herman J: Trauma and Recovery. New York, Basic Books, 1992

Herman JL, Perry JC, van der Kolk BA: Childhood trauma in borderline personality disorder. Am J Psychiatry 146(4):490–495, 1989

Herzog DB, Keller MB, Lavori P, et al: The prevalence of personality disorders in 210 women with eating disorders. J Clin Psychiatry 53:147–153, 1992

Horton PC, Louy J, Coppolillo HP: Personality disorder and transitional relatedness. Arch Gen Psychiatry 30:618–622, 1974

Hudziak JJ, Boffeli TJ, Kreisman JJ, et al: Clinical study of the relation of borderline personality disorder to Briquet's syndrome (hysteria), somatization disorder, antisocial personality disorder, and substance abuse disorders. Am J Psychiatry 153(12):1598–1606, 1996

Jordan J, Kaplan A, Miller J, et al: Women's Growth in Connection: Writings from the Stone Center. New York, Guilford, 1991

Kernberg O: Borderline personality organization. J Am Psychoanal Assoc 15:641–685, 1967

Kernberg O: Severe Personality Disorders: Psychotherapeutic Strategies. New Haven, CT, Yale University Press, 1986

Khantzian EJ: The self-medication hypothesis of addictive disorders: focus on heroin and cocaine dependence. Am J Psychiatry 142(11):1259–1264, 1985

Koenigsberg HW, Kaplan RD, Gilmore MM, et al: The relationship between syndrome and personality disorder in DSM-III: experience with 2,464 patients. Am J Psychiatry 142(2):207–212, 1985

Kopacz DR, Janicak PG: The relationship between bipolar disorder and personality. Psychiatric Annals 26(10):644–650, 1996

Kurtz JE, Morey LC: Negativism in evaluative judgments of words among depressed outpatients with borderline personality disorder. J Personal Disord 12(4):351–361, 1998

Labbate LA, Benedek DM: Bedside stuffed animals and borderline personality. Psychol Rep 79(2):624–626, 1996

Links PS, Steiner M, Boiago I, et al: Lithium therapy for borderline patients: preliminary findings. J Personal Disord 4(2):173–181, 1990

Livesley WJ, Jackson DN, Schroeder ML: A study of the factorial structure of personality pathology. J Personal Disord 3:292–306, 1989

Livesley WJ, Jackson DN, Schroeder ML: Factorial structure of traits delineating PDs in clinical and general population samples. J Abnorm Psychol 101:432–440, 1992

Livesley WJ, Jang KL, Vernon PA: Phenotypic and genetic structure of traits delineating personality disorder. Arch Gen Psychiatry 55:941–948, 1998

Lobel L: A study of transitional objects in the early histories of borderline adolescents. Adolescent Psychiatry 9:199–213, 1981

Loranger AW: The impact of DSM-III on diagnostic practice in a university hospital. Arch Gen Psychiatry 47:672–675, 1990

McGlashan TH, Grilo CM, Skodol AE, et al: The collaborative longitudinal personality disorders study: baseline Axis I/II and II/II diagnostic co-occurrence. Acta Psychiatr Scand, in press

Morris H, Gunderson JG, Zanarini MC: Transitional object use and borderline psychopathology. Am J Psychiatry 143(12):1534–1538, 1986

Nace EP: Substance use disorders and personality disorders: comorbidity. Psychiatric Hospital 20(2):65–69, 1989

Nadelson T: False patients/real patients: a spectrum of disease presentation. Psychother Psychosom 44(4):175–184, 1985

Paris J: Antisocial and borderline personality disorders: two separate diagnoses or two aspects of the same psychopathology? Compr Psychiatry 38(4):237–242, 1997

Perry JD, Perry JC: Conflicts, defenses, and the stability of narcissistic personality features. Psychiatry (in press)

Plakun EM: Distinguishing narcissistic and borderline personality disorders using DSM-III criteria. Compr Psychiatry 28:437–443, 1987

Reich J, Bostler H, Yates W, etal: Utilization of medical resources in persons with DSM-III personality disorders in a community sample. Int J Psychiatry Med 19:1–9, 1989

Rinsley DB: A comparison of borderline and narcissistic personality disorders. Bull Menninger Clin 48(1):1–9, 1984

Robins LN: Deviant Children Grow Up. Baltimore, Williams & Wilkins, 1966

Rogers JH, Widiger TA, Krupp A: Aspects of depression associated with borderline personality disorder. Am J Psychiatry 152(2):268–270, 1995

Ronningstam E, Gunderson J: Differentiating borderline personality disorder from narcissistic personality disorder. J Personal Disord 5(3):225–232, 1991

Sansone RA, Sansone LA, Fine MA: The relationship of obesity to borderline personality symptomatology, self-harm behaviors, and sexual abuse in female subjects in a primary-care medical setting. J Personal Disord 9(3):254–265, 1995

Siever LJ, Davis KL: A psychobiologic perspective on the personality disorders. Am J Psychiatry 148:1647–1658, 1991

Silverman JM, Pinkham L, Horvath TB, et al: Affective and impulsive personality disorder traits in the relatives of patients with borderline personality disorder. Am J Psychiatry 148:546–554, 1991

Stern J, Murphy M, Bass C: Personality disorders in patients with somatization disorder: a controlled study. Br J Psychiatry 163:785–789, 1993

Stone MH: The Fate of Borderline Patients. New York, Guilford, 1990a

Stone MH: Treatment of borderline patients: a pragmatic approach. Psychiatr Clin North Am 13(2):265–285, 1990b

Swartz M, Blazer D, George L, et al: Estimating the prevalence of borderline personality disorder in the community. J Personal Disord 4:257–272, 1990

Tyrer P, Gunderson J, Lyons M, et al: Special feature: extent of comorbidity between mental state and personality disorders. J Personal Disord 11(3):242–259, 1997

Westen D: Towards a revised theory of borderline object relations: contributions of empirical research. Int J Psychoanal 71:661–693, 1990

Westen D: Divergences between clinical and research methods for assessing personality disorders: implications for research and the evolution of Axis II. Am J Psychiatry 154:895–903, 1997

Westen D, Moses MJ, Silk KR, et al: Quality of depressive experience in borderline personality disorder and major depression: when depression is not just depression. J Personal Disord 6(4):382–393, 1992

Widiger TA, Weissman MM: Epidemiology of borderline personality disorder. Hospital and Community Psychiatry 42(10):1015–1021, 1991

Widiger TA, Trull TJ, Clarkin JF, et al: A description of the DSM-III-R and DSM-IV personality disorders with the five-factor model of personality, in Personality Disorders and the Five-Factor Model of Personality. Edited by Costa PT, Widiger TA. Washington, DC, American Psychological Association, 1994, pp 41–58

Widom CS: Child abuse, neglect and witnessing violence, in Handbook of Antisocial Behavior. Edited by Stoff DM, Breiling J, Maser JD, et al. New York, Wiley, 1997, pp 159–170

Winnicott DW: Transitional objects and transitional phenomena. Int J Psychoanal 34:89–97, 1953

Zanarini MC: BPD as an impulse spectrum disorder, in Borderline Personality Disorder: Etiology and Treatment. Edited by Paris J. Washington, DC, American Psychiatric Press, 1993, pp 67–85

Zanarini MC, Frankenburg FR: Emotional hypochondriasis, hyperbole, and the borderline patient. J Psychother Pract Res 3(1):25–36, 1994

Zanarini MC, Gunderson JG: Differential diagnosis of antisocial and borderline personality disorders, in Handbook of Antisocial Behavior. Edited by Stoff DM, Breiling J, Maser JD, et al. New York, Wiley, 1997, pp 83–91

Zanarini MC, Gunderson JG, Marino MF, et al: Childhood experiences of borderline patients. Compr Psychiatry 30(1):18–25, 1989

Zanarini MC, Frankenburg FR, Dubo ED, et al: Axis I comorbidity of borderline personality disorder. Am J Psychiatry 155(12):1733–1739, 1998a

Zanarini MC, Frankenburg FR, Dubo ED, et al: Axis II comorbidity of borderline personality disorder. Compr Psychiatry 39(5):296–302, 1998b

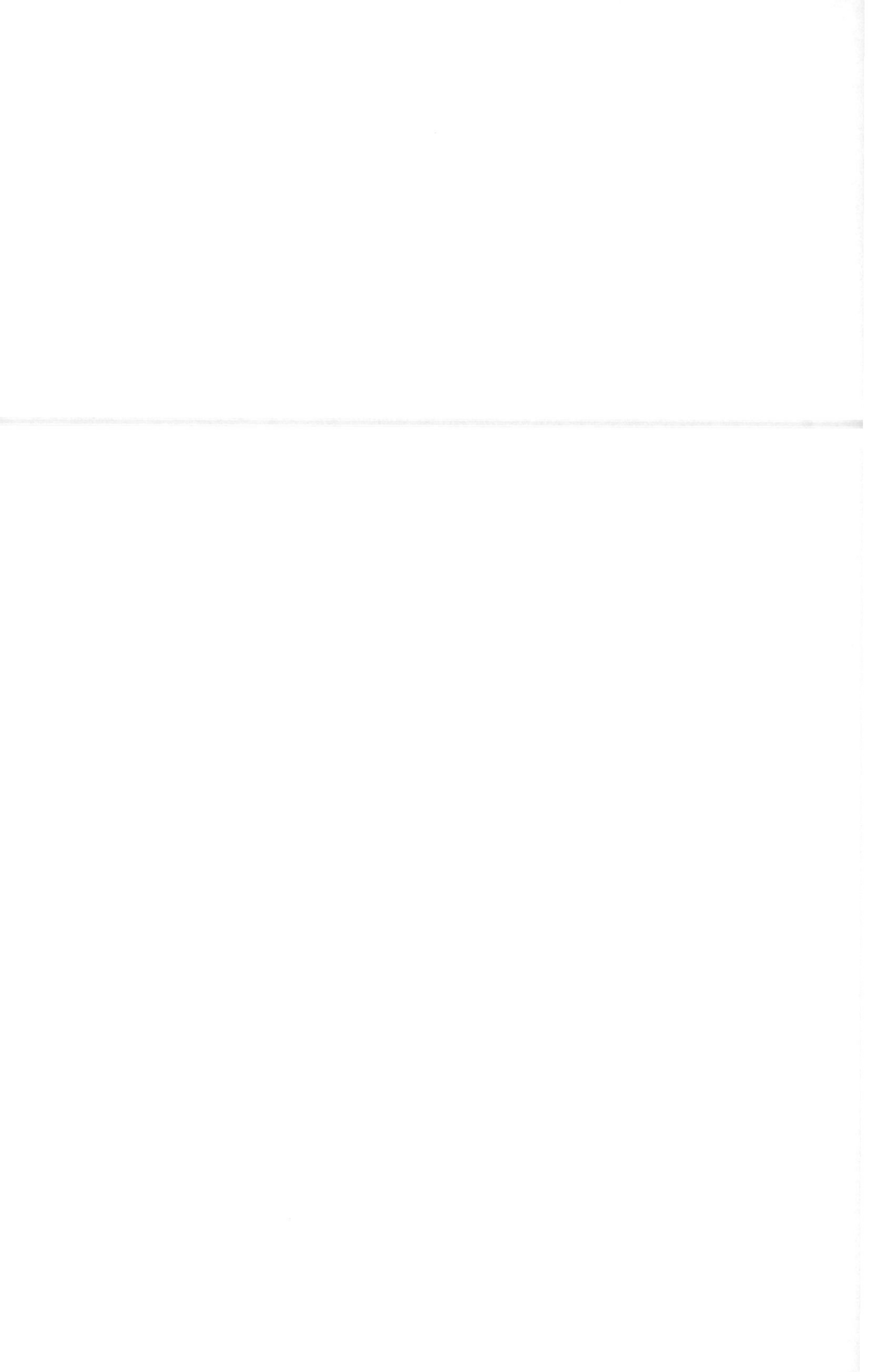

3

Overview of Treatment

Historical Overview

Changes in perspectives on the treatment of borderline patients since the 1970s parallel the larger shifts in psychiatry, in health care services, and (as noted in Chapter 1 of this book) in the diagnostic construct itself. Psychiatry has become more medicalized, health care services have become more diagnosis specific and cost conscious, and the borderline diagnosis has been validated. Psychoanalysts made the initial observations about borderline patients largely on the basis of the uniquely vexing clinical problems these patients created in testing boundaries and in regressing when in unstructured settings. When Kernberg (1968) and especially Masterson (1971, 1972) wrote optimistic reports about the treatability of these patients, they inspired a tide of ambitious long-term, psychoanalytically informed treatments in both inpatient and outpatient settings. As was shown in Figure 1–5, since 1968, 53 books about psychoanalytic psychotherapies have been written, cresting with 19 between 1990 and 1994 (as found in a Library of Congress database search). In institutional settings, most notably in prestigious private hospitals, long-term units devoted to treating borderline patients had developed by the 1980s. Both the psychoanalytic outpatient psychotherapies and these long-term inpatient treatments were based on ambitious hopes for curative changes.

Even as the swell of intensive long-term psychoanalytic treatments was cresting, the excesses, limitations, and narrowness of the approach were being recorded. Many clinicians, including notable analysts (Adler 1981, 1986; H.J. Friedman 1969; Zetzel 1971), felt that long-term institutional care was regressive and that short-term stays had advantages. Others who had worked in long-term settings noted that it often led to intractable control struggles (Gunderson 1984) such as Kaysen (1993) described in her best-selling book *Girl, Interrupted*. In outpatient settings, similar observations occurred. Even psychoanalytic therapies by experts often ended abruptly with the borderline patient's flight (Waldinger and Gunderson 1984), and these therapies were, in any event, economically or logistically unfeasible for all but a few.

Important shifts in psychiatry from a psychoanalytic to a biological paradigm and from a clinical to an empirical base of knowledge changed treatment standards for borderline patients. The foundations upon which ambitious long-term psychoanalytic therapies were built during the 1970s (i.e., compelling theories and expert opinions) were permanently undermined during the 1980s. Those theories and expert opinions were reframed as hypotheses, whose continued implementation would require empirical nourishment. Since the 1980s, empiricism and reliance on standardized diagnostic and outcome measures have established new foundations for testing treatment efficacy. These foundations showed that different treatments may effect changes in different and discrete sectors of psychopathology (e.g., mood, cognition, and behavior). Moreover, the continued growth of biological psychiatry underscored the potential for medications to change symptoms that had often been resistant to psychological therapies. These changes were reflected in a series of controlled medication trials conducted during the 1980s with reliably diagnosed borderline patients. These changes were also reflected in the dramatic decline in new books about treating borderline patients since 1994 (only 5).

In the 1990s, clinical and research attention slowly turned to sociotherapeutic modalities—that is, the role of partial hospital, group, family, and cognitive-behavioral therapies. This change seemed extremely overdue: a dramatic finding of the first comparative study (Gunderson et al. 1975) had been that the social functioning of borderline patients was as handicapped as that of schizophrenic patients—and far worse than that of depressed patients. I believe that this delayed attention to treating the severe social dysfunction of borderline patients stemmed from the resistance to such attention found in most borderline patients themselves. They often actively avoid or react with disdain to talk of vocation or social skills, as if these factors are unimportant. No doubt advances in overcoming such resistance has been pushed by more awareness of deficits, as well as by deinstitutionalization: the rehabilitative needs of these patients was masked within hospitals.

An informed approach to treating borderline patients now involves the thoughtful deployment of multiple modalities. It is in the context of these historical developments in treating borderline patients that modern professionals are confronted with the need for much more complicated treatment planning and the need to integrate the component modalities. In this chapter I offer an overview of the selection and conceptualization of treatment services.

GENERIC THERAPEUTIC PROCESSES AND THE FUNCTIONS THEY SERVE

A conceptual framework about therapeutic processes helps clinicians and patients understand what functions can be served by different therapeutic programs. In this section are described five therapeutic functions: containment, support, structure, involvement, and validation (see Gunderson 1978). The first two of these, containment and support, are often performed unilaterally by staff *to* or at least *for* patients; therefore they are treatments. The latter three are usually performed in collaboration *with* patients, requiring their consent and desire. Table 3–1 summarizes how these functions differ in goals, implementation, and applicability to borderline patients (see also Figure 3–1).

TABLE 3–1. Therapeutic functions

Function	Implementation	Indications
Containment	Level IV (hospital)	Loss of self-control, dangerousness
	Medications	
	Monitoring	
Support	All levels (I–IV)	Low self-esteem, self-care deficits
	Caretaking	
	Attention (all modalities)	
Structure	Levels IV–II (intensive outpatient)	Skill deficits, maladaptive behaviors
	Direction: cognitive-behavioral therapies and psychopharmacology	
	Education—patient and family	
	Contingencies	
Involvement	Levels III (partial hospital)–I (outpatient)	Maladaptive interpersonal relationships, social isolation
	1-to-1 interaction	
	Milieu, group, and family therapies	
Validation	Level I (outpatient)	Identity/self-image problems, intimacy aversion
	Individual psychotherapy: interpretation, empathy	

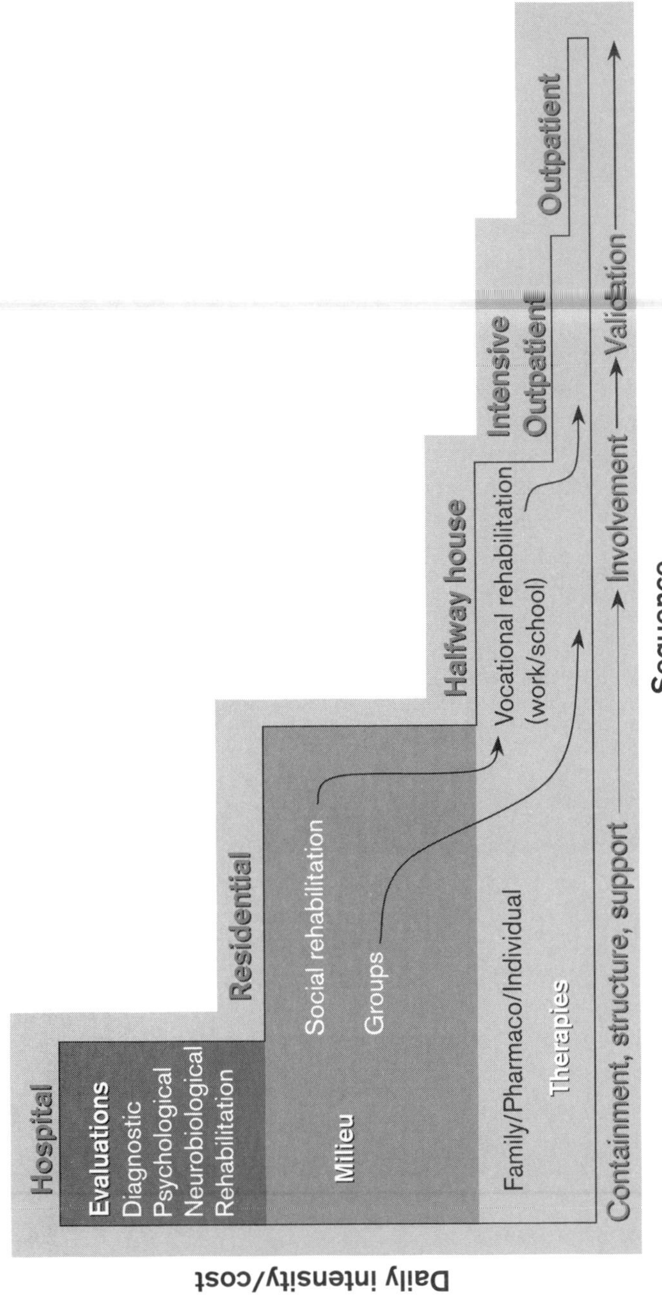

FIGURE 3–1. Multiple modalities and step-down services.

Containment

This process functions to preserve or enhance the physical well-being of people. For borderline patients, containment usually involves securing their safety by provision of asylum from stressful situations, sometimes even with locked doors and supervision, but usually only with monitored food and medications. Containment refers to external imposition of control and is the most concrete form of what Winnicott (1965) referred to as a "holding environment." It alleviates the responsibility for self-control and offers borderline patients a basic form of caretaking. For borderline patients who feel angry about their responsibilities for caring for themselves, too much containment may become habit forming, thereby creating a regressive option that is antitherapeutic. For most borderline patients, the initial relief at containment is followed by fears of being controlled. (Medications often dramatize such a shift: see Chapter 6 of this book.) During the course of successful treatment, borderline patients internalize controls so that by the time they are nearly well, the holding environment can be created and sustained by talking, and by the time they are well, they can create the environment mentally.

Support

This process functions to make patients feel better and to enhance their self-esteem. Support can be given by accommodating patients' limitations (e.g., tutors for those with learning disabilities or clarification for those with poor reality testing). Support is most direct when it consists of assistance with travel or feeding or involves verbal activities such as direction or education. It is most obvious when it consists of praise or reassurance. A very basic supportive technique is validation—affirming the reality of patients' perceptions or the justification for their feelings. (Validation as a technique should be differentiated from validation as a broader therapeutic process, as described below.) Although the absence of significant amounts of support will often evoke attributions of rejection or cruelty in borderline patients, too much support can evoke unrealistic dependency expectations.

For borderline patients, attention is always a critically important supportive process in treatment. Even negative attention is better than inattention. Often borderline patients appeal for direct support through somatic complaints or through their accounts of prior mistreatment. Seeing the borderline patient as handicapped, disabled, or mentally ill is a way to enhance sympathetic responses by staff or by families.

As with containment, support can become less behavioral and more verbal as borderline patients improve. It is, however, a process that is a necessary part of all therapeutic activities throughout treatment. The necessity of this function has sometimes been overlooked in psychoanalytic psychotherapies, but its role with borderline patients has become well documented (Chapter 12 of this book).

Structure

This process functions to make the environment predictable—as simple and repetitious as possible. It involves organizing the patient's time, place, and person. Structure is an impersonal holding, neither invasive nor neglectful. This therapeutic function is served by schedules, clarity of roles and goals, privilege systems, controls, and clear consequences for behaviors. It is most important in addressing the borderline individual's socially maladaptive behaviors, like rages or impulsivity. Structure has particular importance for BPD: its absence invites regression and projection. It is a central component of what the cognitive-behavioral therapies offer (see Chapter 8 of this book) and is usually appealing as well as relieving to borderline patients.

Examples of structure would be a contract regarding wrist slashing that would mandate a visit to an emergency room and one missed therapy session as consequences. More generally, it would mean starting and ending sessions on time, always at the same site, and in the same seats. Within sessions, more structure is desirable early in treatment—for example, consistently recounting reactions to the last visit and to any intervening contacts or consistently reviewing work or health issues.

Involvement

This therapeutic process forces patients to attend to and interact with their interpersonal environment. The process strengthens tolerance and identifies and modifies maladaptive interpersonal traits (e.g., devaluing or idealizing). Examples are development of shared goals and collaboration on treatment planning. All group activities make involvement a central process, especially those where there is discussion of group members' ways of relating to each other. Therapeutic communities as described by Main (1946) and Jones (1952, 1956) made involvement the therapy.

For borderline patients, involvement is facilitated by interpreting symptomatic behaviors as being interpersonally motivated: "You threatened the nurse after your mother failed to call"; "You retreated to bed right after your therapist announced her vacation"; "You avert your eyes whenever I appear disapproving." To return to the wrist-slashing example, the process of involvement would be invoked by interpreting the action as having sadistic or controlling intentions.

Borderline patients generally fear aloneness and hunger for involvement, but its presence usually prompts anxieties. Lewin and Shulz (1996) titled a book *Losing and Fusing* to underscore this dilemma and to give equal attention to the borderline individual's anxieties about too much involvement—his or her intolerance of togetherness. As noted in Chapter 1 of this book, I believe that the fear of losing is a more dominant fear than fear of fusing and perhaps is even part of the core psychopathology in the individual with BPD (see Chapter 13 of this book).

Validation

This therapeutic process affirms and consolidates patients' uniqueness—their individuality. Validation is conveyed by customizing treatment, by one-to-one talks, by attention to patients' past history, and by new learning—encouraging patients to extend themselves into areas of uncertain competence or consequence.

For borderline patients, validation often begins by empathic recognition of their pain and their past misfortunes. (This does not mean affirming that they are victims of malevolence [see Chapters 1 and 11 of this book], only that they suffered from what were "unfair" burdens or stresses.) Validation allows borderline patients to become closer and in time diminishes distrust. The process also underscores their uniqueness and the significance of their life history. It makes them feel understandable, less toxic, and more human—like others.

MULTIPLE MODALITIES AND STEP-DOWN SERVICES: AN OVERVIEW

Whereas virtually all borderline patients require different levels of treatment (see Chapter 5 of this book) and multiple modalities (Chapters 6–10), few will require all levels and all modalities. There are several ways to think about the interactions, complementarity, and sequencing of different modalities of treatment. The usual sequencing of modalities moves from biological therapies to rehabilitative (psychosocial) therapies and finally to psychological (or *intrapsychic*) approaches. As shown in Figure 3–1, the five therapeutic functions discussed above are also offered in progression through the various levels and types of care. The sequencing is anchored by considerations of modalities' usual duration, their expectable costs and benefits, their relative levels of empirical support, and their replicability. In practice, the sequence often involves a shift from the highest level of care (hospital settings) to the lowest (outpatient care) via a series of intermediary step-down services (residential care, day care, etc.). These services and patients' relative length of stay are described in Chapter 5 of this book and schematized in Table 5–1.

Sociotherapies

The most common pair of outpatient modalities (level I in Figure 5–1, this book)—psychotherapy and psychopharmacology—overlook the significant contribution that sociotherapies can make to treating borderline patients. Sociotherapies refer to that middle range of therapies that more directly addresses the observable social impairment and social adjustment issues— the issues that Links (1993) says require a psychiatric rehabilitation model (see Table 3–2). Although the social rehabilitative needs of borderline patients are clearly central to the structured community or milieu therapy aspects of residential (level III) services (as discussed later), most often these rehabilitative needs are inadequately addressed by the time patients begin outpatient care. At present, manual-guided outpatient sociotherapies that were specifically designed for BPD have established their benefits for this population. These are discussed in detail in later chapters: dialectical behavior therapy (DBT) (Chapter 8 of this book), psychoeducational family therapy (Chapter 9), and interpersonal group (IPG) therapy (Chapter 10). These modalities or others that improve social skill and adaptation need to become more central to treatment plans and more available in outpatient clinics.

Generic Sequence of Change

To develop treatment goals and to assess whether existing treatments for borderline patients are making timely progress, it is essential to have an overall conceptual framework for processes of change. Emerging from my own experience (Gunderson 1984) and the research with schizophrenic patients (Hogarty et al. 1997), and buttressed by a review of related literature (Kopta et al. 1994; Lanktree and Briere 1995), a sequence in which changes can be expected

TABLE 3–2. Goals of sociotherapies

Enhance social skills
- Manners
- Listening
- Comfort (e.g., chitchat)

Recognize one's specific interpersonal style
- Tendencies to misattribute
- Typical reactions to praise, criticism, or competition
- Tendencies to disclose (feelings or attitudes) vs. isolate/withdraw vs. deceive/mislead

Goals specific to groups
- Confront undesirable styles
- Diminish aggression and defensiveness
- Enhance disclosure, expression of feelings, and assertiveness

Goals specific to families
- Identify indirect/covert styles of communication
- Enhance communication
- Clarify/modify reinforcement patterns
- Validate/invalidate attributions
- Clarify motives, intentions, and effects

is proposed (Table 3–3). Of particular value is the conclusion by Kopta et al. that, although patients' subjective states can change within weeks, characterological traits and self-concepts cannot be expected to change before a year in therapy.

TABLE 3–3. The framework for expectable changes

Areas of disturbance	Relevant interventions	Expectable time for change
Subjective state	Concerned attention, validation, interpretation	Weeks
Dysphoric feelings	Reality testing, problem solving, pattern recognition	Weeks
Behavior	Clarification of defensive purposes and maladaptive consequences	Months
Interpersonal style	Confrontation, pattern recognition, here and now	6–18 months
Intrapsychic organization	Defense and transference analysis, corrective relationships, real relationships	>2 years

Source. Reprinted from Gunderson JG, Gabbard GO: "Making the Case for Psychoanalytic Therapies in the Current Psychiatric Environment." *J Am Psychoanal Assoc* 47(3):679–704, 1999. Used with permission.

Converging evidence from existing research on schizophrenia supports the general validity of the sequence and timetable for changes suggested here for BPD. With schizophrenic patients, symptom remission, diminished family conflict, and improved social skills function can be accomplished within a year (Hogarty et al. 1986). This treatment still, however, leaves the successfully treated patients interpersonally isolated and anhedonic, thus setting the stage for individual therapies (Hogarty et al. 1997).

Sequence of Expectable Changes for BPD

Figure 3–2 elaborates on the sequence of and approximate timetable for changes that are expectable for successful progress in borderline patients. It is important to recognize that this timetable is schematic—that there are significant variations, depending on the stage from which borderline patients start treatment (e.g., some are very unaware of anger, some are successfully employed).

This account of expectable changes is a variation of my previous efforts (Gunderson 1984; Gunderson et al. 1993; Waldinger and Gunderson 1989) and is revisited elsewhere in this book by accounts of the sequence of therapeutic functions and modalities (in this chapter and Chapter 5 of this book), the sequence of changes in family intervention (Chapter 9), and the sequence of changes within a psychotherapeutic relationship (Chapters 11 and 12). As described previously (Gunderson et al. 1993), the continued growth of knowledge about therapeutic effectiveness for borderline patients depends upon specifying increasingly discrete and more time-limited indices of change in which outcome can be measured. The clinical value of identifying the sequence and timetable for expectable changes is that therapists, patients, and families can recognize that failure to see such changes raises questions about therapeutic effectiveness (see Sidebar 3–1). This does not mean that such therapies are not being beneficial. It means that the question should be raised whether the therapeutic services could be improved. The best way to address these issues is by consultation.

Sidebar 3–1: Can Consumers Judge Progress?

Asking is essential, but consumers often don't do it. Clinicians can expect that increased consumer education and empowerment will magnify the frequency and urgency with which consumers will question answers based on the assumption of authority.

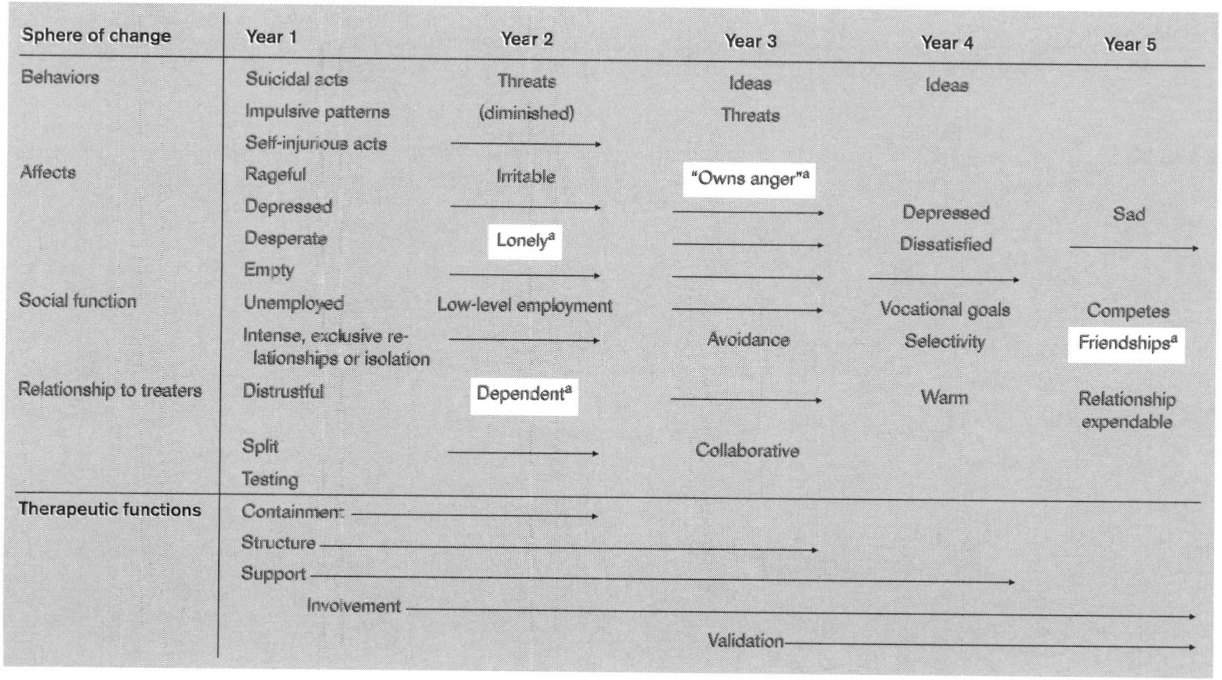

Sphere of change	Year 1	Year 2	Year 3	Year 4	Year 5
Behaviors	Suicidal acts	Threats	Ideas	Ideas	
	Impulsive patterns	(diminished)	Threats		
	Self-injurious acts	→			
Affects	Rageful	Irritable	"Owns anger"[a]		
	Depressed	→	→	Depressed	Sad
	Desperate	Lonely[a]	→	Dissatisfied	→
	Empty	→	→	→	
Social function	Unemployed	Low-level employment	→	Vocational goals	Competes
	Intense, exclusive relationships or isolation	→	Avoidance	Selectivity	Friendships[a]
Relationship to treaters	Distrustful	Dependent[a]	→	Warm	Relationship expendable
	Split	→	Collaborative		
	Testing				
Therapeutic functions	Containment →	→			
	Structure →	→	→		
	Support →	→	→	→	
	Involvement →	→	→	→	→
			Validation →	→	→

FIGURE 3–2. Sequence and timetable for expectable changes in BPD patients during therapy.
Note. Arrows following the spheres of change indicate continution from prior year. Arrows following the five therapeutic functions show the years of treatment in which the functions should be performed.
[a]Particularly notable markers of change.

When progress is obvious, inquiring about it won't be needed. But progress often is not obvious, and treaters often don't go out of their way to volunteer their views on the issue. Therapists, of course, are under no obligation to answer questions about progress. But this doesn't mean the questions shouldn't be asked. If the question comes from the borderline patient, it is often cause for a thoughtful discussion. If the question comes from anyone else, the therapist may feel constraints about confidentiality. These constraints rarely are a real obstacle. Almost always the patient needs reassurance that the therapist's response to others involves only a disclosure of his or her views about progress–views the patient will already have previewed–and not a disclosure of what goes on in sessions.

If therapists too emphatically or categorically say they won't talk about treatment progress, that response will, and should, underscore a consumer's concerns. Consultation is desirable. Most experienced therapists will use such enquiries as opportunities to hear why the patient or the patient's significant others have concerns about progress. Patients may be reassured by the opportunity to address reasons why progress has in fact been disappointing (e.g., missed appointments, substance abuse). Such enquiries from others set the stage for subsequent discussions that will involve the patient. Consumers should become acquainted with the overall sequence of expectable changes, described in this chapter and illustrated in Figure 3–2. With the evolution of more public information and consumer advocacy (see Chapter 13 of this book), clinicians are becoming more comfortable with such discussions.

There are significant variations between patients in how changes in one of the spheres shown in Figure 3–2 affects changes in others (e.g., some patients may become very dependent on their therapist during times when they are unemployed or may become suicidal years after starting treatment when feeling acutely abandoned). Still, the progression of changes is reasonably predictable. This schema is supported in a meta-analysis of the effectiveness of psychosocial therapies for BPD. Perry and Bond (2000) noted that subjective complaints, mood states, and global function improved more in the first year of treatment than did social function and interpersonal relationships. Following are more detailed accounts of what changes involve within each of the four spheres of change shown in Figure 3–2. This figure also shows how these changes relate to the primacy of the different therapeutic functions described above.

Changes Within Four Spheres

Affects

Some negative affect states (anxiety, despair, anger, fears) in borderline patients are among those that can change the soonest. Most notably, the states of desperation or panic engendered by abandonment and aloneness can be dramatically reduced (within hours even) by involvement in an adequate "*holding environment*" (Winnicott's [1965] term, as mentioned previously in this chapter, connoting a situation in which a person feels contained and safe). Although the rapid relief of dysphoric affects has always characterized the borderline patient's response to hospitalization, the relief can be sustained by adequate aftercare treatment or by medications (Chapters 6 and 7 of this book), or sometimes by increased familial supports. Similarly, states of rage will be dramatically reduced by the presence of holding relationships. Here, however, the rages give way to ongoing occurrences of ready irritability and impatience, traits whose change in response to medications or other treatments is not very predictable.

The depressed symptoms of hopelessness, worthlessness, or despair about the future remain intermittent states that can gradually diminish in intensity. Depressed moods may persist or actually become more evident when borderline patients correct the behavioral problems that have served defensive functions. Thus the use of carbamazepine (see Chapter 7 of this book) or DBT (Chapter 8) could change behaviors without improving depressed symptoms. It is a step forward when these depressive mental states become connected to longings for care or feelings of loneliness. Both psychoanalytic partial hospital programs (Chapter 5) and Adler/Kohut self-psychological psychotherapy (Chapter 12) have shown improvements in the first year. Still, persistent dysphoric states typify many borderline patients (Zanarini et al. 1998) and, in my experience, only give way significantly when patients resolve their splitting—that is, when they learn to own their own hostilities comfortably and accept them as an appropriate part of their relationships. The earliest I have seen this occur is in the fourth year of treatment (see Chapter 12 for discussion).

Of all the negative affects typifying borderline patients, emptiness seems to be the most resistant to change. After years with improved functioning, some borderline patients do report that it bothers them less or they feel it less often. This seems to be a gradual process that, in theory, relates to the internalization of good experiences of being cared for, either within intensive therapy or in relationships outside therapy.

Behaviors: Impulse/Action Pattern

This is another area in which medications can help borderline patients. Usually the benefits are not dramatic. As noted in Table 8–1, dialectical behavior therapy (DBT) identifies behavioral changes as the highest priorities for change—for obvious reasons of safety and survival and to sustain the therapy that will, it is hoped, then improve the quality of life. Traditionally, psychodynamic therapies have accorded behavioral change secondary status, believing that self-destructive or suicidal behaviors will diminish by themselves when patients acquire either insight into their motivations or stable relationships. In both types of therapy, the process of behavioral change begins by recognizing—or learning—that behaviors that have been habitual and may have had adaptive functions are counterproductive. This recognition occurs through having unwanted consequences clarified (e.g., being rejected after being too needy) or enacted (being given less attention after cutting oneself), or through learning new coping strategies (see Chapter 8 of this book). The primary targets for behavioral change involve self-destructive behaviors such as cutting, substance abuse, or eating disorders, but others involve alienating behaviors such as yelling, demanding, or withdrawal. Of note, in addition to medications and DBT, psychodynamically based partial hospitals (Chapter 5), and individual therapies (Chapter 12) have also now empirically demonstrated their ability to bring about behavioral change within the first year of treatment.

Social Function: Impairment

The clearest evidence of borderline patients' social impairment is their unemployment rate, a rate similar to that seen in individuals with schizophrenia (Gunderson et al. 1975)—despite apparent social and intellectual abilities that should enable individuals with BPD to do better. Structure is needed to diminish an elaboration of affects or a decreased reality sense (Singer and Larson 1981). The simplest and most common form of structure involves a steady job. But remaining vocationally or otherwise socially dysfunctional has many determinants. Some patients are too impulse-driven; but even when they are not, they often resist attaining employment because it threatens secondary gains (e.g., attention, sympathy, low expectations) and generates abandonment fears as well as fears of failure. To make employment as palatable as possible, low-demand, high-structure work is optimal (see Sidebar 5–2 in this book). At present there has been no documentation of the advantages for vocational performance of any treatment; but, as shown in Figure 3–2, my experience is that job progress should become evident in the course of effective therapies during the second year.

Social impairment in interpersonal relations is also a focus of treatment. An early goal in this area is to develop a network of friendly but somewhat superficial acquaintances. Group living situations may be more feasible than a romance, in which too many needs or expectations are ignited. Of note is that when behavioral problems diminish, many borderline patients become quite socially phobic. To avoid expected rejections, they isolate themselves, even to the point of qualifying for the diagnosis of avoidant personality disorder. True friendships, without dependency but built on shared interests and depth of caring, are triumphs that signal someone as no longer having BPD. Although this may occur by the third year of treatment, I believe it is truly rare before five years.

Relationship With Treaters

More will be said about the relationship with treaters throughout this book, and certainly this aspect of treatment has received extensive coverage in the literature. Initially, borderline patients' relationships with treaters are distrustful or split (i.e., idealized or devalued). Idealization is helpful and can be promoted by validation and the promise of relief from dysphoric moods. The proactive "I can help you" approach offered by psychopharmacologists or cognitive-behavioral therapists exemplifies this validation and promise. More sustained trust can be engendered by reliability, availability, and resilience in the face of testing. Case managers, group leaders, family therapists, and psychopharmacologists, as well as individual therapists, will all need to achieve this type of relationship. Establishing trustworthiness sets the stage for emotional dependency—a good basis for case management, psychopharmacology, or exploratory psychotherapy. The subsequent changes seen in Figure 3–2 are relevant primarily to long-term psychotherapy (Chapter 12 of this book). Even in DBT (Chapter 8), the third-stage targets of increased self-respect and pursuit of individual goals involve intrapsychic changes (Linehan 1993) that are consistent with the overall sequence of changes expectable from both generic and BPD-specific observations about change described in this chapter.

General Principles That Guide the Initial Structuring of Treatment

The following five general points are important in initiating treatments for borderline patients:

Diagnosis

Patients and those they live with should be familiarized with the diagnosis (see Chapter 1 of this book), including its expectable course, responsiveness to treatments, and known pathogenetic factors. Psychoeducational methods are appropriate and are generally welcomed by both patients and their families (see Chapter 8 for a more explicit description of ways to conduct psychoeducation).

Comorbidity

It has become common practice in treating those with BPD to give priority to treating comorbid Axis I conditions, such as substance abuse, depression, PTSD, or eating disorders (see Chapter 2 of this book). However, this practice should be accompanied by offering cautions about the overall prognosis for that Axis I condition. It is useful to anticipate problems and explicitly cite how having BPD usually limits the responsiveness of Axis I conditions to the usual treatments. Still, the partial remission either of the Axis I condition or of BPD can beneficially affect the other condition.

Primary Clinician

It is essential that someone be identified who will assume responsibility for each patient's safety and treatment. This person's role inevitably involves serving as case manager (see Chapter 4 of this book). The role may also include being the patient's psychotherapist, but only if the person has suitable training and the patient indicates an interest in change (see Chapter 11).

Short-Term Goals

Short-term goals establish the task orientation of therapy: it is for the purpose of change. Realistic goals such as diminished suicidality, balancing a checkbook, developing alliances, or structuring time should be targeted with time-limited treatment plans. At the same time, long-term goals (e.g., tolerating aloneness, developing intimate relationships, and achieving career satisfaction) should be encouraged as possibilities.

Least Restrictive Safe Treatment Setting

Identifying the least restrictive safe treatment setting not only is cost beneficial, but also allows the most effective treatment. See Chapter 5 of this book for a discussion of this topic.

TYPES AND SEQUENCE OF THERAPEUTIC ALLIANCE

The concept of a therapeutic alliance helps frame the discussion of both the initial engagement of borderline patients in all forms of therapy and the subsequent longer-term processes of therapies. The concept of alliance has special significance for BPD: at one time, an alliance was considered a prerequisite for dynamic psychotherapy, which, if true, would in theory render many such patients unsuitable for that modality (see Sidebar 3–2).

To guide our usage of the term *alliance,* Table 3–4 adopts definitions of three types that occur sequentially (Greenspan and Scharfstein 1981; Luborsky 1976). Defining roles and goals and establishing a concrete framework for the treatment (schedule, fee, confidentiality) constitutes the earliest form of alliance, the *contractual* alliance (see Table 3–4). It is relevant to all modalities of treatment. To a considerable extent, the problem of dropouts can be diminished by giving special attention to mutually agreed upon expectations for the therapy.

TABLE 3–4. Three forms of therapy alliance

Contractual (behavioral). This form refers to the agreement between patient and therapist on treatment goals and their roles in achieving them. This type can be established in the first session, though it often takes two or three.

Relational (affective/empathic). Emphasized by Rogerian client-centered relationships. This form refers to patient's experience of the therapist as caring, understanding, genuine, and likable. This type develops in the first 6 months.

Working (cognitive/motivational). The analytic model prototype that, as noted, develops as a significant improvement for borderline patients. Here the patient joins the therapist as a reliable collaborator who helps the patient understand her/himself. This type forms gradually but is unlikely to be reliable for several years.

Sidebar 3–2: Myths About Alliance With Borderline Patients

A report provocatively entitled "The Myth of the Alliance With Borderline Patients" was written more than 20 years ago by Adler (1979). In that report, Adler, following L. Friedman (1969), argued that a *working* alliance (as in Table 3–4) develops as an outcome only late in psychoanalytic psychotherapy with borderline patients—so late that they may in fact no longer have a borderline personality. This thesis contrasted with an earlier analytic theorem, that the presence of or capacity for a working alliance was prerequisite to engaging in an exploratory, insight-oriented, transference-based psychotherapy (Greenson 1965; Sterba 1934; Zetzel 1956).

This separation of the alliance from transference has served conceptual purposes, but it is intrinsically mythical. In fact, the ability to observe oneself collaboratively (i.e., while sitting with a therapist, which might be considered evidence of an alliance) is itself based on a transference wherein the patient's suspension of disbelief and suspiciousness is based on acquired expectations about relationships. It is unlikely to be an expectation that has been "earned" by virtue of experience with the therapist. Indeed, a good working alliance within psychotherapy is based on a transference, presumably derived from early childhood experiences, in which there was a secure attachment with sufficient opportunity for self-expression and nonpunitive response that positive expectations of relationship can be operative with a relative stranger (Brenner 1988; Gill 1979; Hoffman 1998; Langs 1976).

The *relational* alliance (discussed in Chapter 12 of this book) is a type that is central to most individual therapies, including cognitive-behavioral types, and is often an important, albeit adjunctive, element of a psychopharmacologist's, family therapist's, or group therapist's functioning.

The *working* form of alliance is the classical psychoanalytic model of alliance. In this mature form, the patient and the therapist are joined by their mutual interest in and attentiveness to a common task, the understanding of the patient. As described in Chapter 12 of this book, the presence of this form evolves slowly and can dramatically disappear in sessions with borderline patients, even years after therapy has begun.

COUNTERTRANSFERENCE

No report about treating borderline patients can fail to note the strong countertransference responses that such patients evoke and the frequency with which those responses are destructive to therapies of all kinds. The classic paper on countertransference hate by Maltsberger and Buie (1974) was written from experience with borderline patients. Gabbard and Wilkinson (1994) provide a comprehensive and clinically valuable guide to this essential topic. So strong is this feature that even the diagnosis itself carries countertransference weight (as described in Sidebar 1–5). A distinction can be made between emotional or attitudinal responses to general characteristics of borderline patients (e.g., neediness or anger) that may determine whether a clinician will want to work with them and the emotional or attitudinal responses that are evoked as an outgrowth of getting involved with a patient. The latter are what can greatly affect whether a clinician's work will prove personally rewarding for the clinician and effective for the borderline patient.

As is evident throughout this book, no clinical role offers a safe retreat from potential transference-countertransference enactments with borderline patients. Having said this, the more central one's responsibilities, the more intensive the contracts, and the more involving one's interactional style, the more likely it is that transference-countertransference problems will arise. Psychopharmacological and cognitive-behavioral interventions enhance early positive transferences by their explicit and structured efforts to relieve subjective distress. Psychoanalytic therapies invite more negative transference in that they emphasize the role of interpretive rather than supportive interventions and in that they invite projections by virtue of their inactivity, neutrality, and encouragement of self-disclosure.

It is an important aspect of caring for BPD patients that clinicians not work alone. The need for supervision, consultation, case discussions, and/or communication with other members of a team are all safeguards against countertransference enactments. These interactions with other clinical professionals also provide a type of supportive relief that transforms such reactions into understandable, commonplace, and clinically valuable experiences. It is not coincidental that the two outpatient therapies with the best empirical support, DBT (Chapter 8 of this book) and Adler/Kohut psychoanalytic therapy (Chapter 12), involve very heavy doses of supervision, consultation, and discussions.

SUMMARY

This chapter offers an overview of the processes, modalities, and levels of care involved in the treatment of borderline patients. The chapter offers clinicians and patients a conceptual infrastructure by which they can organize treatment plans and by which they can determine whether progress is occurring—in essence, a structure for deciding whether a treatment program is well suited to the patient's changing goals and needs. This discussion establishes the road map for the rest of the book, which follows the borderline patient's progress from being severely impaired and suicidal to having conflicts about competition and concerns about capacity for intimacy.

References

Adler G: The myth of the alliance with borderline patients. Am J Psychiatry 1136:642–645, 1979

Adler G: The borderline patient in the general hospital. Gen Hosp Psychiatry 3(4):297–300, 1981

Adler G: Borderline Psychopathology and Its Treatment. New York, Jason Aronson, 1986

Brenner C: Working alliance, therapeutic alliance, and transference, in The Mind in Conflict. New York, International Universities Press, 1988, pp 137–157

Friedman HJ: Some problems of inpatient management with borderline patients. Am J Psychiatry 126(3):299–304, 1969

Friedman L: The therapeutic alliance. Int J Psychoanal 50:139–153, 1969

Gabbard GO, Wilkinson SM: Management of Countertransference With Borderline Patients. Washington, DC, American Psychiatric Press, 1994

Gill MM: The analysis of the transference. J Am Psychoanal Assoc 27(suppl):263–288, 1979

Greenson RR: The working alliance and the transference neurosis. Psychoanal Q 34:155–181, 1965

Greenspan SI, Sharfstein SS: Efficacy of psychotherapy: asking the right questions. Arch Gen Psychiatry 38(11):1213–1219, 1981

Gunderson JG: Defining the therapeutic processes in psychiatric milieus. Psychiatry 41:327–335, 1978

Gunderson JG: Borderline Personality Disorder. Washington, DC, American Psychiatric Press, 1984

Gunderson JG, Gabbard GO: Making the case for psychoanalytic therapies in the current psychiatric environment. J Am Psychoanal Assoc 47(3):679–704, 1999 (discussion 704–740)

Gunderson JG, Carpenter W, Strauss J: Borderline and schizophrenic patients: a comparative study. Am J Psychiatry 132:1257–1264, 1975

Gunderson J, Waldinger R, Sabo A, et al: Stages of change in dynamic psychotherapy with borderline patients: clinical and research implications. J Psychother Pract Res 2(1):64–72, 1993

Hoffman IZ: Ritual and Spontaneity in the Psychoanalytic Process: A Dialectical-Constructivist View. Hillsdale, NJ, Analytic Press, 1998

Hogarty GE, Anderson CM, Reiss DJ, et al: Family psychoeducation, social skills training, and maintenance chemotherapy in the aftercare of schizophrenia, I: one-year effects of a controlled study on relapse and expressed emotion. Arch Gen Psychiatry 43:633–642, 1986

Hogarty GE, Kornblith SJ, Greenwald D, et al: Three-year trials of personal therapy among schizophrenic patients living with or independent of family, I: description of study and effects on relapse rates. Am J Psychiatry 154:1504–1513, 1997

Jones M: Social Psychiatry: A Study of Therapeutic Communities. London, Tavistock, 1952

Jones M: The concept of a therapeutic community. Am J Psychiatry 112:647–650, 1956

Kaysen S: Girl, Interrupted. New York, Random House, 1993

Kernberg O: The treatment of patients with borderline personality organization. Int J Psychoanal 49:600–619, 1968

Kopta SM, Howard KI, Lowry JL, et al: Patterns of symptomatic recovery in psychotherapy. Journal of Clinical and Consulting Psychology 62:1009–1016, 1994

Langs R: The Bipersonal Field. New York, Jason Aronson, 1976

Lanktree CB, Briere J: Outcome of therapy for sexually abused children: a repeated measures study. Child Abuse Negl 19:1145–1155, 1995

Lewin RA, Schulz C: Losing and Fusing: Borderline Transitional Object and Self Relations. New York, Jason Aronson, 1992

Linehan MM: Cognitive-Behavioral Treatment of Borderline Personality Disorder. New York, Guilford, 1993

Links PS: Psychiatric rehabilitation model for borderline personality disorder. Can J Psychiatry 38(suppl 1):35–38, 1993

Luborsky L: Helping alliances in psychotherapy, in Successful Psychotherapy. Edited by Claghorn JL. New York, Brunner/Mazel, 1976, pp 92–116

Main TF: The hospital as a therapeutic institution. Bull Menninger Clin 19:66–70, 1946

Maltsberger JT, Buie DH: Contertransference hate in the treatment of suicidal patients. Arch Gen Psychiatry 30:625–633, 1974

Masterson J: Treatment of the adolescent with borderline syndrome (a problem in separation-individuation). Bull Menninger Clin 35:5–18, 1971

Masterson J: Treatment of the Borderline Adolescent: A Developmental Approach. New York, John Wiley & Sons, 1972

Perry JC, Bond M: Empirical studies of psychotherapy for personality disorders, in American Psychiatric Press Review of Psychiatry, Vol 19. Edited by Oldham JM, Riba MB. Washington, DC, American Psychiatric Press, 2000, pp 1–31

Singer MT, Larson DG: Borderline personality and the Rorschach test. Arch Gen Psychiatry 38(6):693–698, 1981

Sterba R: The fate of the ego in analytic therapy. Int J Psychoanal 15:117–126, 1934

Waldinger RJ, Gunderson JG: Completed psychotherapies with borderline patients. Am J Psychother 38(2):190–202, 1984

Waldinger RJ, Gunderson JG: Effective Psychotherapy With Borderline Patients: Case Studies. Washington, DC, American Psychiatric Press, 1989

Winnicott DW: The Maturational Process and the Facilitating Environment. London, Hogarth Press, 1965

Zanarini MC, Frankenburg FR, DeLuca CJ, et al: The pain of being borderline: dysphoric states specific to borderline personality disorder. Harv Rev Psychiatry 6(4):201–207, 1998

Zetzel ER: Current concepts of transference. Int J Psychoanal 37:369–376, 1956

Zetzel ER: A developmental approach to the borderline patient. Am J Psychiatry 127:867–871, 1971

4

Case Management

The Primary Clinician

EVEN AS THIS BOOK emphasizes that minimal—and certainly optimal—treatment plans for BPD patients require complementary modalities, and thus a coordinated team, it is essential to recognize that some one member of the clinical team needs to assume the primary responsibility for the patient's care. This point needs special emphasis because of the natural and universal tendency for members of a team to want to avoid or reduce negative countertransference reactions or to avoid responsibilities where criticism or liability can be expected. The person who takes on primary responsibility essentially is the final decision maker for the numerous questions that borderline patients pose about who, what, where, and when regarding therapies. Traditionally, this role has been assumed by someone who defines himself or herself as the patient's therapist. However, there are inherent problems in trying to administer the selection and implementation of a therapeutic effort while remaining in the noncontrolling, exploratory, and empathic stance required of therapists who practice psychodynamic psychotherapy.

The clinician who oversees decisions and implements a treatment plan (including delegation of responsibilities), hereafter referred to as the *primary clinician*, must appreciate what is entailed in his or her role, and this role must be explicitly agreed to by other members of the patient's treatment team. For example, the dialectical behavior therapy (DBT) social skills group leader depends on a primary clinician to reinforce the contingencies that therapy requires, the family therapist often needs a primary clinician to manage the patient's crises, and the psychopharmacologist needs a primary clinician to monitor compliance, help assess benefits, and the like. The primary clinician may evolve into a role that is primarily psychotherapeutic, but initially the required responsibilities include administrative functions (e.g., monitoring safety, implementing treatment recommendations) that may in themselves be therapeutic but will often take precedence over traditional psychotherapeutic activities (e.g., self-disclosure, insight, affect recognition).

Qualifications

Any mental health clinician who is experienced with borderline patients and who combines good judgment and a readiness to communicate with others can fulfill the primary clinician role. Even mental health workers without professional degrees who have years of experience in inpatient or residential treatment settings can become very skilled. Nonetheless, the expectable safety issues, the judgment questions around level of care, and the potential legal complications of the required decisions mean that there are definite advantages in having psychiatrists fill this role. Psychiatrists generally have more training in making these judgments (and experience shows that even when their assigned role is modest, they will probably be included in any legal action to collect damages). The psychiatrist's advantages are outweighed, however, when his or her contacts with the patient are limited and an experienced and capable clinician from another discipline, usually a psychologist or social worker, is seeing the patient more intensely, knows the patient better, or has a stronger alliance. Regardless of discipline, no one should undertake the role of primary clinician without significant experience or, in its absence, without ongoing supervision by an experienced clinician.

Responsibilities

As outlined in Table 4–1, the responsibilities assumed by a borderline patient's primary clinician involve complicated clinical judgments. The issue of monitoring safety is the most important and is given extended discussion later in this chapter.

The first task is to establish a *contractual alliance* (as described in Chapter 3 of this book). This is often begun by educating both the patient (Chapter 1) and his or her family (Chapter 9) about the diagnosis. With respect to recommended therapies, the contractual alliance is established

TABLE 4–1. Responsibilities of a primary clinician

Establish a therapeutic framework (a contractual alliance)
Identify needs and develop treatment plan
Level of care (i.e., hospitalization, day or night care, etc.)
Modalities (e.g., group, rehab, family, or cognitive-behavioral therapy)
Comorbidity
Monitor safety
Monitor progress/effectiveness
Use (attendance, involvement)
Benefits (e.g., is patient learning? changing?)
Coordinate therapies
Carry out communication and collaboration
Provide psychoeducation
Between treaters
With those responsible for financing treatment

through discussion with the patient about what roles will be played and what the goals of therapy will be. Both Linehan for dialectical behavior therapy (Linehan 1993) and Kernberg for psychodynamic psychotherapy (Kernberg et al. 1989; Yeomans et al. 1993) recommend an extensive process in which the patient's motivation for the treatment is assessed (and tested) and in which the limits of the clinician's role are elucidated (e.g., contingencies for continuation, unavailability except for true emergencies). These authors make it clear that many borderline patients will be excluded as a result. No doubt such selectivity is important—especially so when conducting research intended to demonstrate the value of therapies. However, this selectivity is not usually available to clinicians who are assigned or referred patients who need to be treated and for whom they are assuming responsibility, including making judgments about the appropriateness of any type of treatment. For primary clinicians, including those who do not assume a psychotherapeutic role (e.g., psychopharmacologists) (see Chapter 6), the development of an alliance is a mandate, not an option.

The primary clinician combines administrative (i.e., management and assessment) tasks with alliance-building therapeutic activities (e.g., engagement, support, and, when necessary, confrontation). Clinicians who accept responsibility for the care of borderline patients during or after a crisis must provide what the patient needs, if possible; these clinicians do not have the privilege of saying, "I offer this type of therapy, and if it isn't suitable, goodbye." At the same time, it requires experience and good judgment to know when a treatment is inappropriate or unworkable. As described throughout this book, it requires skill to manage the tasks of being a primary clinician without enacting transference wishes or fears that cause flight or otherwise undermine the patient's participation in growth-enhancing therapies. Hence, to do these tasks well requires a good understanding of the major borderline issues. Of note (also specified in many places in this book) is the important role of using consultants or of otherwise avoiding the exclusivity that borderline patients often crave—at their own risk.

This book summarizes most of the knowledge upon which primary clinicians can base their recommendations about therapeutic options. The most desirable options are often not accessible (e.g., a well-informed and capable cognitive-behavioral therapist or a halfway house for nonpsychotic patients); the primary clinician then needs to judge whether the available therapies are potentially effective or are likely to make things worse. It is essential for the primary clinician to be aware that any therapy, poorly conducted, is likely to have harmful effects (e.g., increased crises, self-harm, regressions, rages). Thus, it is unwise to triage a borderline patient to therapists who are inexperienced and unsupervised or to clinicians who dislike working with these patients.

It is sometimes hard to know *a priori* whether available therapies can work, and the primary clinician's role involves ongoing assessment of effectiveness. Here too the sequences and time framework for expectable changes described in this book can provide a framework (see, for an overview, the Chapter 3 discussion and Table 3–3, this book). Frequently, the primary clinician's assessment of ineffectiveness becomes very simple—for example, the patient isn't attending groups, the patient keeps abusing his or her medications, the psychotherapist is clinically depressed, the psychopharmacologist is inaccessible. The more serious problems involve implementing the consequences of this conclusion.

Liability Issues

Gutheil (1985, 1989) noted that borderline patients are particularly likely to involve their treaters in liability suits. Without question this is related to these patients' ongoing suicide risks, their tendency to project malevolence, and the fact that borderline patients are usually—and optimally—treated by teams. Psychiatrists usually carry a disproportionate level of liability risk, but the principles that help diminish such risk are relevant to all members of a team. Sidebar 4–1 offers some guidelines on how primary clinicians can conduct their tasks and minimize the dangers of having liability suits. Chapter 6 of this book addresses the more specific liability issues related to *split treatment*—when a psychiatrist assumes primarily a psychopharmacologist role.

Sidebar 4–1: Guidelines to Avoid Liability

Know what usual practices are. If you plan to do anything innovative (e.g., Amytal [amobarbital] interviews, regressive psychotherapy), obtain consultation, and be sure that the patient's consent is informed and documented.

Do not see a patient more than twice a week without having significant prior experience or a qualified (experienced, credentialed) supervisor (see Chapters 11 and 12 of this book).

Use consultants whenever treatment has an extended impasse or the patient is getting worse (develops new behavioral problems, becomes more self-injurious). (See Chapter 12.)

When implementing treatment changes against a patient's wishes (e.g., discontinuing therapy), **seek consultation and document your reasons** (see Chapters 4, 5).

If you are a psychiatrist who is not assuming primary responsibility for monitoring treatment implementation or safety monitoring, 1) be sure the responsible others are credentialed and capable, and 2) explain the agreement about your role to the patient (see Chapters 4, 5).

In the face of significant risk of suicide or violence, suspend any agreements about confidentiality. (See Chapters 4, 8, 10.)

Do not agree to participate in therapies that you believe are unworkable (e.g., seeing an alcoholic adolescent who refuses to enter a day hospital for outpatient pharmacotherapy) without first advising the patient and having his or her significant others accept that your participation is a time-limited trial to determine whether treatment is possible.

RELATIONSHIP MANAGEMENT

With the book entitled *Relationship Management and the Borderline Patient*, Dawson and MacMillan (1993) made a significant contribution to the treatment wisdom for borderline patients. Unlike most books that emphasize ways to interpret or confront borderline patients' relational problems with treaters,

Dawson and MacMillan move into operational ways to sidestep these problems and have borderline patients be responsibly involved in their own treatment—or otherwise not be in treatment at all. Central to their thesis is that the traditional proactive approaches of psychiatrists and institutions (e.g., prescribing, directing, controlling) expected by—indeed, welcomed by—most patients are approaches that provide the materials with which borderline patients destroy their therapies and make themselves worse. Hence, the wise clinician will step back and wait for borderline patients to first identify what they want, even though the clinician's inaction may be protested.

One useful principle of relationship management is that the primary clinician shifts (i.e., "demedicalizes") the focus of discourse from diagnosis, pills, and suicide risk to social competence—for example, employment, budgeting, and self-care. As noted (Chapter 3 of this book), therapies to address social competence issues have been slow to develop.

A second principle involves practicing what Dawson and MacMillan call "no-therapy therapy." Thus, in response to the borderline patient's wish for psychotherapy, a regular time for sessions may readily be offered, but with the caveat that the therapist isn't sure how she or he can be helpful. This "contract" is well suited to primary clinicians. The patient sets the agenda; or, as often happens, concerns about the patient voiced to the primary clinician by others become an agenda. Sessions explicitly are not intended to be therapeutic. The atmosphere is informal; sharing coffee or discussing public events is commonplace. The primary clinician, despite his or her responsibilities (noted in Table 4–1), doesn't pursue these except as they are "forced" on him or her by the patient or by others in the patient's life. Even then, the primary clinician accepts responsibility reluctantly, with explicit statements that he or she will be likely to make mistakes unless the patient provides direction.

In my experience, Dawson and MacMillan's approach is generally useful and is very helpful for orienting trainees whose instincts are to "do things." On the other hand, this approach is more easily implemented within a health-care system where the patient is assigned a clinician than in a system where the patient selects the clinician. In the private-practice sector, Dawson and MacMillan's approach—unless buttressed by explanations for the patient and the patient's significant others—will evoke devaluation and a search for someone who evokes more hope of being helped.

MANAGING SAFETY

Assessing Suicidality

Because of apprehensions about the legal, administrative, and psychological consequences should a suicide occur, mental health professionals feel highly anxious about distinguishing true suicidal intentions from self-harming behavior without lethal intent. In the absence of such a distinction, mental health professionals are likely to assume the worst; this covers their liability and offers the bonus of allowing them to feel that they are fulfilling one of the most dramatic and perhaps alluring roles of a caretaker: saving a life.

The statistics documenting the high rates of suicide (about 9%; see Chapter 1 of this book, section titled "The Behavioral Specialty: Self-Injurious Behavior") can be used to vindicate clinicians who attempt to prevent borderline patients from performing suicidal acts. For primary clinicians, this can mean involuntary hospitalization of patients, but more often it entails decisions such as giving prescriptions for only small quantities of medications, enlisting family members to help monitor patients' suicidality, and making oneself available for crises. From another perspective, the statistics documenting the low percentage of suicidal acts that are serious attempts vindicate clinicians who are primarily concerned about the secondary gain and manipulative intentions related to borderline patients' self-destructive acts. Interventions by these clinicians are typically directed toward diminishing the secondary gains from self-destructive acts by, for example, staying uninvolved with hospitalizations or being unavailable between sessions. On balance, the statistics about borderline patients' suicidality offer little comfort.

Of only modest additional help are a series of studies examining predictors of suicidality in borderline patients (see Chapter 1 of this book, section titled "The Behavioral Specialty: Self-Injurious Behavior"). These studies indicate that greater severity (i.e., more criteria for BPD met or more impairment) or comorbid depression or substance abuse enhances the likelihood of suicide. These general impressions have not received uniform or strong support. The painful truth is that a clinician working with borderline patients must make thoughtful judgments about their suicidality that takes into consideration the patients' motives and intentions, access to lethal means, the complexity of the patients' relationship to significant others, including oneself, and the past responses from those others, including oneself. From a medicolegal point of view, clinicians making these judgments should document their considerations of such issues.

A Preventive Stance

Primary clinicians should early and often advise borderline patients that the clinicians view suicidal acts as dangerous distractions from the patients' work—that of attaining a better life. To make this message meaningful, it is essential that—while never ignoring any hints of suicidality—they do not proactively look for evidence of it. This approach contrasts with the approach used in DBT, in which the therapists systematically inquire about self-destructiveness at the start of each session (see Chapter 8 of this book). On the other hand, I do think that the recurrence of suicidality should be assumed and specifically predicted whenever the borderline patient is about to lose some source of support. The latter is an essential aspect of the first year of treatment (phase 2 of psychotherapy; see Chapter 12), because it gives an essential meaning to the patient's ideas, impulses, or behaviors—a response to feeling insufficiently cared for. Interpretation of this meaning can then allow discussion of alternative, more adaptive responses (much as DBT therapists do).

Two embellishments of this simple stance can often be useful. The first is to suggest that suicidality is motivated by anger, not depression. The second is to link patients' history of counterdependence to family dynamics, where wanting to be cared for was unacceptable—thence, extreme behaviors and illness became the vehicle for getting needs met. When the clinician is proactive with such interpretations—often presented in an educational way—borderline patients will hear that their anger or their wishes for care are understandable feelings that can be talked about.

Responding to "Feeling Unsafe"

In conjunction with increased awareness in the current mental health community about the prevention of suicide, patients have increasingly been advised to talk about suicidal ideas or impulses—rather than acting on them. In this context, patients will now report that they "feel unsafe." The following vignette illustrates the issues that this development requires a primary clinician to manage:

Vignette

Ms. A was a 28-year-old woman who began treatment while hospitalized for an overdose. Her primary aftercare clinician, also her therapist, had seen her once weekly while she attended an interpersonal group (IPG) and attempted to reenter graduate training.

Two weeks after discharge from the hospital, she called the primary clinician at 11:00 P.M. on a weeknight:

Patient (in a weak voice): I'm sorry to call, but I've been feeling strange, unsafe, out of control.
Therapist (waits, then asks): When did this start?
Patient: I don't know. . .I've been getting worse for awhile.
Therapist (no response).
Patient: You're not saying much.
Therapist: I'd like to help, but I'm unclear about what I can do. Did you have some ideas?
Patient: No.
Therapist: Hmm.
Patient: What does that mean?!
Therapist (no response).
Patient: I guess you can't help me.
Therapist: That's what I was thinking.
Patient: Then what should I do?
Therapist: I do hope you will take good care of yourself and make use of the emergency services if necessary.

Of note in this vignette are the clinician's modest expressions of curiosity or alarm, but equally modest, albeit reassuring, expressions of concern. The clinician seems aware that the patient could be in danger of self-harm but doesn't ask for reassurance that she won't act on such impulses. The clinician appears confident that, should the patient need more active help, she knows how to obtain it. This assumption contrasts with the practice of *contracting for safety* (see Sidebar 4–2). Not noted in this vignette is that the therapist had trouble getting to sleep after the call. It is notable that this fact (trouble sleeping) was told the patient in the following session. This example illustrates some of the general principles related to monitoring safety in borderline outpatients shown in Table 4–2.

Sidebar 4–2: Is Contracting for Safety Safe?

There are many borderline patients—probably most—who, although capable of distorting reality, would find it abhorrent to knowingly lie, especially to anyone who appears caring. Thus has evolved the practice of contract-

TABLE 4–2. Guidelines for management of safety

During a crisis

1. *Express concern* after the patient alerts you to suicidal or other safety issues.
2. *Allow patients to ventilate.* It will relieve tensions around suicidality.
3. *Avoid taking actions* to prevent potential suicidal behaviors when possible:
   a. Ask patients to be explicit about wanting help.
   b. Ask patients to be explicit about what help they hope you can offer.
   c. Assume, unless told otherwise, that the patient can use community-based emergency services.

After the crisis

1. *Follow up* by discussing all safety issues, including their effect on you, within the context of scheduled appointments.
2. *Actively interpret the nonspecific reasons* that can and did provide relief—for example, the perception of being cared for.
3. *Identify the infeasibility* of depending upon your being constantly available; work on problem solving about available alternatives.
4. *Actively address* the patient's anger toward you whenever it becomes apparent.

ing for safety,[1] in which clinicians ask patients for reassurance that they will not harm themselves, formally inviting them to be explicit about this, sometimes even writing it out. This procedure encourages patients to remain safe to uphold the honor of their promise once given; it is also an exercise that affirms the clinician's concern and acts as a deterrent to impulsive action. Hence its popularity.

What's the downside? First, special conditions are required before contracting for safety is appropriate. The contracting borderline patients must have a value system that values honesty or keeping their word. Alternatively, even patients who lack these values may perceive their clinician as so "good" (for example, not motivated by interest in asserting control) that they would not want to betray the clinician's trust. Another condition that allows contracting to help is that contracting patients must be sufficiently reflective to control self-destructive impulses. When these conditions are met, the contract will help secure a holding environment: the patients will be safer.

But even when the conditions discussed above exist, there can be a more subtle downside to contracting for safety. Contracting will alter (I think damage) the process of establishing a psychotherapeutic *working* alliance (see Chapter 3 of this book). Alliances for treatment–the contrac-

[1] Contracting for safety is very different from contracting for therapy, although the latter may include expecting patients to take care of safety issues (see, for example, Plakun 1994 or Kernberg et al. 1989).

tual and relational forms—are created to keep an illness at bay, and these can rest on a businesslike, explicit verbal agreement. A working therapeutic alliance (as needed for dynamic psychotherapy) depends on a patient's commitment to change and growth. Contracting for safety implicitly moves the act of preventing self-destructiveness into the therapy: the therapist is actively trying to become a barrier to self-destructive behaviors. By this activity, the therapist enacts a borderline patient's powerful transference wish for the therapist to be the patient's protector and caretaker. Such a transference, once established, is hard to undo and is easily disrupted by the inevitable vicissitudes of the relationship. Thus, the patient may agree to contract for safety as a way to please the idealized therapist; but the contract itself, once made, reifies the therapist's transference role as an omnipotent protector. Thus, because the clinician is ready to have the patient's life rely on the contract, the patient's idealized transference can become intensified. Because of this intensified transference, the patient's inevitable subsequent disillusionments with the therapist may be all the more dangerously life threatening.

Is contracting for safety safe? It depends.

Of course, the type of clinician response shown in the last vignette does not always get the same type of response from the patient. In that vignette, the patient fortunately seemed somewhat reflective, wanting a discussion. Other principles identified in Table 4–2 are illustrated by a different version of that vignette. In the version following, the therapist's responses evoke an angrier, more threatening response:

Vignette

Patient: I'm sorry to call, but I've been feeling strange, unsafe, out of control.

Therapist (waits, then asks): When did this start?

Patient: I don't know. . .(Irritably): How the hell can I think about that?! Didn't you hear me say that I feel unsafe, out of control?! I'm standing here with a bottle of pills.

Therapist (waits, then): You need me to respond to the fact that you're at risk?

Patient: Yes!

Therapist: This is a crisis?

Patient: Yes!

Therapist: How can I help?

Patient: I don't know! You're the fucking doctor, you should know.
Therapist: I wish I did.
Patient: Are you telling me you don't know how you can help me?!
Therapist (no response).
Patient: Is that what you're saying?!
Therapist: I hope you won't hurt yourself.
Patient (starts weeping): Oh God, I just don't know what to do. I feel so awful.
Therapist: I know you do. I can hear that.
Patient: It all started yesterday. . .(begins to narrate a detailed recounting of the intervening events).

In this instance, the patient's desperation and anger move the therapist to address more directly the patient's at-risk behaviors. Even here, however, he enlists the patient in articulating that she is in a crisis and in identifying how she wants him to respond. As is usually the case, she as a borderline patient has trouble saying what is wanted. Unspoken is the fact that she wants concerned attention. Also unspoken is what the primary clinician should know in this situation: that if the patient is given license to ventilate, the immediate danger of self-harm will dissipate. After the exchange in this vignette, the therapist slept comfortably.

In the session following the exchange above, the therapist insisted, against the patient's protests, on discussing what had transpired. He identified how "surprisingly angry" the patient had become when he didn't immediately express concern for her safety and when he said he didn't know what she wanted him to do to help.

Patient (irritably): I'm sorry for getting so angry, but it was a crisis. I guess you've never been through what I go through.
Therapist (sidestepping her anger): When you began to talk about what was bothering you, that seemed to have helped.
Patient: Yes, it really did. I appreciated that you listened.
Therapist: That was most interesting to me. What seemed to help was just having someone listen. I didn't do anything. How can that be?

The patient then discussed how rare it had been to have someone listen to her. The therapist used this exchange to educate the patient about theory, suggesting that some people (with BPD) get overwhelmingly panicked when they don't have someone available to offer comfort and that such people find aloneness intolerable. That led to a discussion of the patient's living situation and alternative sources of comfort. He added that, although he was glad to have proved useful, it was dangerous for her safety to depend upon his availability. Moreover, providing comfort wasn't a function he could serve too often without disrupting his own life. (He thereby actively drew attention to his own limits, as opposed to setting limits on the patient—as detailed in the later section of this chapter titled "Boundaries, Violations, and Setting Limits.")

RESPONDING TO RECURRENT SUICIDALITY: THE "PRINCIPLE OF FALSE SUBMISSION"

Encounters with borderline patients who voice active suicidal intentions present other problems. Frequently, the borderline patients who voice such intentions have histories of chronic suicidality and multiple attempts. For clinicians, this history makes it hard to judge the seriousness of the intentions and creates moral and ethical dilemmas (Fine and Sansone 1990; Frances and Miller 1989). The clinician usually feels that questioning the seriousness of the patient's suicidal intentions could magnify the likelihood and lethality of an attempt. Beyond this, the clinician will know that hospitalizations—the usual response to suicidality—can rarely address the underlying causes for the suicidality and might in fact actually perpetuate the borderline patient's allegations of suicidality (as a result of the secondary gains of being rescued, getting attention, and avoiding the problems of living in the community).

Vignette

Ms. B was a 35-year-old disheveled, agitated, overweight single woman who appeared for her first clinic appointment. She promptly stated that she was grateful to "now have a therapist," and that she had needed one for 3 years. Even as the evaluating clinician felt uneasy about the role assigned by the patient, she went on to say she felt very suicidal. In response to the clinician's inquiries, she reported that she had been suicidal "off and on for many years" and had already had 31 hospitalizations.

Clinician: What has caused you to become suicidal now?
Patient: I don't know; what difference does it make? (now becoming irritated and defensive)

Clinician: Has anything happened in your life recently? (Clinician is skeptical about the patient's lethality and hoping to isolate specific events that can be addressed but already feeling highly anxious about the patient's volatility and potential flight.)

Patient: All I know is that I visited my parents and became very upset and had to leave. No, I don't know why. No, they didn't say anything. Yes, it's happened before, and last time I nearly killed myself.

Clinician: What happened?

Patient: I drank a quart of vodka, and then took any fucking pills I could find. . .I would have been dead if my landlord hadn't noticed that the TV was on all night.

Clinician (now convinced that the patient is dangerous, but still feeling coerced into suggesting hospitalization): Are you feeling that way again?

Patient: I just want to get control of myself. If I can't, I'm going to slash my neck. This time I don't want to fail.

Clinician: Would you like to go into the hospital?

Patient: Yes, I need to.

This vignette illustrates a not unusual situation, a relatively unknown patient presenting with agitation and suicidal ideation, and a not unusual intervention, the patient getting hospitalized. This is done despite the clinician's doubt about the seriousness of the intention and despite an expectation that another hospitalization (in Helene's case, the 32nd!) is unlikely to help and may even be reinforcing a self-defeating pattern. The clinician will usually feel coerced, manipulated, and helpless. Still, in the absence of alternatives that can as surely safeguard the patient, he is doing the right thing by suggesting hospitalization.

In a thoughtful disquisition on this borderline-specific dilemma, Behnke and Saks (1998) argue that an extended informed-consent process (using contracting in DBT as an example in which the patient commits to treatment goals) can redirect such patients' intentions. This is true for patients soliciting treatment, a situation in which clinicians have the choice of saying they cannot help an unmotivated patient. But the dilemma stated in the previous paragraph was felt very acutely by Ms. B's clinician, who did not have the choice of turning down the patient's request for help. The problem for the field of therapeutic jurisprudence is whether the law can protect clinicians who keep such patients out of hospitals—basing their decision on the patient's welfare and acknowledging what Maltsberger (1994) referred to as a "calculated risk" of death—rather than hospitalizing the patient because it protects the clinician's welfare. Having identified the problem, Behnke and Saks could offer no remedy.

My own approach to this situation starts by making the dilemma explicit. I tell patients such as Ms. B that hospitalization would be the safest option, but that it is not likely to be helpful and will probably be harmful to her longer-term welfare. I explain that hospitalization involves inviting others to assume control of their life and that this can discourage their learning self-control. Moreover, I say that for many patients such "rescues" become a way of feeling cared for and that being hospitalized feels like being adopted, though that's not actually what hospitalizations mean. I tell these patients, "To me, offering hospitalization to you primarily represents a way to avoid my being legally liable should you commit suicide. I actually believe the more caring response would be to try to keep you out of a hospital despite the potential risk to me." I then tell them that in my judgment the best way to proceed would be to take the time needed to see why they are recurrently suicidal and to develop a treatment plan that addresses those reasons. Patients are often unsurprised by such statements, and a different negotiation then occurs, as seen in the following vignette:

Vignette

Patient: Are you saying that you really think it's a mistake to go into the hospital?

Clinician: Not if you'd otherwise kill yourself, but if you stay alive you'd be better off without it.

Patient: Are you saying you won't put me in a hospital?

Clinician: No, of course not. It would be "suicidal" *for me* to try to prevent a potentially suicidal patient like you [note that therapist does not question her suicidal potential] from entering a hospital if they want to [note that therapist moves action into area of *their* wanting]. It's just that I don't believe it will be good for you. If you were to make a suicide attempt after leaving here, it could be difficult for me personally and professionally; potentially, I could even be sued. So if you tell me that you intend to kill yourself, that's very powerful. Then in you have to go. But, if you go, don't go thinking I've done what I think is the right thing for you—or that it's because I care for you. It doesn't mean either of these things. I would think you are just hoping for an adoption.

This is the *principle of false submission.* By ostensibly giving the patient what he or she wants but disarming it of its meaning, the cycle of repeated admissions can be broken. This will not usually happen the first time: the patient will almost always go into the hospital on hearing this exchange. But the action now has a different meaning: now the patient is going because he or she *wants* to go, not because the doctor said so. When this is followed up on and reinforced by others on the patient's treatment team, it diminishes the treaters' sense of being manipulated or coerced by the patient and breaks down the patient's fantasies of rescue or love. The therapist "gives in" but robs the patient of much of the expected satisfaction.

In Ms. B's case, I would want to involve the patient's family and her previous treaters in the decision about being hospitalized. Such involvements take time and may for practical reasons prove unfeasible, but the principle behind advocating this process is to underscore the clinician's wish to do the right thing, and this involvement will encourage the patient to consider alternatives. With my patients, ultimately I declare that I agree to their going into the hospital only because they "insist" on it (now moving "want" into "insist" to underscore their agency, but still carefully avoiding suggesting that it is because they are in my view suicidal). This helps move the discourse from medical necessity into the patient's agency. In essence, this approach extends the principles described earlier by Dawson and MacMillan (1993).

Implementing Changes

When implementing changes in treatment of a borderline patient, the primary clinician must proceed with sensitivity and caution. It is easy to unwittingly evoke a response in which the borderline patient desperately or defiantly clings more tightly to the ineffective therapy. The mechanism for this angry resistance to a proposed change often involves evoking a split, whereby the primary clinician is seen as cruelly depriving the patient rather than trying to help. Therefore, the way in which the need for change is communicated to a patient is very important. Autocratic announcements will usually evoke resistance, but even when accepted, they can be harmful because they do not improve the patient's self-awareness about his or her needs or about the ways in which these needs can be communicated. Certainly, recommendations for change—especially if they involve changes to less intensive services—should be accompanied by empathic anticipation that the changes will be difficult. Giving "you can do it" assurances causes borderline patients to feel that the therapist is minimizing their difficulties. It is also of critical importance that the primary clinician initiate communications with the collaborating member(s) of the therapy team, and with the patient, to ensure that everyone is aware of and involved in all treatment planning. Most clinicians who like working with borderline patients learn to do this quite comfortably; clinicians who are hesitant about addressing problems usually avoid this sector of psychiatry.

BOUNDARIES, VIOLATIONS, AND SETTING LIMITS

Boundaries refers to the agreed-upon differentiation of the patients' and the clinicians'/therapists' roles. Both patients and clinicians are capable of boundary transgressions—that is, stepping out of their roles. When this is done behaviorally (e.g., having lunch together or giving stock tips), it is called a boundary violation. Without doubt, transgression by either patient or clinician is likely to evoke the transgression of the other.

Although many of the pioneering psychoanalytic leaders practiced what would now be considered boundary violations (Gutheil and Gabbard 1993), the acceptable norms of practice are now better established. Still, departures from these norms are most likely to occur on the part of therapists who are working with borderline patients (Gutheil 1989). Because professionals' consciousness about boundaries is so tinged by concerns about professional ethics and liability, discussion of this issue runs the risk of increasing therapists' anxieties about liability. This in turn can cause therapists to adhere rigidly to "professionalism" and decrease their willingness to get deeply involved with borderline patients. On the other hand, increased consciousness about this topic may underscore the importance of extensive supervision, use of consultants, and attention to countertransference.

Clinicians are often warned that borderline patients do not respect the boundaries of a professional relationship and that, as a result, clinicians need to be prepared to set limits. Indeed, Colson et al. (1986) noted that the psychotherapies with the most negative outcomes in the Menninger Psychotherapy Research Project were those in which therapists were content to interpret acting-out behaviors without setting limits. Table 4–3 identifies a sequence of responses that usually sidestep the necessity of setting limits. Limits are sometimes valuable, but usually they reflect impatience or fearfulness on the part of therapists who are uninformed about or do not trust the process described in this table. It can be very difficult to insist that patients talk about the meaning behind their undesirable behaviors, but this discussion remains the cornerstone of prevention and resolution of boundary violations.

Central to the process described in Table 4–3 is that the clinician recognize his or her own limits. These limits should be compatible with compassion and with accepting a responsible role in monitoring patient safety. But, having said this, it must be added that limits should also be compatible with the clinician's personal and professional welfare. When they are at risk, the limits should be introduced as originating in oneself (steps 4 and 5 in the table). Being clear that it is the clinician's limitation, while remaining empathic about the patient's wishes, rather than hostile, is almost always accepted by borderline patients.

TABLE 4–3. Sequential responses to boundary violations

The therapist's responses to boundary violations should be as follows. Possible phrasings of responses appear in parentheses:

1. Identify it as a problem *after* it occurs. ("Let's talk about. . . ")
2. Investigate what the patient *wants*. Don't assume the behavior was based on *"needs."* ("I was unclear how you hoped I could help.")
3. Validate how that wish is understandable. ("Yes, I could see how that would help you.")
4. Discuss how the behavior can be harmful to the therapy or the therapist. ("I do find it troubling because. . . .")
5. Apologize for one's limitations. ("I wish I [could give, be] what you want.")
6. If the behavior recurs under circumstances when points 4 and 5 have been discussed—that is, when the therapist's disapproval has been established—inquire why. ("Did you misunderstand? Are you angry? Did you want me to disapprove?")
7. Note that whatever motivated the recurrence should be discussed, not enacted, for therapy to benefit the patient.
8. If it still recurs, set a limit—preferably when the limit setting can be processed, not when the patient is angry.

Splits, Splitting, and the Principle of Split Treatment

Splitting is a term used to describe both an interpersonal and an intrapsychic phenomenon. Within psychoanalytic terminology it refers to a defensive process identified by Melanie Klein (1946) as originating early in life that allows a child to ignore or dissociate *(split off)* negative hostile perceptions of their needed other, thereby preserving a "good," albeit distorted, representation (a *part object*) of that other. Within the larger mental health community, this defense became identifiable by the borderline patient's tendency to perceive others in dichotomous, "all-good" or "all-bad" terms and then to treat others very differently (idealized or devalued, respectively), depending on which side of the internal split they occupied. Because of this tendency to split, prior generations of clinicians have been warned to beware of splitting lest they develop antagonistic views toward the member(s) of a treatment team who are on the opposite side of the patients' split, or lest they otherwise get involved in countertransference enactments (Gabbard 1989, 1994).

As described elsewhere (Gunderson 1984), the splitting between objects is not simply a product of the borderline patients' *splits*—that is, their projections—but is predictably based on whether the other is in fact frustrating or supportive. Such projections are well suited to the recipients (i.e., are based on real characteristics of the objects). As such, splitting refers to an interpersonal as opposed to an intrapsychic process. Moreover, such splits otherwise serve desirable functions within treatment teams by helping borderline patients grow aware and tolerant of both frustrations and support ("kisses and kicks"). The critical issue is that members of a treatment team recognize that whether they are providing frustration or support (or *being seen* as providing them), the other component is necessary and desirable for others to provide. Unfortunately, when clinicians are aware that validating borderline patients' projections of badness (i.e., agreeing with their devalued view of another treater) can lead to splits, this awareness can lead members of teams to bond together by invalidating the borderlines' attributions (i.e., being protective about the other treater's goodness). Such responses negate the partial reality of the borderline patients' perceptions. Moreover, the idea that, to prevent splits, staff members need to protect each other against negativity confers too much power on the patients' hostility. This too is harmful.

The *principle of split treatment* is that, despite the dangers of splitting, treatment plans for borderline patients should routinely involve at least two treaters, two modalities, or any two components. When coordinated, two components in a treatment can provide a container for the splits and projections that keep the borderline patient in treatment. To be specific, split treatment means that patients receive two different and, in some respects, independent services. Whatever the components (e.g., hospital and psychotherapist, psychopharmacologist and family therapist, or primary clinician and self-assessment group), the governing principle is that having two relatively independent but complementary therapies allows the inevitable frustrations with any particular treatment to be contained without necessitating flight (see Sidebar 5–1). Borderline patients' inability to experience frustrations without assigning malevolence and taking angry or fearful flight is the reason why they so frequently drop out of therapies (Waldinger 1987). This is why selecting appropriate psychotherapeutic techniques relates to a borderline patient's level of care (see Sidebar 4–3). When they have a second component to discuss their frustrations with, they retain a "good object" who will urge them to voice their complaints to the frustrating therapist (psychopharmacologist, group leader, etc.) rather than leave.

Sidebar 4–3. How Psychotherapeutic Technique Relates to Level of Care

The function of containing splits has often been performed by the staff of inpatient units who have helped borderline patients appreciate the more benign significance of what the patients often experienced as "angry" and "cruel" interpretations, confrontations, or frustrations from their psychotherapists. It is not accidental that Kernberg's (Kernberg 1968; Kernberg et al. 1989) advocacy of these techniques (see Chapter 11 of this book) arose from experience working at the Menninger Clinic, where long-term (level IV) containment was then being provided. In contrast, Adler (1986), who worked in his level I private office with a short-term hospital backup, became a champion for validating and empathic interventions. Similarly, the successful outpatient therapies advocated by Linehan (1993) and Stevenson and Meares (1992) emphasize these more supportive techniques.

The usual setting in which the advantages of split treatment are met is by the combination of a psychopharmacologist and a psychotherapist (usually a psychologist; see Chapter 6 of this book), with one or the other serving as the primary clinician. The containing function of split treatment is, I believe, one reason why DBT had such a low dropout rate (16%; see Chapter 8). Linehan (1993) nicely operationalized the response that clinicians/therapists should make when confronted about the alleged failures, cruelties, and so forth of the other "bad" therapy. The "good" therapist should *neither agree with the patient nor defend the other*—simply encourage the borderline patient to express complaints directly to the object of the complaints. Split treatments are advantageous to borderline patients if provided by knowledgeable and mutually respectful clinicians. If not, they may be harmful and may increase liability risks (see Sidebars 4–1 and 6–3).

SUMMARY

To clarify and simplify the process of clinical decision-making, someone needs to be clearly identifiable as a borderline patient's *primary clinician*, sometimes referred to as *case administrator*. The person in this role may also fill other roles, but insofar as the borderline patient still requires limits, safety interventions, or unwanted confrontations, it is difficult for the primary clinician also to serve as a patient's dynamic psychotherapist until the patient progresses into a second phase of treatment (see Chapters 3 and 11 of this book). The role of primary clinician is compatible with being a patient's cognitive-behavioral therapist or psychopharmacologist. Central to a primary clinician's tasks is the ability to communicate with the patient's significant others (both family and treaters) and to make good clinical judgments about whether a patient is progressing or is safe and, if not, to implement solutions effectively. A stance about safety issues that involves much inquiry and minimal action is suggested.

REFERENCES

Adler G: Borderline Psychopathology and Its Treatment. New York, Jason Aronson, 1986

Behnke SH, Saks ER: Therapeutic jurisprudences: informed consent as a clinical indication for the chronically suicidal patient with borderline personality disorder. Loyola Law Review 31(3):945–982, 1998

Colson D, Lewis L, Horwitz L: Negative effects in psychotherapy and psychoanalysis, in Above All Do No Harm: Negative Outcome in Psychotherapy. Edited by Mays D, Franks C. 1986

Dawson D, MacMillan HL: Relationship Management and the Borderline Patient. New York, Brunner/Mazel, 1993

Fine MA, Sansone RA: Dilemmas in the management of suicidal behavior in individuals with borderline personality disorder. Am J Psychother 44(2):160–171, 1990

Frances AJ, Miller LJ: Coordinating inpatient and outpatient treatment for a chronically suicidal woman. Hospital and Community Psychiatry 40(5):468–470, 1989

Gabbard GO: Splitting in hospital treatment. Am J Psychiatry 146:444–451, 1989

Gabbard GO: Treatment of borderline patients in a multiple-treater setting. Psychiatr Clin North Am 17(4):839–850, 1994

Gunderson JG: Borderline Personality Disorder. Washington, DC, American Psychiatric Press, 1984

Gutheil TG: Medicolegal pitfalls in the treatment of borderline patients. Am J Psychiatry 142(1):9–14, 1985

Gutheil TG: Borderline personality disorder, boundary violations, and patient-therapist sex: medicolegal pitfalls. Am J Psychiatry 146(5):597–602, 1989

Gutheil TG, Gabbard GO: The concept of boundaries in clinical practice: theoretical and risk-management dimensions. Am J Psychiatry150(2):188–196,1993

Kernberg O: The treatment of patients with borderline personality organization. Int J Psychoanal 49:600–619, 1968

Kernberg O, Selzer M, Koenigsberg HW, et al: Psychodynamic Psychotherapy of Borderline Patients. New York, Basic Books, 1989

Klein M: Notes on some schizoid mechanisms. Int J Psychoanal 27:99–110, 1946

Linehan MM: Cognitive-Behavioral Treatment of Borderline Personality Disorder. New York, Guilford Press, 1993

Maltsberger JT: Calculated risks in the treatment of intractably suicidal patients. Psychiatry 57(3)199–212, 1994

Plakun EM: Principles in the psychotherapy of self-destructive borderline patients. Journal of Psychotherapy Practice and Research 3(2):138–148, 1994

Stevenson J, Meares R: An outcome study of psychotherapy for patients with borderline personality disorder. Am J Psychiatry 149(3):358–362, 1992

Waldinger RJ: Intensive psychodynamic therapy with borderline patients: an overview. Am J Psychiatry 144(3):267–274, 1987

Yeomans F, Selzer M, Clarkin J: Studying the treatment contract in intensive psychotherapy with borderline patients. Psychiatry 56(3):254–263, 1993

5

Levels of Care

Indications, Structure, Staffing

In this chapter I offer condensed statements about the indications for deploying four different and decreasingly intensive levels of care: IV, hospital; III, residential/partial hospital; II, intensive outpatient; and I, outpatient (see Figure 5–1). Experienced clinicians know that the capability of programs on levels IV and III (hospital and residential programs) to help borderline patients varies greatly. This chapter may help those who administer or develop such services to provide them more effectively. With each decrement in level of care, the need for borderline patients to have specialized (i.e., BPD-specific) services is increased. The responsibility for borderline patients' making significant and enduring changes usually rests with therapies residing in outpatient (level I) settings. Yet whether outpatient (level I) services can be effective may depend on whether the borderline patient's behavior has been contained and whether his or her capacity to recognize feelings has been developed within residential/partial hospital (level III) or intensive outpatient (level II) services. The growth in clinical experience since the borderline diagnosis was established has shown that effective therapies at any level of care require modifications of traditional modalities. Helping to increase staff knowledge about BPD by talks or reading material at all levels of treatment can alter attitudes in ways that help these patients (S. A. Miller and Davenport 1996).

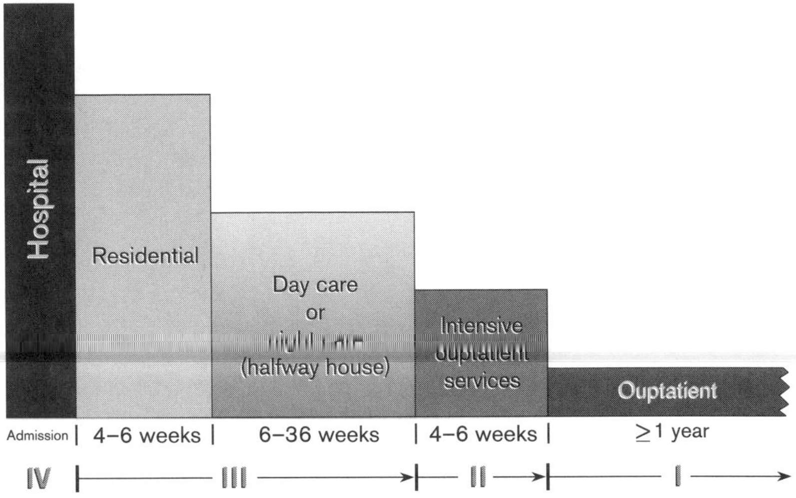

FIGURE 5–1. Levels of care for borderline personality disorder patients.

SELECTING OR CHANGING A LEVEL OF CARE

Discussion of each level of care in the chapter includes descriptions of the structures, staffing, and clinical processes that best serve the needs of borderline patients. Table 5–1 summarizes some aspects of this with special reference to the five basic therapeutic processes described earlier (see Chapter 3 of this book). It is important in selecting the appropriate level of care to appreciate that it is primarily a consideration of what level of support and structure a patient needs. Although this chapter suggests that all borderline patients progress by moving sequentially through all levels of care, this process is rarely feasible and, fortunately, is rarely necessary. Most borderline patients use brief hospitalizations (level IV) for crises but otherwise remain in outpatient (level I) care. Still, the presence and use of the intermediary levels (III and II) offer social rehabilitative opportunities that are highly beneficial options for many more patients than now receive them. The absence of either of these intermediary levels of care extends the amount of time needed at the hospital level. Similarly, stays in residential/partial hospital (level III) programs need to be greatly extended either in the absence of an intensive outpatient service (level II) or in the absence of the skilled professional help needed for level I care. Hence, health care systems that do not have all the levels available will be cost ineffective (Quaytman and Sharfstein 1997).

TABLE 5–1. The four levels of care

Level	Type and its components	Goal and its components	Expectable length of stay[a]	Process[b]
IV	**Hospital**	**Crisis management**	2–10 days	C
	Medication	Assessments		
	Psychoeducation	Treatment planning		
III	**Residential/partial hospital**	**Social rehabilitation**		
	Night	Daily living skills	2 wks–3 mo	C, St, Su
	Day	Social skills	2 wks–6 mo	St, Su, I
		Alliance building (relational)	2 wks–6 mo	St, Su, I
II	**Intensive outpatient**	**Social (behavioral) adaptation**		
	Self-assessment group	Socialization	1–3 mo	St, Su
	Case management	Anticipation, planning	6–18 mo	St, Su, I
	Dialectical behavior therapy	Impulse/affect control	6–12 mo	St, Su
	Family prescription	Alliance building (relational)	2–6 mo	St, Su, I
I	**Outpatient**	**Psychological growth**		
	Group prescription	Interpersonal skills	1–2 yr	I
	Psychotherapy	Intrapsychic change	1–6 yr	I, V
		Alliance building	6 mo–4 yr	St, I, V

Note. Each goal component is aligned with the expectable length of stay for that goal (in the next column to the right), as well as with the processes involved in the goal component (in the column furthest right). Type components do not relate one for one to the goal components, lengths of stay, or processes.

[a]Lengths of stay are estimates based on the author's experience when the appropriate step-down level of care is available.

[b]C = containment; Su = support; St = structure; I = involvement; V = validation (see Chapter 3 of this book for explanation of terms).

The unavailability of any one level of care is also clinically ineffective; the general principle is that it is never good to have a patient in a level of care higher than is needed. This is easier in principle than in practice, because it is expectable that, whether borderline patients know it or not (or whether they need it or not), they prefer a safe, secure, familiar haven, and most have angry or regressive reactions to any step-down in level of care, even if they have urged such a step.

Because of these predictable reactions, it is absolutely essential that administrators hold steady with expectations of patients and that key treaters (i.e., primary clinicians and/or therapists) remain constant, moving with the patient across levels of care. Step-downs offer excellent opportunities for clinical staff in all roles to help borderline patients realize and accept that they want more nurturance, caretaking, and attention than they might otherwise know they do or might otherwise wish to acknowledge. This is one of the central psychological themes for borderline patients in the early phase of treatment, no matter what the level of care or the type of modality.

Level IV: Hospital Treatment—Makes Therapy Possible

Until the 1990s, long-term hospitalizations were feasible and even desirable options for treating borderline patients. Although there remains a role for long-term hospitalizations (at least 6 months), the indications for it are rare (see Sidebar 5–1). Since this option is now rarely available, the following discussion focuses on short-term stays, which are both more common and usually more beneficial (Gunderson 1984; Nurnberg and Suh 1978; Sederer and Thorbeck 1986; Silk et al. 1994).

Sidebar 5–1: Is Long-Term Hospitalization Desirable for BPD?

Long-term hospitalizations (meaning a minimum of 6 months and usually a year or more) have become infrequent, largely as a result of the cost consciousness of the managed care environment. Yet there is evidence from Henderson Hospital in England that borderline patients selected for long-term (1-year) hospitalization do get better in such settings, and that their improvement is positively correlated with the length of stay (Dolan et al. 1997). About 43% of the patients showed significant improvement on a borderline symptom self-report, compared to about 18% of an otherwise comparable sample who were referred but did not receive funding. Moreover, without question, long-term hospitalization of the borderline patient is often desirable for the patient's significant others, who otherwise feel too responsible for the patient's safety and health. Specifically, it will often seem desirable for parents or spouses to have their family member with BPD treated apart from the family to avoid their being exposed to the patient's disruptive or dangerous behaviors. Long-term hospitalizations have also had benefits for academic programs, because trainees can learn to understand and manage borderline patients within a contained environment that has a preestablished team structure.

When long-term hospitalizations were more available, they were in my experience rarely useful for borderline patients: too much containment led to a regressive dependency or a paranoid combativeness. It proved unrealistic to hope that analysis of either of these negative reactions could have much meaning as long as the nonspecific factors of being held, taken care of, and given unsolicited attention were sustained.

Exceptions to the generally negative effects of long-term hospitalization can occur with exceptional patients or exceptional hospital treatment conditions. The exceptional borderline patients for whom long-term hospitalizations is desirable include those in need of functions in loco parentis–specifically, adolescents with chaotic or excessively punitive home environments. Another group for whom long-term hospitalizations can help are patients whose failure to control their impulses is sufficiently frequent and dangerous that the initial task of learning self-control requires many months of containment. The exceptional hospital treatment conditions involve a clinical administration that can give–or insist on–privileges for the patients to engage in activities that allow their longings for attention and dependency to be meaningfully awakened, identified, and understood. Long-term hospital units typically become so inner-directed and totalitarian that it is very difficult to do this. The apparent success reported at Henderson Hospital was attributed to a therapeutic community (Jones 1952) that was nonauthoritarian and expected the borderline patients to be actively involved in decisions and self-governance. This makes sense, but it clearly requires skilled staff. The issues of dependency and attention will usually be better addressed by the structures and off-unit options of partial hospital (level III) or even less containing (level II or I) programs.

Within the framework of the borderline patient's overall treatment, hospitals serve as the place for initiating or changing therapies or for managing crises. Whereas patients without personality disorders who are in crisis can benefit from a community outreach intervention that avoids hospitalization, hospitalization may have some added benefits for those with a personality disorder (Rosenbluth and Silver 1992; Tyrer et al. 1994). Almost all borderline patients do best with brief 1- to-2-week hospitalizations. It is wise to establish this time frame at the point of admission to discourage regressive, idealized, or dependent attachments (Sederer 1991). Longer stays in a hospital usually do not occur because of their therapeutic value, but because appropriate step-down services (levels III or II) are unavailable (Lewin and Sharfstein 1990). The importance of graduated and careful discharge planning is brought home by the observation that many suicides occur just after discharge or just before a mandatory discharge (Kullgren 1988).

Vignette

Ms. C was a 28-year-old female with a history of substance abuse and promiscuity who has been prescribed increasing doses of tranquilizing and sedating medications. She presented herself to her state mental health department caseworker as affectively blunted and mentally dull. She angrily dismissed outright, or failed to follow through on, all treatments arranged by her caseworker. It was unclear whether her obtunded mental state was due to misuse of her prescriptions. Hospitalization was recommended to adjust medications, evaluate her problems (e.g., hostility, missed appointments) with her psychiatrist and caseworker, and assess whether her divorced parents can offer more consistent supports, including possibly residence.

Goals: Contain Patients for Safety, Assessments, and Treatment Planning

The containment (see Chapter 3) offered by hospitalization (level IV) offers opportunities to do evaluations and treatment interventions that would be impossible elsewhere. Following are the major goals and the usual time required for meeting them:

- *Crisis interventions.* Hospitalization is responsive to acute suicidal or violent dangers. (2–6 days)
- *Extensive neurological or psychological evaluations.* These evaluations are more easily coordinated in, and for some borderline patients may be feasible only in, hospital settings. (2–6 days)
- *Development of a treatment plan and personnel.* Such plans usually require arranging for continuity through appropriate step-downs and through assessing the suitability of new therapy personnel. An essential part of these processes is to identify the primary clinician (see Chapter 4 of this book)

who will be responsible for the patient's treatment (3–14 days). For primary clinicians, an essential first step is to define roles and goals, i.e., establish a "contractual alliance" (see Chapters 3 and 11), and to contract with the patient about participation in aftercare services.
- *Changes in prior therapies.* These changes are often indicated, but they may require expert consultation and the introduction of new therapists. If the changes are considered undesirable by the patient, working through resistance may be possible only in the hospital, where the options for flight from the proposed changes are reduced (3–14 days). Hospitalizations may allow therapists to review prior impasses or establish a clearer treatment framework for their ongoing work (Chapter 11). For many borderline patients, hospitalization serves as an environment to evaluate medication benefits and to initiate medication changes (Chapter 6).

Structure

To establish the businesslike, practical orientation that allows the goals above to be reached efficiently, it is useful to have clarity and simplicity in the inpatient units' structures. This means a clear hierarchy, fixed roles, and consistent policies. Each patient needs to have a case manager/coordinator who processes the patient's wishes and the administrative decisions. The administratively responsible psychiatrist during the hospitalization needs to assess the patient, preside over treatment plans, delegate tasks, and prescribe medications. A social worker or the coordinator/case manager needs to assess with the patient what are the available social supports, especially family, and involve these support persons in planning aftercare. Psychoeducation of families can begin (see Chapter 9 of this book). Family meetings can serve to improve communication and avoid incendiary responses; both of these processes may be useful in establishing a viable aftercare plan and may even help to prevent future hospitalizations (Lansky 1989).

Note that short-term hospital programs should not offer community meetings or group therapies that encourage cohesion or bonding. Rather, groups oriented toward coping, crisis management, and psychoeducation are more valuable.

Staff

The ideal staff within hospital programs are comfortable but impersonal about setting limits, recognize (preferably even enjoy) but do not enact provocations, and keep a focus on the patients' community living situations and needs rather than on their in-hospital behaviors. Although staff can be selected with these attitudes in mind, often the development of the desirable approach is acquired only by considerable experience. This means that units should consciously avoid having too many inexperienced staff and should actively inculcate the attitudes discussed above for those who are new. The primary danger with inexperienced staff is that they are often hesitant to engage borderline patients actively in focusing on their aftercare and their situational crises.

Generic inpatient units are capable of fulfilling very well the goals of hospitalization suitable for borderline patients, but the staff of such units need to be attuned to the special needs of borderline patients for clear structure, treatment goals, and leadership and staff supervision or meetings to safeguard against splits. Generic units that are too medically oriented or too organized around the low-stimulus needs of psychotic patients will be likely unwittingly to foster staff hostility toward the emotional and time demands typically made by borderline patients. At best, hostility may result in strict limits and early discharges, but this is less than optimal. Units that do not welcome the challenges posed by borderline patients are likely to aggravate the problems they dread.

Level III: Residential/Partial Hospital Care—Basic Socialization

Level III includes residential care per se, meaning round-the-clock psychiatric services in settings that are less intensively monitored and less restrictive than hospitals. Level III also includes two divisions: day care alone and night care (usually a halfway house). These types of level III services offer sufficient holding of the patient to reduce suicidality to a degree that allows extramural activities (Stone 1990). During the period borderline patients spend in level III, they establish a *contractual* alliance with their primary clinician by defining and agreeing on roles and goals and begin work on a *relational* alliance with the primary clinician and/or with a therapist (see Chapter 3 of this book for discussion of types of alliance). This is also a placement in which the medication changes introduced during hospitalization, or during recent outpatient upheavals, can be stabilized and both the benefits and the usage of medication can be monitored. For patients in full residential care, it is critical for the patient's primary clinician or case manager to actively help the patient arrange for room and board (night care) if he or she will be staying in day care, or to help arrange for structured community activities that will enable him or her to leave day care while continuing to need night care. As noted in Table 5–1, the primary goals of level III services involve social rehabilitation.

Vignette

Arthur was a 16-year-old boy who lived with his mother and used both head banging and violence (breaking dishes, threatening to strike her) to intimidate and control her. His mother's retreat into excessive use of anxiolytics escalated his threats to the point that he threatened her with a knife. School counselors impressed by his aptitude and likability but concerned by his deteriorating school performance identified a need for a consistent, structured living situation to enable him to get to school on time, to help him control his anger, and to help his mother develop better coping strategies. His mother and his therapist agreed enthusiastically. An adolescent residential program that could allow him to commute to school proved unavailable, so he went to a halfway house with young adults.

Goals

- *Teach or stabilize daily living skills (eating, sleeping, hygiene, etc.).* The need for this goal varies, as does the optimal approach to achieving it. Most borderline patients need consistent monitoring and education about the importance of eating and sleeping in regular patterns. Sleep medications may prove useful for many who have trouble getting to sleep because of fearfulness.
- *Initiate vocational rehabilitation.* This goal is typically the most likely to be overlooked. Borderline patients don't introduce it or welcome it. Young or inexperienced staff have little consciousness of its value and importance. Program administrators or primary clinicians usually determine whether it is addressed.

  An important component of level III services is the availability of vocational rehabilitation services. The feelings and actions of borderline patients so often preoccupy clinical staff that they overlook enduring impairments in social function (see Sidebar 5–2).

Sidebar 5–2: Vocational Counseling: Should He or She Return to School, Pursue a Career, or Become a Caregiver?

Returning to School

A common problem concerns the young borderline patient whose self-destructiveness has necessitated a hospitalization that interrupts a school term. Often, especially if school performance was fine or if the student says he or she wants to return to school, it becomes reflexive to support a return. After all, the education itself is a valuable asset, and the threat of being set apart (as well as lagging behind) one's peers is significant. Unfortunately, returning to school virtually never succeeds if the youth's parents or treaters agree reflexively, and especially if they appear to be optimistic. Returning to school occasionally succeeds when the parents or treaters are explicitly opposed but yield to the youth's insistence. Their resistance may show that the self-destructive behaviors are taken seriously and conveys concern for the youth's welfare above his or her achievements. Support for returning to school fuels the borderline patient's fears that his or her caretakers want to expel or abandon him or her. For parents or treaters to "forbid" a return may be a relief to some patients—primarily to those who welcome a prolonged and regressive return to dependency and flight from autonomy. To others, being forbidden may simply amplify rebellious, defiant behaviors and a sense of alienation from "overcontrolling," anti-independence authorities.

Returning to school, especially when the person has had prior school problems, should always be preceded by holding down a steady job. This is the way to determine whether the person with BPD has motivation, concentration, conscientiousness, ability to accept external authority, and willingness to complete what may at times be undesirable tasks. These are prerequisites to be able to succeed in school, and they should be established in a context that doesn't involve competition or the fear that advancement means separation or autonomy.

Seeking a Job

When borderline patients have been out of the work or school marketplace for a sustained period of time—6 months or more—the reentry (or entry) should be gradual. A general principle is that this process should begin with a job that does not test their capabilities and that does not have too many implications for their eventual career (and subsequent independence). This means that the initial job placement should be carefully attuned to their past work experience, aptitudes, and long-term goals. For the 30-year-old who hasn't previously held a paying job, it is better to start as a volunteer. For the future dress designer, it is better to start as a clothing salesclerk than as a designer's aide. For the son who was expected to take over his father's business, it may be better to work alongside a supportive friend or relative. It may be beneficial for a son or daughter who has an underinvolved parent to work with or for that person.

Becoming a Caregiver

Many BPD patients will want to pursue or return to work that involves caregiving functions. It is wise to caution them that such work is invariably stressful for people who themselves need caretaking and/or who perceive that they haven't gotten adequate care in the past. If patients nevertheless insist on this field, encourage them to move slowly: plants before pets before people. Certainly, the ability to assume responsibility for a pet is a useful indicator of aptitude. Here too there is a hierarchy: start with fish, go to rodents, then cats, and finally dogs. For those who insist on pursuing the delivery of people services, the likelihood of success will be inversely related to the likelihood of negative (hostile or critical) feedback and the level of responsibility. Thus, working with people who have dementia is better than working with adolescents, and working as an aide is better than working as a nurse.

- *Identify/modify gross maladaptive behavioral (impulse control) and interpersonal (affect recognition/tolerance) traits.* To identify maladaptive behaviors and traits requires that staff of the residential program repeatedly clarify for BPD patients, or confront them about, aspects of themselves that are dysfunctional and undesirable (e.g., behaviors that are attention seeking; traits like maladaptiveness that prevent them from achieving their goals, such as being praised or preventing rejections). This is done in order to make behaviors or traits ego-dystonic that have previously been ego-syntonic (e.g., bullying, hiding feelings, or procrastinating). In the vignette above, the mother's behavioral responses to Arthur's tyranny were unwittingly positive reinforcement, the modification of which could be initiated.

Staff

To facilitate attachment, identification, and transferences, it is desirable for the staff of level III services to have a mixture of gender, age, levels of experience, and even attitudes (see discussion of splitting, Chapter 4 of this book). Regular staff meetings are needed in order to facilitate communication, examine countertransference, address splits, retain focus on goals, assess progress, and provide education, and develop a case formulation (a way of understanding the sources and meaning of the patients' symptoms).

As in hospitals (level IV), each patient needs a staff case manager/coordinator, preferably a full-time nonprofessional mental health worker, whose responsibility is to implement the treatment plan, monitor progress, and help patients address the how-to issues of coping with daily life and goal attainment. This person needs to be in regular communication with the patient's primary clinician (usually the therapist) to implement or change treatment plans. When, as is usually the case, the level III service has its own administrative personnel, the case manager/coordinator needs to clarify whether or when the patient's primary clinician/therapist defers decision-making authority to the program administrator. This, I think, should depend on the expected length of stay: for residential stays of less than 1 month, the primary clinician/therapist is best left in charge; for longer residential stays, the program administrator should at least share authority. Failure to clarify these roles often renders the level III care useless, if not harmful.

The meetings of staff coordinators with patients should be frequent, brief, and as needed, not sit-down "pseudotherapy" (inviting disclosure of secrets or expression of feelings) sessions. When patients are very angry or frustrated by the case manager's message or style, they can and should know who his or her supervisor is and be encouraged to take up the problem there. This is the *principle of triangulation*. It means that borderline patients who are in institutional treatment should always—or at least in the early phases of treatment—have an identifiable means of appealing their case. This prevents splits, diffuses rage, and offers useful holding and learning opportunities. Within level III or IV programs, the program administrator can perform this function if there are problems with a primary clinician/therapist. Similarly, the primary clinician/therapist can perform this function when there are problems with the program administrator.

Structure

Group Meetings

The most important structures of residential/partial hospital programs involve group meetings. These can be divided into those for the entire community and more focused or time-limited types. Community meetings are for all patients and staff, whereas the group therapies with staff leadership are for patients assigned by virtue of their problems, and recreational/expressive groups are elective.

- *Community meetings.* Typically scheduled in mornings to maximize attendance by patients and staff, these meetings help establish a sense of community among patients by focusing on ward administrative issues, such as policies or disruptive events, and inviting discussion of feelings or opinions. I believe there are advantages in 1) having such meetings three or more times a week, 2) making attendance mandatory for everyone who is not in seclusion and who has no authorized non–hospital-based activities (e.g., a job interview), and 3) having meetings led or co-led by the clinician in charge of the unit. The effectiveness of the long-term inpatient unit at Henderson Hospital in England rested heavily on this form of therapeutic community, emphasizing patients as collaborators (Dolan et al. 1997). In level III programs, the lower level of external containment requires more staff leadership.
- *Group therapies.* Membership in a group will be based on whether the group's goals have relevance to patients, and thus assignment is not controlled by the group leaders. These groups should meet three times a week to allow cohesion and depth. Because of the potential for borderline patients to overwhelm psychotic patients, it is usually best not to put the two groups together. All groups in day- or night-care settings require active, directive affect and anxiety-controlling leadership. Traditional topics for these groups include family issues, vocational issues, skills of daily living, and increasingly the use of social skills training modules from dialectical behavior therapy (DBT) or other structured directives (see Chapter 8 in this book).
- *Recreational/expressive groups.* Participation in these groups is often elective. They invite borderline patients to be active participants. Recreational outlets, such as exercising, cooking, carpentry, or even attending community events enhance social skills and encourage the development of friendships over a common task. The expressive (e.g., collage, pottery, dance) groups can enhance self-esteem and offer opportunities for symbolic communication of conflicts and hopes. Because of the emotional expressiveness invited, the leaders of such activities need to encourage verbalization and to be alert to the potential loss of control.

Day Care/Night Care: Partial Hospital (Day) or Halfway House (Night)

It should be noted that day services and night services are not all—or necessarily—connected to hospitals and therefore should not all be referred to as partial hospital services, except in the sense that they are clearly a transitional level of care between hospital and outpatient care. Transition from full residential care to either day care or night care alone is best initiated by 1) advising patients that the transition will be difficult insofar as they will miss their supports and will need to assume added responsibilities for themselves and 2) encouraging them to make the transition on a trial basis, since to suggest that transitions are irreversible will beget angry, panicky behavioral responses. (For borderline patients needing this level of care, learning to contain and verbalize their responses will often become an indicator that this level of care is no longer needed.)

Day care (living in the community while receiving structured treatment 3 or more hours a day for 3–5 days each week) is the usual step-down from residential (day and night) care. It allows the social rehabilitation goals of the day program to continue. Day care alone is for patients who have a reasonable place to live, meaning they are safe from lethal, self-destructive acts and are able to take care of the basic tasks of self-care like eating, sleeping, and responsibly using medications. The clinical value of a long-term, well-organized day hospital program has impressive empirical support (see Sidebar 5–3). Most day treatment programs are offered for too brief a period to achieve social rehabilitation goals. Stabilization can be achieved in a matter of weeks, but social learning requires at least a month and usually a minimum of 2–6 months.

Sidebar 5-3: Empirical Support for a Psychoanalytic Day Hospital

Welcome confirmation of the clinical effectiveness of a day hospital program has come from the English team of Bateman and Fonagy (1999). Forty-four BPD patients were randomly assigned to receive 18 months of day hospital service or to receive "general hospital" care. The latter control condition involved as-needed use of hospital and day services with medications and community/outpatient follow-ups. In contrast, the experimental condition provided a more continuous care system in which medications were used in conjunction with psychoanalytically oriented group psychotherapy three times a week, psychoanalytically oriented individual psychotherapy (by nurses, occupational therapists, or psychiatrists) once a week, and expressive therapy of a psychodrama type once a week. These specific modalities were coordinated in daily staff meetings, senior psychotherapy consultation, and periodic case conferences.

The 22 patients in the day hospital condition showed significantly more improvement than the 19 control patients (3 dropped out due to suicidality) in depressive symptoms, suicidal and self-destructive acts, number of hospital days (reduced), and social and interpersonal functioning.

These advantages were already evident by 6 months, and these distinctions grew at the 12- and 18-month assessments. In follow-up on the 38 study subjects 18 months after the treatments, those who were in the day hospital program continued to show improvement, whereas the 16 control subjects did not (A. Bateman and P. Fonagy, "Follow-up of Psychoanalytically Oriented Partial Hospitalization Treatment of Borderline Personality Disorder," unpublished manuscript, February 2000). The investigators concluded that the initial 18 months of treatment set in motion longer-term rehabilitative changes.

This study is notable in that, like the better-known study of DBT (see Chapter 8 of this book), it demonstrates very impressive benefits from a coherent and well-informed approach to borderline patients when compared with the usual treatment offered to such patients. The symptomatic and interpersonal benefits from the partial hospital treatment seem considerably stronger than those observed after a year in DBT. Whether this observation is due to the psychodynamic focus of this treatment (as opposed to DBT's behavioral focus), or to sample differences, or to the considerably greater intensity and longer duration of the therapy, are empirical questions yet to be answered.

Although less specific to borderline patients, a 4-month day treatment program at the University of Alberta Hospital showed confirmatory results. That program is a psychodynamically based therapeutic community, with emphasis on group therapies, that is designed to treat patients with personality disorders. Piper et al. (1993) showed that 60 patients treated in this program had significantly better outcomes than 60 waiting-list control subjects in four areas: interpersonal functioning, symptoms, self-esteem, and satisfaction with their lives. These gains were sustained on follow-up 8 months later. Although supportive of Bateman and Fonagy's conclusions, this study only involved 14 BPD subjects, whose outcomes were not broken out. This limits the ability to generalize the otherwise optimistic results by Piper et al., insofar as a study done at the Ulleval Hospital in Oslo indicates that it is likely that this subgroup would probably be less responsive than those with other diagnoses (Wilberg et al. 1998).

For Bateman and Fonagy, the next major outcome study that is needed should compare the benefits of their day hospital program with those that can derive from an intensive outpatient service (i.e., level II, to be described later in this chapter). I heartily agree; I also add the caveat that less than 18 months in day treatment is, in my experience, often possible and almost certainly desirable if patients can step down into an adequately intensive and coordinated outpatient service (level II).

Night care (usually in a halfway house) is important for BPD patients who are able to work or go to school but who do not have sufficient supports or are otherwise unable to take care of themselves at night. This is symptomatic of the intolerance of being alone (Chapter 1) that makes solitary living unacceptable. This problem means that the need for night care can extend for considerable periods. The night care function is often performed by community-based halfway houses or cooperative apartments, but enlightened residential (day and night) programs will offer this as a step-down. Under the rare circumstances when there exists the possibility of choosing between (in descending order of capability of holding) an on-site residential step-down service, an off-site halfway house, or an off-site cooperative apartment, the selection should be based on the patient's expected tolerance—the least monitored choice being best. To make such a selection requires an understanding of the patient's ego functioning, level of community supports, and relationship to the treating agencies. For counterdependent patients, it may be better to "recommend" a more monitored setting than is actually needed. For regressive patients prone to act for secondary gains, it may be better to "recommend" less monitored settings (i.e., level II or even level I) than is judged to be needed. In both instances, the eventual compromise may be what works best.

Level II: Intensive Outpatient Care—Behavioral Change

The intensive outpatient (IOP) level of care is for patients who are able to manage some social role, such as some part-time school or work, and who have adequate room and board. This level of care is relatively new, is still often unavailable, and in my experience, is highly beneficial for many borderline patients, either as a direct step-down from hospitalization or as a step-up from outpatient care. Dialectical behavior therapy involving 5 hours of treatment per week and a system of coverage that contains crises should be classified as a specific type of IOP care (see Chapter 8 of this book). It successfully diminishes hospitalizations. There is no question in my mind, although still no empirical evidence, that IOP type of care (other than DBT) greatly reduces the need for residential/partial hospital programs, in much the same way as residential/partial hospital programs can reduce the need for hospitalizations. The success of these programs depends on their offering sufficient holding to counter regressive flights and to support sustained community living. As noted by Smith et al. (G. Smith, A. Ruiz-Sancho, and J. G. Gunderson, "An Intensive Outpatient Program for Treatment of Borderline Personality Disorder," unpublished manuscript), this holding function is directly related to the degree to which the case is coordinated via frequent communications between the clinical team members. In the absence of good, preferably standardized, communications, hateful rivalries can form between patients who share clinic therapists.

Links (1998) has reviewed studies in which patients with personality disorders have received a type of IOP care called *assertive community treatment* (ACT). ACT uses proactive interventions involving visits to the patient's place of residence, with a focus on assistance with the tasks of daily living and in vivo counseling about relationships and work. Only the original study of ACT by Stein and Test (1980) had a large enough cohort of patients with personality disorders (26) to examine their outcomes. That study showed diminished use of hospitals, better compliance with treatment, and decreased legal problems. Links concluded that ACT has potential for BPD patients, but that this model of IOP care, like the one being described and advocated in this chapter, awaits empirical testing.

Vignette

Ms. D was referred for treatment because the small town she lived in had no psychiatric facilities. Her primary care physician thought that hospitalization would provide the containment needed so that she could make use of medications and psychotherapy, with which she was noncompliant, and could terminate her bulimic and rageful behaviors, which were "destroying her family." During the intake interview, it was apparent that Ms. D was frightened of hospitalization. She protested that it wasn't necessary, that she could live with her aunt, and that the only reason she saw for relocating to Boston was that it could offer opportunities to become a dancing instructor. It was recommended that she come to daily self-assessment groups and have an extended psychiatric evaluation. During the next week, it became apparent that she could responsibly use the program, that instruction in dancing could be arranged, and that living with her aunt stabilized what was an 8-year pattern of bulimia.

Goals

- *Vocational.* Enlist in needed training and/or obtain work (see Sidebar 5–1).
- *Interpersonal.* Recognize anger and dependent needs as part of self and others.

- *Behavioral.* Improve abilities to contain impulsive expressions of feelings or attitudes or impulsive acts.

Components

Figure 5–2 diagrams the components of level II outpatient services and the relative lengths of time during which patients participate. Discussion of the nonpharmacological components follows.

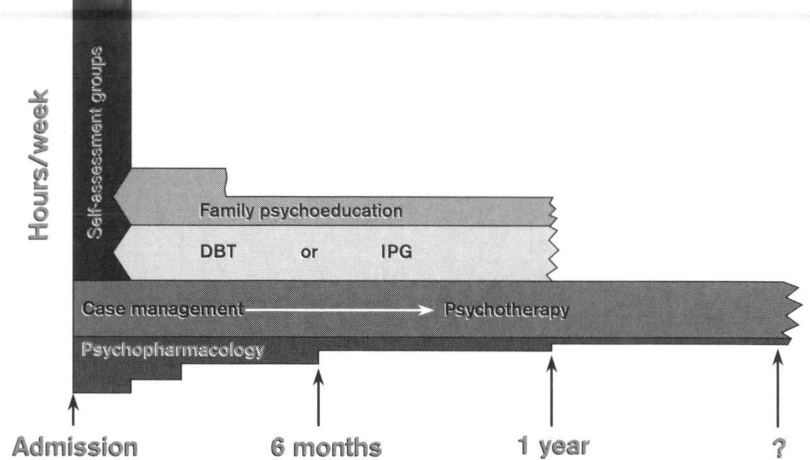

FIGURE 5–2. Borderline personality disorder outpatient services.

- *Self-assessment groups.* Such groups, available every day (a minimum of at least three times a week), are the backbone of an IOP service. They function well for as few as 3 patients and as many as 10. The group leader needs to be an experienced clinician who is comfortable with both group dynamics and crisis interventions. Coleadership, as with other groups having predominantly borderline members, serves to diminish burdens and countertransference enactments and to assure continuity. Participants' attendance is flexibly arranged: they can come as often as every weekday or as little as once a week. They should expect to remain from 2 weeks to 8 weeks. Crises are referred to the patient's primary clinician.

These groups provide a social network, since most members will be dealing with similar immediate issues of transition into community living. The frequency of meetings allows participants to become familiar quickly with the details of each other's current lives. Common issues include the attitudes encountered on returning to families or co-workers, feelings related to losing prior supports (e.g., school peers or treatment staff), and the difficulties involved in working with new mental health staff and new therapeutic modalities.

Groups meet daily, but participants attend with variable and usually gradually diminishing frequency. Each group begins with a go-around, in which each participant reports on recent events or plans about which they receive feedback from others. Because members all have one foot in community living, they are vigilant to signs of retreat or regression in one another. Groups meet for an hour, preferably in the early morning or late afternoon so as to minimize conflicts with work or school responsibilities.

- *Case management.* At the IOP level of care, the clinician responsible for the patient's care, the primary clinician/therapist, needs to be active and direct in administrative decisions. There is no longer a separate administrative structure such as exists on levels IV and III. Now the primary clinician, in principle, is responsible for implementing plans, assessing safety, communicating with family, seeking consults, and changing the treatment (including shifts in level of care). In practice this is often not done well, either because 1) the primary clinician/therapist is not geographically present and immediately accessible or because 2) he or she may be trying to establish a role as a dynamic therapist who can see the patient's behavioral problems as a subject for interpretation rather than for management. Both of these problems can lead to splits by the patient.

  Leaders of self-assessment groups will encounter occasions when they need to inform the primary clinician about what actions are needed. Sometimes this isn't possible, and they themselves need to get involved in crisis management. The primary clinician can actively help a patient anticipate problems and select coping methods that are adaptive. Usually, borderline patients at this level of care are able to do psychotherapeutic work such as identifying feelings and how they relate to current issues, including the clinician/therapist's functioning. Either the primary clinician should be able to accommodate and conduct such work, or a psychotherapist needs to be added (see Chapter 10 of this book).
- *Other activities.* The minimal essential components of IOP care are self-assessment groups and the case management/therapy activities cited above. Preferably, these are complemented by functions that introduce and stabilize the longer-term modalities that patients will need for continued progress when they enter level I (outpatient) care. This level of care is particularly suited to family interventions designed to identify and diminish

the triggers that lead to crisis (see Chapter 9 of this book). As noted, the staff who offer level I services needs to include someone who can do psychotherapy. In addition, a second collaborating and complementary modality (in accord with the principle of split treatment, discussed in Chapter 4) is best initiated while the patient is still attending self-assessment groups. Either a DBT social skills training group or an interpersonal group (IPG; see Chapter 10) is an ideal complement to psychotherapy. Other group options that can begin as part of the IOP level are vocational rehabilitation, family issues, or either trauma or alcoholism recovery groups. Finally, this is an excellent time to get involved in self-help organizations (e.g., Alcoholics Anonymous or Overeaters Anonymous) or community organizations (e.g., churches or volunteer groups).

Level I: Outpatient Care—Interpersonal Growth

Outpatient care (level I) is where critically important changes in interpersonal and intrapsychic functioning can occur. For most borderline patients, the first year also involves continued work on significant behavioral problems; but at the outpatient care level this continued work takes place concurrently with the development of a relational alliance with the primary clinician/therapist (see Chapter 12 of this book). A major function of the primary clinician is to facilitate the patient's transition from a higher level of care (usually level IV, but often from level III or II) to the less intensive outpatient care. This process begins by identifying a suitable second modality to accompany the primary clinician/therapist's ongoing work. At this level of care the split treatment (Chapter 4) often involves the combination of a psychiatrist overseeing medications and another mental health professional doing psychotherapy. When a psychiatrist is doing both of these tasks, the second modality should include a social rehabilitative component—cognitive-behavioral therapy (see Chapter 8) or an interpersonal therapy group (see Chapter 10) and/or some continuation of family involvement (see Chapter 9). These therapies ideally begin while the patient is still in a higher level of care.

Vignette

Ms. E, a 28-year-old single woman, returned to live with her mother and stepfather after a year's absence, during which she lost the job for which she'd relocated. She had lost her job because of absences necessitated by four hospitalizations for suicidal impulses. Her hospital psychiatrist had referred her for aftercare. At intake she noted that, since returning, she had gotten a new job and her suicidality had diminished. She was hesitant to relate these changes to returning home insofar as she reported long-standing conflicts with her mother. She also reported that her problems are related to several romances that "ended badly" because of her "losing her own identity" (e.g., opinions, interests) and that were followed by a progressive reluctance to socialize because of fears of rejection. Her ability to work and her history of nonpromiscuous romances were judged to be strengths that should be encouraged. It was recommended that Ms. E begin once-weekly psychodynamic therapy and an interpersonal group (IPG; see Chapter 10 of this book). She was encouraged to have her parents read materials about BPD (see Chapter 9) to better understand her problems.

The outpatient level of care is the most extended. It is also the most unpredictable in its expectable duration. This is true because the motivation for change, the vicissitudes of life, and the goals and skill of the outpatient therapists are so variable. As described in Chapter 12, this is the level of care where basic personality change is sometimes possible over a period of years.

SUMMARY

This chapter describes distinctions in the goals, functions, structures, and lengths of stay for four levels of care that can be appropriate for borderline patients. Most clinical sites do not offer the intermediary levels of care (III and II), yet are still able to do well for many borderline patients. But for those who need a prolonged social rehabilitative experience (e.g., many adolescents and those with sustained dangerous habits such as substance abuse), the absence of levels III or II is costly and ineffective. The principle of *split treatments* (Chapter 4 of this book) is again introduced, meaning that two complementary forms of treatment can diminish flight and enhance effectiveness by containing splits.

In the background of the discussion about levels of care is the need for a primary clinician/therapist, who works in conjunction with those responsible for administering services or modalities to make thoughtful judgments about 1) what level of care a borderline patient needs, 2) when it is time to change that level, and 3) who facilitates these changes. Moreover, the clinician who will be part of the patient's longer-term outpatient care, preferably along with others (e.g., DBT group leader, family therapist), should anticipate that any changes to lower levels of care will be experienced as losses and should therefore be prepared to help borderline patients put the related issues of abandonment and dependency into words. Borderline patients need to be involved in reaching judgments about levels of care, but until the need for such services is over, it is incompatible with their psychopathology to expect them to make these wise judgments for themselves.

References

Bateman A, Fonagy P: The effectiveness of partial hospitalization in the treatment of BPD: a randomized controlled trial. Am J Psychiatry 156:1563–1569, 1999

Dolan B, Warren F, Norton K: Change in borderline symptoms one year after therapeutic community treatment for severe personality disorder. Br J Psychiatry 171:274–279, 1997

Gunderson JG: Borderline Personality Disorder. Washington, DC, American Psychiatric Press, 1984

Jones M: Social Psychiatry: A Study of Therapeutic Communities. London, Tavistock, 1952

Kullgren G: Factors associated with completed suicide in borderline personality disorder. J Nerv Ment Dis 176(1):40–44, 1988

Lansky MR: The subacute hospital treatment of the borderline patient: management of suicidal crisis by family intervention. J Clin Psychiatry 11:81–97, 1989

Lewin R, Sharfstein SS: Managed care and the discharge dilemma. Psychiatry 53(2):116–121, 1990

Links PS: Developing effective services for patients with personality disorders. Can J Psychiatry 43:251–259, 1998

Miller SA, Davenport NC: Increasing staff knowledge of and improving attitudes toward patients with borderline personality disorder. Psychiatr Serv 47(5):533–535, 1996

Nurnberg HG, Suh R: Time-limited treatment of hospitalized borderline patients: considerations. Compr Psychiatry 19(5):419–431, 1978

Piper WE, Rosie JS, Azim HFA, et al: A randomized trial of psychiatric day treatment for patients with affective and personality disorders. Hospital and Community Psychiatry 44:757–763, 1993

Quaytman M, Sharfstein SS: Treatment for severe borderline personality disorder in 1987 and 1997. Am J Psychiatry 154(8):1139–1144, 1997

Rosenbluth M, Silver D: The inpatient treatment of borderline personality disorder, in Handbook of Borderline Disorders. Edited by Silver D, Rosenbluth M. Madison, CT, International Universities Press, 1992, pp 509–532

Sederer LI (ed): Inpatient Psychiatry: Diagnosis and Treatment, 3rd Edition. Baltimore, MD, Williams & Wilkins, 1991

Sederer LI, Thorbeck J: First do no harm: short-term inpatient psychotherapy of the borderline patient. Hospital and Community Psychiatry 37(7):692–697, 1986

Silk KR, Eisner W, Allport C, et al: Focused time-limited inpatient treatment of borderline personality disorder. J Personal Disord 8(4):268–278, 1994

Stein LI, Test MA: Alternative to mental hospital treatment. Arch Gen Psychiatry 37:392–397, 1980

Stone MH: Multimodal therapy: applications to partial hospitalization in the light of long-term follow-up of borderline patients. International Journal of Partial Hospitalization 6(1):1–14, 1990

Tyrer P, Merson S, Onyett S, et al: The effect of personality disorder on clinical outcome, social networks, and adjustment: a controlled clinical trial of psychiatric emergencies. Psychol Med 24:731–740, 1994

Wilberg T, Friis S, Karterud S, et al: Outpatient group psychotherapy: a valuable continuation treatment for patients with borderline personality disorder treated in a day hospital? a 3-year follow-up study. Nordic Journal of Psychiatry 52(3): 213–221, 1998

6

PHARMACOTHERAPY

Clinical Practices

HISTORY

The role of psychotropic medications for borderline patients was extremely peripheral to discussions of these patients' treatment in the 1970s, when psychoanalytic perspectives predominated. The role of these medications began to be actively explored in the early 1980s as a result of the existence of standardized criteria and reliable assessments, the medicalization of psychiatry, and a growing appreciation for the value of medications for other disorders. The initial considerations about medications reflected the question of whether BPD was an atypical form of another disorder, schizophrenia (see Chapter 2 of this book). The issue of whether BPD was an atypical form of schizophrenia was originally examined by Brinkley et al. (1979), whose pioneering but noncontrolled account encouraged use of low-dose neuroleptics. The issue rapidly switched to the boundary of BPD with depression in response to provocative accounts by Akiskal (1981), Klein (1975, 1977), and Stone (1979) (Chapter 1). All three of these psychiatrists had clinical and empirical experiences suggesting that BPD was an atypical form of depressive disorder that might prove responsive to antidepressant medications. The initial series of controlled studies investigating these boundaries suggested that the response of borderline patients to antipsychotics or antidepressants was not as impressive as would be expected were BPD an atypical offspring of either of these parent conditions (Cowdry and Gardner 1988; Goldberg et al.

1986; Soloff et al. 1986). These studies did, however, show that both types of medication can be helpful in BPD and thereby opened up an exciting and still ongoing era of pharmacotherapeutic optimism.

Even as the early projects made it clear that neither traditional antipsychotics nor antidepressants offered very strong answers to the question of "borderline to what," these medications also revealed some more specific, surprising, and important results. For example, the studies by Cowdry and Gardner (1988) and Soloff et al. (1989) showed that antipsychotics were as effective in diminishing depression as were antidepressants. A second finding was that the dramatic effects that the first few weeks of hospitalization can have on reducing presenting symptoms made it impossible to discern the effects of medications initiated in that context (see Chapters 1 and 2 of this book) (Siever and Davis 1991; Soloff et al. 1989). A third finding was that borderline patients' judgments about the benefits of a medication could differ dramatically from judgments made by professionals. Medications most favored by borderline patients appeared actually to make them worse, in the judgment of others, whereas the type of medication they disliked most was judged most beneficial by others (Cowdry and Gardner 1988). A fourth finding is that although many types of medications could be helpful, no type proved consistently beneficial.

Overall Role of Medications

Whereas a previous generation of clinicians worried about whether, or under what circumstances, medications should be added to therapy, such concerns (for better or for worse) are now rare. Even in the 1980s, only about 10% of psychiatrists treated borderline patients without medications (Cole et al. 1984; Pope et al. 1983; Skodol et al. 1983; Soloff 1981; Waldinger and Frank 1989a; Zanarini et al. 1988). Such treatment is now truly rare. For many psychiatrists, the question has become whether it is ever reasonable to forgo pharmacotherapy. Undervaluation of medications is unlikely, and many psychiatrists even consider it unethical to withhold drugs. As a group, psychologists are only slightly less prone to advocate their use. In a recent sample selected from many clinical sites in four northeastern cities, 90% of borderline patients had received psychotropic medications—a significantly higher percentage than in a sample with major depression (Bender et al., in press).

Medication effects are hard to assess in borderline patients, for three very basic reasons:

- First, many of the symptoms that are the targets of medications are very dependent on context (Chapter 1). As a result, psychiatrists who lack experience with borderline patients can easily attribute too much benefit to medications (e.g., hospitalized patients whose depression disappears), or too little (e.g., discharged patients who cut themselves), when patients' symptoms are really the product of predictable changes in their level of care.
- The second reason why assessing benefits is difficult involves their use as vehicles for projection. It is very easy for borderline patients to attribute changes in their moods to their medication. If they feel bad, the medications offer an easily discernible and less painful explanation than, for example, the patients' being rejected. More will be said about this.
- The third reason is that medications are rarely, in my experience, dramatic in their effectiveness. Their effect is almost always partial and modest.

Sidebar 6–1: Listening to Prozac: Can SSRIs Cure BPD?

Peter Kramer's best-selling book *Listening to Prozac* (Kramer 1993) reported that selective serotonin reuptake inhibitors (SSRIs) changed the personality (i.e., the attitudes, expectations, level of energy, and overall mood) of his patients. His report raised the expectations of many patients—and their psychiatrists too. High expectations are also encouraged by drug trials that report borderline patients who stop meeting criteria for the diagnosis after only 1–2 months of taking medications.

Alas, Kramer's hopeful message is not borne out by listening to borderline patients. Medications can decrease the frequency of symptomatic acts and affects so that DSM criteria can appear to have remitted. Thus medications appear to have affected borderline *personality.* These changes are not insignificant, and the prescribing psychiatrist can easily exaggerate the benefits. Still, the more core personality features of impulsivity, misattributions, and pathological object relations await other means of intervention.

There remains hope that Kramer's optimistic message might one day be fulfilled, but the type of medication for curing BPD has not yet been developed.

If a borderline patient responds dramatically, by becoming essentially nonborderline as a result of medications, the borderline diagnosis was probably mistaken (see Sidebar 6–1). This clinical impression is confirmed by Paul Soloff (personal communication, January 2000), the investigator who has performed the most drug trials, and is further confirmed by the experience gained from observing the course of large numbers of borderline subjects during prospective longitudinal studies. Such experience is illustrated by the following vignette:

Vignette

A 30-year-old obese married woman, with a highly dependent relationship on her husband (she called him four times daily), was diagnosed as borderline when she began self-mutilating activities. They occurred in the context of the couple's having decided, at the husband's urging, to apply for adoption. Eight months later, having been on an SSRI, she no longer met DSM-IV (American Psychiatric Association 1994) criteria for BPD. Indeed, she had stopped cutting, was working full-time, and had ceased needing excessive reassurances from her husband. This remission originally was thought by her psychiatrist to exemplify a medication cure (like those that can be seen with depression or anxiety disorders). On closer examination, the patient's recovery did not actually begin until four months after starting the SSRI—too long a delay to assume that the SSRI accounted for the changes. Moreover, the improvements began shortly after she and her husband decided to withdraw the adoption application.

This vignette illustrates the temptation to credit medications with changes that might better be understood by examining life events. The patient may well have had BPD, but the reasons for her regression and recovery are unlikely to be explained by her serotonin metabolism.

Because medications are primarily intended to reduce subjective distress (i.e., symptoms considered undesirable to the patient) and help contain behavioral problems (often considered undesirable by others), they are a type of intervention that can have relatively rapid and desirable effects (see Chapter 3 of this book on the sequence of change). Medications may also help with longer-term and later goals of treatment. In my experience, medications are often, perhaps even usually, helpful for borderline patients. But, in the absence of knowledge about long-term risks and benefits, and in the presence of the very real dangers of misuse, it remains clinically and scientifically important to recognize that we lack empirical justification for our usual practices.

The overall role of medications in the long-term care of borderline patients still remains uncertain. Beyond their usual, but often uncertain, helpfulness, the continued proliferation of new types of medications fuels the hope that their role may become more significant and certain. Moreover, as is pointed out throughout this chapter, the role of medications is not static; it can be expected to change as borderline patients get better.

GETTING STARTED

An important role of psychopharmacology involves its usefulness in engaging and allying BPD patients and their families in treatment. By first anchoring BPD psychopathology within medicine and biology, the psychopharmacological approach underscores the "illness" (see Chapters 1, 3, and 11 of this book). This approach usefully diminishes unrealistic expectations that the patient can willfully "get over it." A survey reported by Waldinger and Frank (1989) shows that most borderline patients feel pleased and impressed by the doctors who prescribe and that 92% of the psychiatrist/therapists believed that prescribing strengthened the alliance. Anchoring BPD within medicine and biology also prompts a less defensive, more supportive posture by families regarding treatment (see Chapter 9). Moreover, this approach conveys a proactive and hopeful attitude about diminishing immediate symptoms that, if not oversold, is always welcome and helps establish the relational alliance (Chapter 3) needed for longer-term goals involving psychological change (Chapter 12). However, it is also critically important to convey to borderline patients and their families the overall *limitations* of expectable benefits from medications in order to set the stage for appropriate (i.e., multimodal) treatment (see Sidebar 6–2). Pfohl and colleagues' survey of clinicians (B. Pfohl, K. Silk, C. Robins, M. Zimmerman, and J. Gunderson, "Attitudes Towards Borderline PD: a Survey of 752 Clinicians," unpublished data, May 1999) indicates that most psychopharmacologists have a realistically modest view of the role of medications in the overall treatment of BPD.

Sidebar 6–2: "I Don't Know If It Will Help"

An interesting alternative to the approach to psychopharmacology presented here comes from Dawson and MacMillan (1993). In their "no treatment treatment," they advocate not suggesting, recommending, or promoting any medication, but rather actively discussing their past experience with medications and providing borderline patients with existing knowledge so that the patients decide whether and what medications to use–without influence. This approach clearly has advantages in sidestepping control/authority/compliance struggles and emphasizing the patient's responsibility in assessing benefits.

The problem with this approach is that experienced psychopharmacologists usually have informed opinions about what medications to use and whether benefits can be expected. For them this approach is disingenuous.

The second problem is that the reluctance to assume a doctorly role at the outset of treatment bypasses the alliance-building effects of the clinician's recommending medications and may offer insufficient holding for some borderline patients and their families. Third, this approach requires that patients be more proactive and thoughtful than might be realistic. For example, depressed borderline patients may get some relief from medications that allow them to *then* become more curious and active.

The Prescribing Psychiatrist's Role

With the Borderline Patient

It is important for the prescribing psychiatrist to begin by clarifying what the patient can expect from him or her (as noted above), as well as from medications. Regarding the expectable benefits of medications, important messages to convey to patients appear in Table 6–1. The overall message is to proactively guard against too high expectations and to proactively insist on the borderline patient's collaboration in selecting targets for treatment and on his or her being an alert, well-informed consumer. These guidelines establish an atmosphere of pragmatic empiricism not unlike that advocated for cognitive-behavioral therapies (see Chapter 8 of this book).

As the Primary Clinician (Psychiatrist/Therapist)

If the prescribing psychiatrist is also the primary clinician (i.e., therapist), his or her role among treaters working as a team is not usually a problem. Moreover, the psychiatrist in this role has the opportunity for more frequent and longer appointments, necessitated by his or her expanded role and consequent greater knowledge of the patient's contextual factors (e.g., forthcoming exams or separations). This position on the team offers the psychiatrist enormous

TABLE 6–1. Guidelines for psychopharmacological treatment

1. Medications can be helpful, but their overall role is adjunctive. They should not be expected to be curative of BPD. Convey cautious optimism about expectable benefits.
2. Require the patient's collaboration in identifying target problems/symptoms that medications might reasonably benefit, e.g., stabilizing affects, undesirable behaviors, or distorted perceptions.
3. Outline the expectable time course by which benefits might occur.
4. Inform the patient about the possible adverse side effects and about alternative medications. This helps patients to be active in decisions and more frankly communicative.
5. Encourage the patient to read about whatever medications are prescribed.
6. Stress that effects are hard to evaluate and enlist the patient as an ally in this process. Indeed, encourage the patient to view this as a research process in which you will learn together whether, and what, medications can help.
7. Because noncompliance is common, stress the necessity for meticulous and responsible usage to evaluate effectiveness.

benefits in assessing the role of medications, and it can also offer an excellent opportunity to explore the meanings assigned to the medications.

The downside of the prescribing psychiatrist's also serving as the therapist is that the transference arising from the directive caretaker role can become more heated. Too, if unsuccessfully explored, this more intense transference can increase the likelihood of misuse of medications (e.g., noncompliance, overdosing). As will be discussed, the transference to the prescribing therapist can also influence the borderline patient's apparent responsiveness to the medications and the therapist's prescribing behavior. Waldinger and Frank (1989b) note that when the prescribing psychiatrist is also offering psychotherapy (i.e., when the psychiatrist is the primary clinician, as described in Chapter 4 of this book), medication abuse takes place about 50% of the time. The important empirical question remains whether this rate is higher or lower when the medications are prescribed by someone who does only pharmacotherapy (in the arrangement often called *split treatment*).

As a practical matter, the issue of medications is often set apart to be dealt with in the first or last 10–15 minutes of sessions. Obviously, the need to devote time to this issue should diminish considerably over a period of 2–4 months unless problems with compliance or usage persist. Such persistence may be an indication for splitting the treatment.

As the Psychopharmacologist Only (Split Treatment)

It is increasingly normative for psychiatrists to split treatment responsibilities with other mental health professionals who conduct the psychotherapy. This practice stems from the cost-saving mandate of managed care—saving ostensibly by limiting the amount of time psychiatrists spend with patients. This practice, in turn, is diminishing the training, experience, and comfort that many psychiatrists have in filling other roles, most notably psychotherapy. When the prescribing psychiatrist's role does not include being the borderline patient's primary clinician (i.e., therapist), there will usually be a less intense relationship, but psychological splitting of the treaters (into "good" and "bad") is more easily enacted.

It often becomes complicated to establish and maintain a clear definition of what the psychopharmacologist's responsibilities are. Problems are often due to unstated role expectations. One of the psychopharmacologist's responsibilities, easily neglected when he or she is not the patient's primary clinician, is to communicate and discuss interventions with whoever is responsible for the patient's overall care (the primary clinician)—often the individual psychotherapist. This communicative role is especially necessary when medications are being changed and the effects of those changes need to be monitored. Communication is equally important for assessing whether changes in a patient's symptoms are related to the prescribed medications. For example, the isolated psychiatrist acting as psychopharmacologist only might attribute too much benefit to drugs for the patient whose depression disappears after a boyfriend moves in, or too little benefit to drugs because that same borderline patient resumes cutting after the boyfriend moves out. In both instances the patient's symptom changes are really the product of changes in interpersonal life.

A second complication involves coordination of roles and responsibilities around safety issues. Because the prescribing psychiatrist is often the legally (i.e., medically) responsible member of a team, a crisis plan needs to be developed that includes him or her in assessing safety and in making decisions about changing the patient's level of care (see Sidebar 6–3). In any event, the psychopharmacologist needs to clarify how and when he or she can be contacted for medication questions.

Sidebar 6–3: Liability Hazards of Split Treatment

Psychiatrists whose responsibilities are confined to psychopharmacological management and who, as a result of managed care incentives or personal preference, see their borderline patients only briefly, often have disproportionate legal responsibilities and liability risks. They often represent the deep-pocket member of the treatment team. The APA's *Guidelines for Consultative, Supervisory, or Collaborative Relationships With Nonmedical Therapists* (American Psychiatric Association 1980) states that the psychiatrist must spend sufficient time to ensure that proper care is given and warns against psychiatrists' being used as figureheads (Annotation 5, Section 3). Psychiatrists therefore should recognize that most liability exposure is due to negligence of two kinds. The first involves communication that is inadequate to ensure that the psychiatrist understands and approves of what the teammates are doing. The second involves inadequate involvement in decisions about changes in the treatment plan. This may mean only the psychiatrist's approval, but it does mean that the nonphysician primary clinician needs to clear decisions with the psychiatrist.

Gabbard (2000) notes that *explicit* discussion and agreement between the prescribing psychiatrist and other clinicians (usually the therapist) is the best defense against liability. Explicitly, both should have the following:

1. Adequate liability insurance
2. Competence and credentialing in the treatment they provide
3. An agreement about whether the psychiatrist has supervisory responsibility
4. The patient's agreement that patient and therapist will discuss changes or concerns with each other

The disproportionate liability risk of psychiatrists is increasing their fears about getting involved with borderline patients. The real implication of these risks is that the greater the involvement with and knowledge about a patient a psychiatrist has, the less the psychiatrist's liability risk. Still, greater knowledge about the patient will not necessarily diminish the risk associated with a psychiatrist's need to know and approve of the practices employed by others who are members of a borderline patient's team.

SYMPTOM CHASING

Symptom chasing with borderline patients can, at its worst, involve multiple nonsustained medication trials in pursuit of alleviating a patient's transitory, dramatized symptoms. It results in little relief of the underlying problems impelling the patient's complaints and in little learning about whether medications could be useful. It may further result in a patient who is chronically overmedicated.

At its best, though, symptom chasing is a reasonable extension of the pragmatic, empirical approach cited above. The prescribing psychiatrist should be aware that the borderline patient's needs for medication change over time. The patient who is overly constricted but intermittently explosive may profit from a regimen different from the one he or she will need later in treatment, when he or she may be depressed and fearful of abandonment. Within an even more transient time frame, the borderline patient who is reentering school may have needs for sleeping medications or anxiolytics that were previously unnecessary and may in a few months be again unnecessary. This is good psychopharmacological practice. It is responsive to the patient's changing needs, and it sustains an ongoing collaborative alliance.

Attitudes, Meanings, and Attributions

Table 6–2 identifies the dichotomous (split) thinking about both the medication and the prescribing doctor that borderline patients often bring to bear when medications are prescribed. Psychopharmacological interventions should be accompanied by an awareness of such possibilities. This table chronicles what Koenigsberg (1994, 1997) described as the important meanings that borderline patients can attribute to medications. These attributions confound a patient's compliance and also a clinician's interpretation of the actual value of the medications. When positive meanings are attributed to medications, as is most often the case, this reaction should be accepted gratefully by the clinician, but watched carefully lest it inflate the patient's evaluation of benefits. When negative attributions about drugs are present, they need to be taken seriously. The patient's subsequent report of side effects or lack of benefit will be colored by this kind of attribution.

First and foremost in the patient's thinking are the issues that involve *control*. One fear is that medications will take control of the patient's mind—a fear that is worst in borderline patients who have felt exploited by prior caretakers. Closely related is the fear that by taking medications, the borderline patient will feel too controlled by the therapist. A patient who is very distrustful may passively be noncompliant or even deliberately store the medications for possible overdosing. Since noncompliance and overdosing may occur as often as half the time (Waldinger and Frank 1989a), it is very important that psycho-

TABLE 6–2. Dichotomous attitudes of BPD patients that affect medication usage

	Positive attributions	Negative attributions
About medications	I'm ill; meds are needed.	Meds are irrelevant.
	Meds reduce pain.	Meds control mind.
	Meds can cure.	Meds are addictive, cause disability.
About prescriber	He or she has medical training.	M.D.'s are only interested in illness.
	He or she wants to alleviate suffering.	He or she's not interested in getting involved.
	He or she will do everything possible.	He or she doesn't think therapy helps.
	I can depend on him or her.	He or she wants to control me.

pharmacologists initiate medications cautiously, actively inquiring about how a suspicious or quiet patient feels about these issues, and being particularly respectful of the patient's hesitations or concerns. Under these circumstances, it is particularly important for a prescribing psychiatrist who is not a patient's therapist to have close communication with others who know the patient better.

Transference-Countertransference Issues

Despite the fact that psychopharmacologists often try to define a quite narrow and limited role for themselves as a way to maintain a cool, professional relationship, they too are vulnerable to the same intense countertransference responses to borderline patients (see Table 6–3) that psychotherapists are familiar with: being overinvolved in alleviating patients' pain (i.e., in "rescuing") or being overly frustrated by patients' resistances (i.e., becoming angry). Rescuing is the more common hazard, impelled by the doctorly role of psychopharmacologists. In wanting to alleviate suffering, they become objects of idealizing transferences. That idealization can further encourage their wish to be helpful, which further encourages idealization, which encourages more ambitious, special efforts to help, and so on.

Often impelled by a focus on treating depressive symptoms, psychopharmacologists may embark on extensive searches for curative changes, which they have unwittingly joined their idealizing borderline patients in believing may be possible. The countertransference issue is that of ignoring how all

TABLE 6–3. Three common transference-countertransference enactments

Wary, worried prescribing evokes hostile, secretive usage.
Solicitous attention evokes increased dysfunction (including being noncompliant) and exacerbates symptom complaints.
Medicalization of the patient's problems (i.e., telling a patient that he or she has a biological or brain disease) can encourage the patient to feel not at responsible for symptoms.

these prescriptive activities enact the borderline patient's transference wish to retain the doctor's caretaking attention. Such doctors may respond to their perception of the patient's needing them by assuming an increasing, and increasingly inappropriate, role in the patient's life within—or even outside—treatment.

Vignette

A 35-year-old BPD patient gained 75 pounds while taking lithium plus divalproex (Depakote), amitriptyline, perphenazine (Trilafon), and fluoxetine (Prozac). There was little evidence of improvement, but the patient was grateful for her psychopharmacologist's earnest, kindly, responsive care. Her mother sought out the doctor to complain that as a result of the medications her daughter was increasingly dazed, somnolent, and short of breath. The psychiatrist recognized that this could be due to medications but did not believe he could discontinue any of them without risking the patient's increased suicidality. Moreover, the patient always protested efforts to diminish her regimen. On her way to the ensuing appointment, the patient fell, was too weak to move, and was eventually taken to an emergency room. She died of pulmonary emboli.

Another common transference-countertransference enactment occurring around medications arises when prescribing psychiatrists are too wary of borderline patients. Undue wariness arises when the prescribing doctor's countertransference involves viewing borderline patients as primarily deceitful, litigious, and angry. Of course borderline patients can be any of these, but such qualities are far less likely to become significant problems when clinicians are aware of such apprehensions but are discerning in assessing them. Wariness leads to overly cautious prescribing and inadequate efforts to build an alliance. Borderline patients are sensitive to what they perceive as withholding, dislike, or distrust, and their resentment sets the stage for noncompliance or misuse.

Psychiatrists who devalue psychosocial therapies can conceptualize BPD as either being biological (and amenable to medication) or otherwise being untreatable. This thinking can create a split with other treaters and aggravate the split within the borderline patient's mind about his or her accountability (i.e., the medicalization can cause patients who feel overly responsible for symptoms to feel they are not at all responsible) (see Bolton and Gunderson 1996). This represents another of the common countertransference issues (see Table 6–3). The usually innocuous and beneficial informalities, such as self-disclosures, gifts, or sharing coffee, take on much more meaning for borderline patients than an unsuspecting clinician may anticipate (see Chapter 11). Medications multiply, side effects occur, and the prescribing doctor can respond either by mounting more heroic efforts (e.g., Amytal [amobarbital] interviews) or by coming to dread the patient's next appointment. When the prescribing doctor's increasingly desperate efforts to help fail, he or she may try to withdraw too quickly and without explanation or referral.

CONTRAINDICATIONS/DISCONTINUANCE

When a borderline patient is being prescribed four or more psychotropic medications, it often signifies the absence of identifiable effectiveness. With the growth of augmentation strategies, this conclusion now has more exceptions, but multiple medications should always be a concern when working with BPD patients. Be cautious about changing medications until effects are clarified. For psychiatrists without special expertise, the prescription of more than four medications or the absence of clear benefits after several trials warrants seeking expert consultation. Such consultations are almost always desirable if a patient breaks through the inhibiting and muting effects of his or her psychopharmacological blanket with a relapse requiring a higher, more intensive level of care. The outcome of such consultations, when a borderline patient has already been on a heavy medication regimen for a long enough duration, is typically that the consultant advises a fresh start with trials of single medications.

Remarkably, despite the wide agreement that medications are adjunctive and that they frequently offer only modest and uncertain benefits, there are no guidelines, or even literature, about when to conclude that usage is contraindicated or should be discontinued. The exception here is the finding by Soloff et al. (1993) that the value for neuroleptics wanes rapidly and they can therefore be discontinued after 6 weeks without harm. In effect, however, the lack of advice or discussion means that, in the current era, a patient who receives a borderline diagnosis will be given medications. And, once medications are started, given their positive transferential significance (i.e., their role as transitional objects that connect them with a powerful caretaker), it can be very difficult to discontinue the medications, even if they are not helpful (Adelman 1985). In preliminary analyses, my colleague Mary Zanarini (personal communication, April 1999) has documented that 2, 4, and 6 years after an index hospitalization, 90% of her borderline sample were taking medications at all three assessments and that nearly half were taking three or more medications at all three times. In practice, the only times that exceptions arise are if the patient expresses a fairly sustained or vehement wish to discontinue.

It is not uncommon to be able to diminish without problems the number of medications on which borderline patients are maintained. At the least, efforts to diminish maintenance medications offer a useful way to clarify the relative advantages of continuation versus discontinuation.

Vignette

A 26-year-old single woman had started taking paroxetine (Paxil) during her initial hospitalization 4 years previously. After about 2 years during which she had resumed work and tapered her other outpatient care to ongoing group therapy, the dose of 40 mg/day was reduced to 20 mg/day. Though she was stable on this dose, she was increasingly disturbed by how her taking paroxetine was used by her family as a reason to see her as weak and to question or discount her judgments. Indeed, she had reason to think her emotionality and her readiness to discuss problems rendered her the healthiest member of the family. She wondered, "Could I be normal?" She wanted to discontinue the medication. With her doctor's agreement, the dose was lowered to 10 mg/day. She felt more, including more readily becoming tearful, but her feelings seemed to be appropriately responsive to circumstances. After 2 months, she went from 10 mg to none. In about 10–14 days, her "sadness increased." She began to feel empty. Her life seemed to lack substance or value. Feeling desperate and like a failure, she renewed a dose of 10 mg/day and began to notice a change in 4 days. Within a week, she had stopped crying without good reason and her work again was a source of personal satisfaction.

It is possible to taper off a patient's medications altogether, but in practice, tapering is rarely prompted by prescribing psychiatrists. A significant number of borderline patients can, however, get by comfortably using prn hypnotics or anxiolytics when they have progressed to what is called phase 3 issues (Chapter 11). It isn't clear to me that these medications are needed, but they clearly play a reassuring role. Sometimes, borderline patients can get well enough or are suspicious enough about whether medications are helpful that they will purposely stop taking them. Borderline patients who develop new coping mechanisms, forgo regressive flights, and/or have otherwise gained ego strength, resilience, or maturity may exchange these traits for the ego-buttressing functions that medications have otherwise served. Notably, it is more often the patient than the prescribing psychiatrist who has the courage or optimism about his or her ability to live with less medication. Less medication allows a patient to feel more and makes him or her feel more like a normal person.

Often, the issues of discontinuing medication are confounded by a history of Axis I diagnoses about which the current psychiatrist has only secondhand knowledge. If the patient was prescribed the medications for an alleged Axis I disorder, a psychiatrist is often hesitant to discontinue them even if there is good reason to doubt their value. Adding to the doubts seeded by an unclear history and the current absence of an Axis I condition is the fact that Axis I diagnoses in a managed care environment, where short evaluations and short-term treatments are mandated, are often made for reasons of expedience (Zimmerman and Mattia 1999). In the absence of empirically based guidelines, psychiatrists must balance what patients want with their own judgments about what the risks and benefits of medications are. Twenty years ago, the risk with borderline patients was that the benefits of medications would be underestimated; now the risk is that their benefits will be overestimated.

SUMMARY

The routine and long-term prescription of multiple psychoactive medications that are usually of modest and sometimes of uncertain benefit is a reality of modern psychiatric practice for borderline patients. This is so despite the likelihood of misuse and the potential for long-term dependency. Although it is not unethical to treat borderline patients without medications, the widespread impression about their likely value renders it unwise to treat patients without assessing whether they can benefit from medications. Once they are initiated, it is always wise to consider—and then reconsider—whether the expected benefits are actually being derived. The evaluation of medication effectiveness remains tied to the subjective responses of both patients and doctors. For this reason, skilled psychopharmacology requires a psychotherapist's appreciation of the meanings attached to the pills as well as those attached to the prescriber. The prescribing psychiatrist is subject to the same transference-countertransference problems that beset psychotherapists. A pragmatic, empirical approach, consultations, cautious optimism, and actively engaging the borderline patient as a co-investigator sets the stage for meaningful trials—*and* reduced risks.

References

Adelman SA: Pills as transitional objects: a dynamic understanding of the use of medication in psychotherapy. Psychiatry 48(3):246–253, 1985

Akiskal HS: Subaffective disorders: dysthymic, cyclothymic, and bipolar II disorders in the "borderline" realm. Psychiatr Clin North Am 4(1):25–46, 1981

American Psychiatric Association: Guidelines for Consultative, Supervisory, or Collaborative Relationships With Nonmedical Therapists. Washington, DC, American Psychiatric Association, 1980

American Psychiatric Association: Diagnostic and Statistical Manual of Mental Disorders, 4th Edition. Washington, DC, American Psychiatric Association, 1994

Bender DS, Dolan RT, Skodol A, et al: Treatment utilization by patients with personality disorders. Am J Psychiatry, in press

Bolton S, Gunderson JG: Distinguishing borderline personality disorder from bipolar disorder: differential diagnosis and implications. Am J Psychiatry 153(9):1202–1207, 1996

Brinkley J, Zeitman S, Friedel R, et al: Low-dose neuroleptic regimens in the treatment of borderline patients. Arch Gen Psychiatry 36:319–326, 1979

Cole JO, Salomon M, Gunderson J, et al: Drug therapy in borderline patients. Compr Psychiatry 25(3):249–254, 1984

Cowdry RW, Gardner DL: Pharmacotherapy of borderline personality disorder: alprazolam, carbamazepine, trifluoperazine, and tranylcypromine. Arch Gen Psychiatry 45(2):111–119, 1988

Dawson D, MacMillan HL: Relationship Management and the Borderline Patient. New York, Brunner/Mazel, 1993

Gabbard GO: Combining medication with psychotherapy in the treatment of personality disorders, in Psychotherapy for Personality Disorders. Edited by Gunderson JG, Gabbard GO. (In Review of Psychiatry, Vol. 19. Edited by Oldham JM, Riba MB.) Washington, DC, American Psychiatric Press, 2000, pp 65–94

Goldberg SC, Schulz SC, Schulz PM, et al: Borderline and schizotypal personality disorders treated with low-dose thiothixene versus placebo. Arch Gen Psychiatry 43(7):680–686, 1986

Klein D: Psychopharmacology and the borderline patients, in Borderline States in Psychiatry. Edited by Mack I. New York, Grune & Stratton, 1975, pp 75–92

Klein D: Psychopharmacological treatment and delineation of borderline disorders, in Borderline Personality Disorders: The Concept, the Syndrome, the Patient. Edited by Hartocollis P. New York, International Universities Press, 1977, pp 365–384

Koenigsberg HW: The combination of psychotherapy and pharmacotherapy in the treatment of borderline patients. J Psychother Pract Res 3:93–107, 1994

Koenigsberg HW: Integrating psychotherapy and pharmacotherapy in the treatment of borderline personality disorder, in Session: Psychotherapy in Practice 3:39–56, 1997

Kramer P: Listening to Prozac. New York, Viking Penguin, 1993

Pope HG Jr, Jonas JM, Hudson JI, et al: The validity of DSM-III borderline personality disorder: a phenomenologic, family history, treatment response, and long-term follow-up study. Arch Gen Psychiatry 40(1):23–30, 1983

Siever LJ, Davis KL: A psychobiologic perspective on the personality disorders. Am J Psychiatry 148:1647–1658, 1991

Skodol AE, Buckley P, Charles E: Is there a characteristic pattern to the treatment history of clinic outpatients with borderline personality? J Nerv Ment Dis 171(7): 405–410, 1983

Soloff P: Pharmacotherapy of borderline disorders. Compr Psychiatry 22:535–543, 1981

Soloff PH, George A, Nathan RS, et al: Progress in the pharmacotherapy of borderline disorders. Arch Gen Psychiatry 43:691–697, 1986

Soloff PH, George A, Nathan S, et al: Amitriptyline vs haloperidol in borderlines: final outcomes and predictors of response. J Clin Psychopharm 9(4):238–246, 1989

Soloff PH, Cornelius J, George A, et al: Efficacy of phenelzine and haloperidol in borderline personality disorder. Arch Gen Psychiatry 50(5):377–385, 1993

Stone M: Contemporary shift of the borderline concept from a sub-schizophrenic disorder to a subaffective disorder. Psychiatr Clin North Am 2:577-594, 1979

Waldinger RJ, Frank AF: Clinicians' experiences in combining medication and psychotherapy in the treatment of borderline patients. Hospital and Community Psychiatry 40(7):712–718, 1989a

Waldinger RJ, Frank AF: Transference and the vicissitudes of medication use by borderline patients. Psychiatry 52(4):416–427, 1989b

Zanarini MC, Frankenburg FR, Gunderson JG: Pharmacotherapy of borderline outpatients. Compr Psychiatry 29(4):372–378, 1988

Zimmerman M, Mattia JI: Differences between clinical and research practices in diagnosing borderline personality disorder. Am J Psychiatry 156:1570–1574, 1999

7

PHARMACOTHERAPY

Selection of Medications

INTRODUCTION

The existing body of research that guides the selection and combination of medications is remarkably limited, given the extent of their usage (Chapter 6). Moreover, as noted by Waldinger and Frank (1989a), the frequency of misusage, discontinuation, over- or underdosing, and disregard for warnings adds to the inherent difficulties of evaluating effects. Kelly et al. (1992) found that 46.2% of 97 borderline subjects left in the midst of a 22-week controlled trial. Those who left tended to be the more severely impaired (i.e., those with more prior hospital days, anger, impulsivity, and substance abuse). This finding highlights the risk of generalizing from the results of efficacy (i.e., from randomized controlled trials [RCT]). What can be safely said is that a rational, empirically based approach is available.

OVERVIEW

The breadth of psychopathology seen in borderline patients makes them suitable targets for a broad range of medication types. Their selection can be usefully guided both by whether the prominent symptoms are behavioral, mood, or cognitive (as detailed in Table 7–1) and by a slowly growing body of empirical evidence (Siever and Davis 1991; Soloff 1998).

TABLE 7–1. Targets for pharmacological intervention

Behavior	Mood	Cognitive functioning
Impulsivity	Volatility	Projection
Recklessness	Overly sentimental	Ideas of reference
Promiscuity	Irritable	Suspiciousness
Bingeing or purging	Labile	False attributions
Self-mutilation	Happy/sad	Distractibility
Substance abuse	Hostile/loving	Looseness
Organization	Hypersensitive	Perception
Shoplifting, excessive spending	Intensity	Depersonalization
Aggressiveness	Rageful	Derealization
Rages/temper tantrums	Painfully depressed	Body image distortions
Violence	Agitated	Strange ideas/beliefs
Threats		Clairvoyance
Vandalism		Telepathy
Fights		Flashbacks
		Hypnagogic phenomena

By dividing their problems into these three domains of psychopathology, there is now a reasonable, empirically anchored rationale to selecting which class of medication to use—a rationale that improves the consistency and predictability of drug response.

Soloff (1994, 1998) and Siever (Kirrane and Siever 1998; Siever and Davis 1991) try to distinguish the stable underlying neurobiological vulnerabilities on which medications can be expected to work. Such vulnerabilities or dispositions have traditionally been thought to be constitutional (i.e., temperamental). But we are increasingly aware that neurobiological vulnerabilities may be acquired from early or severe environmental experiences. In either event, Soloff and Siever have pioneered efforts to identify the components of borderline psychopathology that are responsive to medications.

Oldham (1999) proposed a model for identifying the type of borderline psychopathology that can be expected to benefit from psychotropic medications that is inversely related to the degree of benefits expected from psychosocial therapies (see Figure 7–1). Oldham perceives a more important role for medications in BPD patients with heavily affective, impulsive, and aggressive symptoms and a correspondingly lesser role for those with predominantly dependency and internal emptiness as symptoms. Oldham is doubtlessly correct that borderline patients with the more severe symptoms will benefit most from the available array of medications. But, as described throughout this book, I would see Oldham's phenomenological subtypes as reflecting either

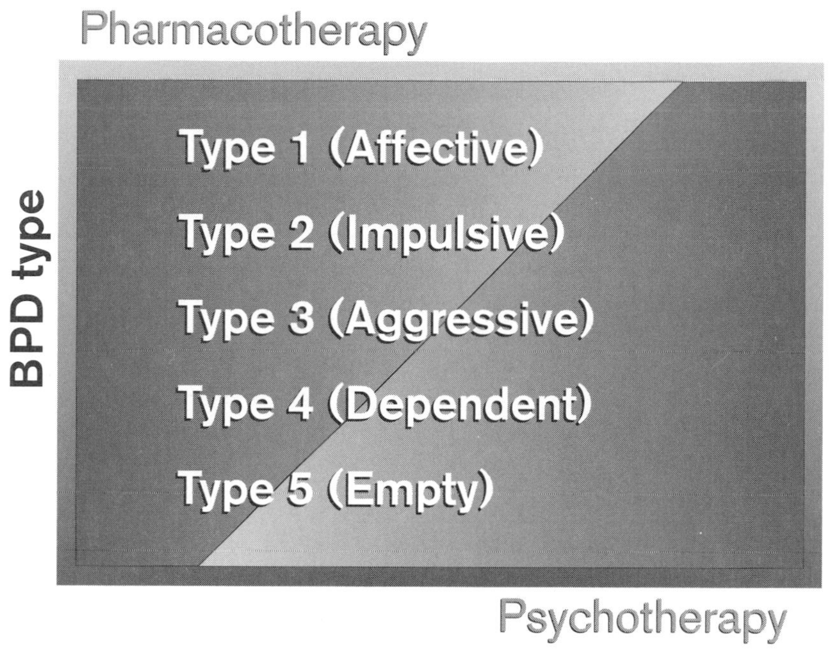

Pharmacotherapy

BPD type

Type 1 (Affective)

Type 2 (Impulsive)

Type 3 (Aggressive)

Type 4 (Dependent)

Type 5 (Empty)

Psychotherapy

FIGURE 7–1. Model for BPD patients of the degree of benefits to be expected from psychotropic medications relative to that to be expected from from psychosocial therapies. *Source.* Reprinted from Oldham JM: "Integrated Treatment Planning for Borderline Personality Disorder," in *Integrated Treatment of Psychiatric Disorders.* Edited by Kay J (Review of Psychiatry Series, Vol 20; Oldham JM, Riba MB, series eds.). Washington, DC, American Psychiatric Press, 2001. Used with permission.

1) different phases of treatment (early phases having subjective distress and behaviors as targets and later phases targeting interpersonal patterns), or 2) different levels of severity (more severe being affective/impulsive and less severe being lonely/empty).

Table 7–2 is my summary of the literature from the 20 years since drug trials were started. It shows that virtually every class of medications has been shown to have a role. What it does not show is that when any one class of medication is given to a representative sample of BPD patients, the benefits prove inconsistent and not very predictable. In general, as summarized in Table 7–2, the behavioral arena is best addressed by selective serotonin reuptake inhibitors (SSRIs) or anticonvulsants (e.g., carbamazepine, valproate), the mood area by SSRIs or monoamine oxidase inhibitors (MAOIs), and the cognition area by antipsychotics. Worth highlighting is that short-acting benzodiazepines, alprazolam (Xanax) in particular, are a class of medications that, al-

TABLE 7–2. Medication efficacy in borderline personality disorder

Medication type	Mood	Impulsivity/self-destructiveness	Cognitive/perceptual	Self-image/interpersonal roles
MAOI	++	?	?	+
SSRI	++	++	±	+
TCA	+	+/−	+/−	±
Antipsychotic	+	+	+	±
"Atypical"	+	+	+	?
Anticonvulsant	+/−	++	+	±
Benzodiazepine[a]	±	−	?	±
Lithium	+	+	?	?

Note. MAOI = monoamine oxidase inhibitor; SSRI = selective serotonin reuptake inhibitor; TCA = tricyclic antidepressant. ++ = usual/clear improvement; + = possible/mild improvement; +/− = can improve or worsen; ± = no effect; − = some worsening.
[a]These impressions relate to short-acting variants only.

though often welcomed by borderline patients—who claim that they are useful, even needed—have observed effects often involving aggressive behaviors that are highly problematic for others (Gardner and Cowdry 1985). In the discussion that follows, my judgments about medications are anchored by the empirical evidence (for reviews see Bornstein 1977; Soloff 1994, 1998; Trestman et al. 1998) but also integrate observations from clinical practice. Observations from clinical practice are unfortunately still very important, since, as discussed in Chapter 6, the RCT evidence is limited, and no studies examine the role of multiple drug regimens over long periods.

Comorbidity and Differential Diagnostic Considerations

I can add little to the rationale offered by Soloff for addressing the inherently blurred boundaries between borderline personality disorder psychopathology and that of adjacent Axis I disorders:

> The neurobiology of personality dimensions transcends our definitions of Axis I and II disorders. The categorical definitions that separate Axis I and II are statistical constructs and are not based on etiology or neurobiology. By targeting personality dimensions for pharmacotherapy, we are making the basic assumption that closely related symptoms in Axis I and Axis II disorders may share a common etiology in neurotransmitter physiology. For ex-

> ample, we assume that the pathophysiology of mild thought disorders in Axis II patients may be related to the same dysfunction found in more severe thought disorders of Axis I patients. Similarly, disinhibition of affect and impulse may be mediated by a common neurotransmitter in BPD and some bipolar disorders. Severity and other disease factors clearly separate the clinical disorders; however, the common elements of pathophysiology suggest the possibility of shared responsiveness to medication. This principle remains the most rational guide for pharmacotherapy trials in the PD patient. (Soloff 1998, p. 197)

If differentiation from schizotypal personality disorder or schizoaffective disorder is unresolved, the primary medication should be with neuroleptics. If differentiation from bipolar I or II disorder is unresolved, either clonazepam (Klonopin) or an atypical antipsychotic is indicated. If sedation is desired, phenothiazines like thioridazine (Mellaril) or chlorpromazine (Thorazine) may be preferable. Although the general contraindication for short-acting benziodiazepines has been noted in this chapter, it is nonetheless true that a surprising number of BPD patients have sufficient social anxiety or panic attacks (McGlashan et al., in press; Zanarini et al. 1998) that anxiolytic medications warrant a trial. Clonazepam (Klonopin) in particular is a long-acting anxiolytic agent that may be less subject to abuse or negative, i.e., impulse-disinhibiting, effects. Monitoring the effects of these medications should rely not only on the borderline patient's usual positive report of subjective relief, but also on the observations of those who can testify to the potential increase in undesirable impulsive behaviors. It bears repeating, however, that clinicians cannot expect that good pharmacological treatment of a coexisting Axis I disorder will resolve the borderline patient's problems in living. In a study of 160 borderline patients, this occurred only twice (J. G. Gunderson, unpublished data, August 2000).

SELECTIVE SEROTONIN REUPTAKE INHIBITORS: THE USUAL STARTING POINT

The use of SSRIs as the medications of choice is supported by their relatively low toxicity and side effects and the relatively strong empirical support for their effectiveness (Coccaro and Kavoussi 1991; Coccaro et al. 1989; Cornelius et al. 1991; Kavoussi et al. 1994; Norden 1989; Salzman et al. 1995). Standard doses are usually effective, and benefits should be evident in 1–4 weeks. Because of the importance of the advantages of the SSRIs (their broad range of effects and their relative safety), this class of medications should not be given up on readily (see Figure 7–2). If the first SSRI had a partial or unclear response (which is usually the case), augmentation is usually the best step to take next.

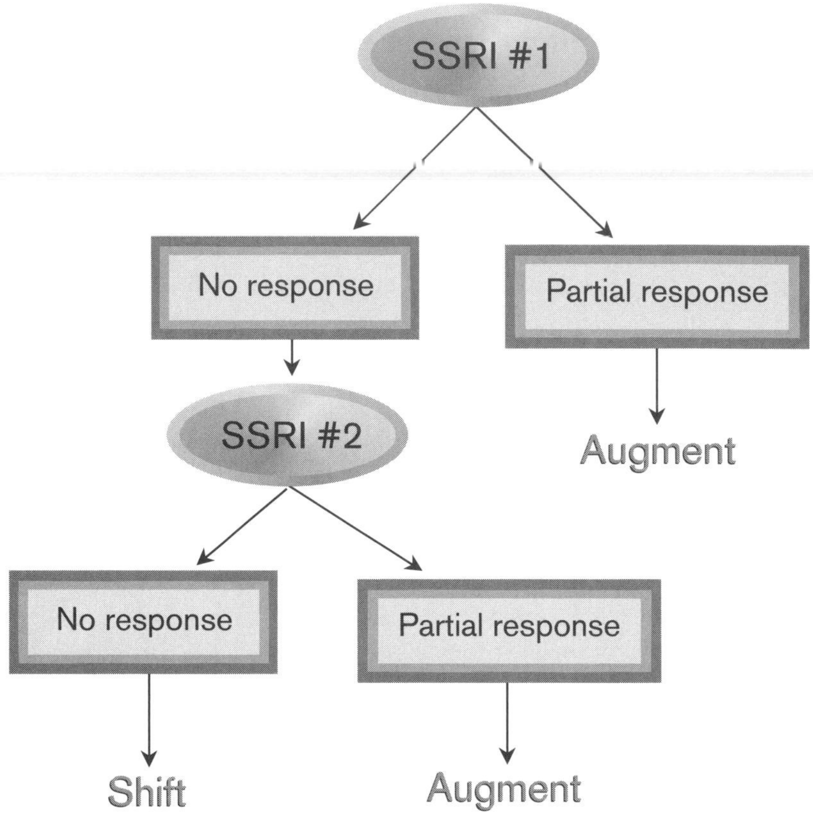

FIGURE 7–2. Protocol for use of selective serotonin reuptake inhibitors with BPD patients.

Recommendations for augmentation of the SSRIs are based on clinical impressions and still lack empirical support. As discussed below, the selection of the augmenting medication should be based on whether the patient's persisting symptoms are primarily behavioral, mood, or cognitive. If the patient had no response to the initial SSRI (with augmentation), then, as Soloff (1998) recommends, a second SSRI trial should be commenced. Failure to respond to one type does not predict failure with another. Although Markowitz et al. (1991) have data indicating that some borderline patients are responsive only to very high doses of an SSRI (140–200 mg fluoxetine or its equivalent), the increase of dosages to such very high levels should be undertaken only after both augmentation strategies and shifts to other medications have failed.

A potentially significant warning note about this otherwise liberal endorsement for using SSRIs is sounded by Teicher et al. (1990), who identified a few cases where use of fluoxetine seemed to aggravate intense suicidal ideation.

BEHAVIORAL SYMPTOM RESISTANCE TO SSRIs

When BPD patients with behavioral problems characterized as impulsive or aggressive (see Table 7–1) do not respond well to adequate trials of SSRIs, clinicians should, as noted in Figure 7–3, augment them with a mood stabilizer or anticonvulsant. Despite the fact that lithium has received some empirical support (Links et al. 1990; Sheard et al. 1976), this research primarily illustrates that its effects are limited. Valproate (Depakote) has some empirical support (Hollander et al. 1996; Stein et al. 1995; Wilcox 1995), and, in my experience, is usually preferable. It has the advantages of fewer side effects, less toxicity, and easier administration—important advantages for BPD patients. When aggressive or impulsive behavioral problems do not respond to the combination of an SSRI and either valproate (Depakote) or lithium, then a third approach, a trial of carbamazepine (Tegretol), an anticonvulsant, is indicated (Gardner and Cowdry 1986a). This medication's effectiveness needs special monitoring, since even BPD patients who appear to achieve the best behavioral control from it often do not like taking it—perhaps because it results in feeling more depressed (Gardner and Cowdry 1986b). This may validate the psychodynamic prediction that the borderline patients' impulsive behavioral problems serve the defensive role of keeping depressive thoughts and feelings out of awareness.

MOOD SYMPTOM RESISTANCE TO SSRIs

When BPD patients with mood instability/intensity problems (see Table 7-1) do not respond well to SSRIs alone, augmentation with anxiolytics such as buspirone or a long-acting benzodiazepine such as clonazepam (Klonopin) are often the best option (Figure 7-3). Yet antipsychotics should be considered. Thioridazine (Mellaril) and haloperidol (Haldol) have been

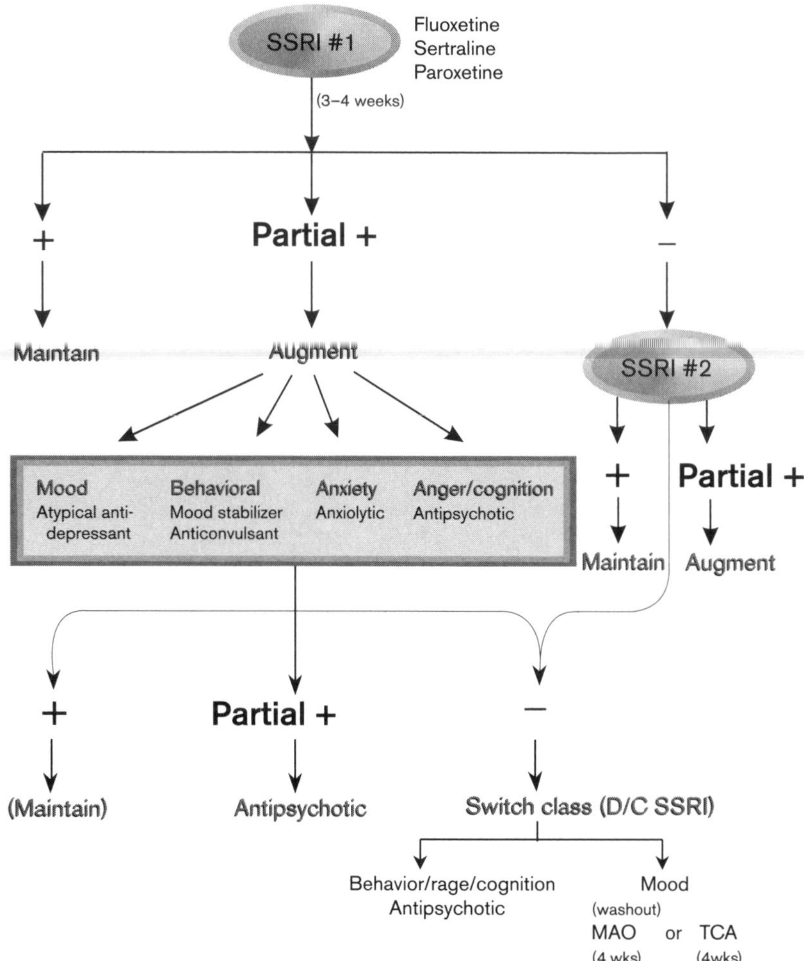

FIGURE 7–3. Algorithm for BPD patients with primary mood or behavioral problems.

shown to have similar effects in reducing depressive symptoms in BPD patients, as have some antidepressants (e.g., amitriptyline) (Soloff et al. 1989; Teicher et al. 1989). Three important—and not uncommon–situations in which it may be preferable to augment with antipsychotics (rather than anxiolytics) are as follows: 1) mood problems largely involving rage (or other excesses of hostility or aggression), 2) coexisting significant cognitive problems (e.g., paranoia; severe, psychotic-like free-floating anxiety), or 2) when sedation/tranquilizing is desirable. Even low doses of antipsychotics should demonstrate value within 1 week. When antipsychotic medications seem useful, the lowest dosage should be determined, and the patient should have a trial without them after 4 to 6 weeks, because their effectiveness may have expired (Cornelius et al. 1993).

For BPD patients who have major mood problems that are not responsive to SSRIs (with augmentation as noted above) and who do not have the indications for taking an antipsychotic noted above, a trial of another class of antidepressant is indicated. Because of their potential toxicity and side effects, non-SSRI antidepressant trials should be undertaken with caution for most BPD patients because of the risk of noncompliance or overdosing. Use of the monoamine oxidase inhibitor (MAOI) antidepressants has some empirical support (Cowdry and Gardner 1988; Parsons et al. 1989), but effectiveness may depend on relatively high doses, and of course these medications should be given only to patients who can be expected to conform to the required dietary restrictions. In effect, this excludes most borderline patients. Nonetheless, this class of medications may be suitable for borderline patients whose internal personality organization is still unstable but whose self-endangering behaviors have remitted or who have stably allied with an ongoing therapy (phase 3 or phase 4 in ongoing psychotherapies; see Chapters 3 and 11 of this book). For such well-behaved BPD patients, the benefits of MAOIs are sufficiently advantageous that they might be introduced even before an SSRI. The tricyclic antidepressants (TCAs) may benefit some depressed BPD patients, but rarely is this benefit dramatic. Moreover, the high lethality of TCAs in overdose and their potential for increasing agitation or irritability (i.e., behavioral problems) (Soloff et al. 1986) consign this class of medications to a minor role for BPD patients.

COGNITIVE SYMPTOMS

BPD patients with severe symptoms in the cognitive-perceptual area (see Table 7–1) are the only ones for whom it is not desirable to begin with SSRIs. For this group, the major choices lie between the more empirically supported traditional neuroleptics (Goldberg et al. 1986; Kutcher et al. 1995; Leone 1982; Serban and Siegel 1984) such as trifluoperazine (Stelazine), perphenazine (Trilafon), or haloperidol (Haldol), or the class of atypical antipsychotics like risperidone (Risperdal), olanzapine (Zyprexa), and clozapine (Clozaril). As shown in Figure 7–3, these medications can benefit a broad range of symptoms. Generally low doses can be effective, and benefit will be evident within days or at most weeks. Because of the potential side effects of long-term usage and the general value of reevaluating the ongoing effects of these medications, discontinuation trials are recommended.

A word more is deserved about the emerging clinical role of the atypical antipsychotics. Experienced psychopharmacologists, basing their judgments on clinical experience and preliminary research findings (Bendetti et al. 1998; Frankenburg and Zanarini 1993; Jensen and Andersen 1989) believe these medications may be particularly useful for borderline patients who are more refractory and self-mutilative. Studies currently under way should show whether this hope is borne out.

Summary

Truly significant advances have been made toward a rational means of selecting medications. The SSRIs have emerged as the cornerstone for most treatments. Nonetheless, there remains a woeful lack of good empirical data that could validate the effectiveness of the proposed practices and could allow clinicians to progress confidently through the suggested algorithms. While the field awaits the much-needed expansion of an empirical base for practice, the prescribing psychiatrist must remain humble, pragmatic, and vigilant about the issues described in Chapter 6. The promising role that medications already play in treatment can be expected only to grow in specificity and effectiveness.

References

Bendetti F, Sforzini L, Colombo C, et al: Low-dose clozapine in acute and continuation treatment of severe borderline personality disorder. J Clin Psychiatry 59(3):103–107, 1998

Bornstein RF: Pharmacological treatments for borderline personality disorder: a critical review of the empirical literature, in From Placebo to Panacea: Putting Psychiatric Drugs to the Test. Edited by Fisher S, Greenberg RP, et al. New York, John Wiley & Sons, Inc, 1997, pp 281–304

Coccaro EE, Kavoussi RJ: Biological and pharmacological aspects of borderline personality disorder. Hospital and Community Psychiatry 42(10):1029–1033, 1991

Coccaro EE, Siever LJ, Klar HM, et al: Serotonergic studies in patients with affective and personality disorders. Arch Gen Psychiatry 46:587–599, 1989

Cornelius JR, Soloff PH, Perel JM, et al: A preliminary trial of fluoxetine in refractory borderline patients. J Clin Psychopharmacol 11(2):116–120, 1991

Cornelius JR, Soloff PH, Perel JM, et al: Continuation pharmacotherapy of borderline personality disorder with haloperidol and phenelzine. Am J Psychiatry 150(12): 1843–1848, 1993

Cowdry RW, Gardner DL: Pharmacotherapy of borderline personality disorder: alprazolam, carbamazepine, trifluoperazine, and tranylcypromine. Arch Gen Psychiatry 45(2):111–119, 1988

Frankenburg FR, Zanarini MC: Clozapine treatment of borderline patients: a preliminary study. Compr Psychiatry 34(6):402–405, 1993

Gardner DL, Cowdry RW: Alprazolam-induced dyscontrol in borderline personality disorder. Am J Psychiatry 142(1):98–100, 1985

Gardner DL, Cowdry RW: Positive effects of carbamazepine on behavioral dyscontrol in borderline personality disorder. Am J Psychiatry 143(4):519–522, 1986a

Gardner DL, Cowdry RW: Development of melancholia during carbamazepine treatment in borderline personality disorder. J Clin Psychopharmacol 6(4):236–239, 1986b

Goldberg SC, Schulz SC, Schulz PM, et al: Borderline and schizotypal personality disorders treated with low-dose thiothixene vs placebo. Arch Gen Psychiatry 43(7): 680–686, 1986

Hollander E, Grossman R, Stein DJ, et al: Borderline personality disorder and impulsive-aggression: the role for divalproex sodium treatment. Psychiatric Annals 26(7, suppl):S464–S469, 1996

Jensen HV, Andersen J: An open, noncomparative study of amoxapine in borderline disorders. Acta Psychiatr Scand 79(1):89–93, 1989

Kavoussi RJ, Liu J, Coccavo EF: An open trial of sertraline in personality disordered patients with impulsive aggression. J Clin Psychiatry 55:137–141, 1994

Kelly T, Soloff PH, Cornelius J, et al: Can we study (treat) borderline patients? attrition from research and open treatment. J Personal Disord 6(4):417–433, 1992

Kirrane R, Siever LJ: Biology of personality disorders, in The American Psychiatric Press Textbook of Psychopharmacology, 2nd Edition. Edited by Schatzberg AF, Nemeroff CB. Washington, DC, American Psychiatric Press, 1998, pp 691–702

Kutcher S, Papatheodorou G, Reiter S, et al: The successful pharmacological treatment of adolescents and young adults with borderline personality disorder: a preliminary open trial of flupenthixol. J Psychiatry Neurosci 20(2):113–118, 1995

Leone NF: Response of borderline patients to loxapine and chlorpromazine. J Clin Psychiatry 43(4):148–150, 1982

Links PS, Steiner M, Boiago I, et al: Lithium therapy for borderline patients: preliminary findings. J Personal Disord 4(2):173–181, 1990

Markowitz PJ, Calabrese JR, Schulz SC, et al: Fluoxetine in the treatment of borderline and schizotypal personality disorders. Am J Psychiatry 148(8):1064–1067, 1991

McGlashan TH, Grilo CM, Skodol AE, et al: The Collaborative Longitudinal Personality Disorders Study: baseline axis I/II and II/III diagnostic co-occurrence. Acta Psychiatr Scand (in press)

Norden MJ: Fluoxetine in borderline personality disorder, in Prog Neuropsychopharmacol Biol Psychiatry 13(6):885–893, 1989

Oldham JM: Treatment for borderline personality disorders, in Integrated Treatment. Edited by Kay J (Review of Psychiatry Series; Oldham JM, Riba MB, series eds.). Washington, DC, American Psychiatric Press (in press)

Parsons D, Quitkin FM, McGrath PJ, et al: Phenelzine, imipramine, and placebo in borderline patients meeting criteria for atypical depression. Psychopharmacol Bull 25(4):524–534, 1989

Salzman C, Wolfson AN, Schatzberg A, et al: Effect of fluoxetine on anger in symptomatic volunteers with borderline personality disorder. J Clin Psychopharmacol 15(1):23–29, 1995

Serban G, Siegel S: Response of borderline and schizotypal patients to small doses of thiothixene and haloperidol. Am J Psychiatry 141(11):1455–1458, 1984

Sheard MH, Marini JL, Bridges CI, et al: The effect of lithium on impulsive aggressive behavior in men. Am J Psychiatry 133:1409–1413, 1976

Siever LJ, Davis KL: A psychobiologic perspective on the personality disorders. Am J Psychiatry 148:1647–1658, 1991

Soloff PH: Is there any drug treatment of choice for the borderline patient? Acta Psychiatr Scand (suppl 379):50–55, 1994

Soloff PH: Algorithm for pharmacological treatment of personality dimensions: symptom-specific treatments for cognitive-perceptual, affective and impulsive-behavioral dysregulation. Bull Menninger Clin 62:195–214, 1998

Soloff PH, George A, Nathan RS, et al: Progress in pharmacotherapy of borderline disorders: a double-blind study of amitriptyline, haloperidol, and placebo. Arch Gen Psychiatry 43(7):691–697, 1986

Soloff PH, George A, Nathan S, et al: Amitriptyline versus haloperidol in borderlines: final outcomes and predictors of response. J Clin Psychopharmacol 9(4):238–246, 1989

Stein DJ, Simeon D, Frenkel M, et al: An open trial of valproate in borderline personality disorder. J Clin Psychiatry 56(11):506–510, 1995

Teicher MH, Glod CA, Aaronson ST: Open assessment of the safety and efficacy of thioridazine in the treatment of patients with borderline personality disorder. Psychopharmacol Bull 25(4):535–549, 1989

Teicher MH, Glod CA, Cole JO: Emergence of intense suicidal preoccupation during fluoxetine treatment. Am J Psychiatry 147:207–210, 1990

Trestman RL, Woo-Ming AM, deVegvar M, et al: Treatment of personality disorders, in The American Psychiatric Press Textbook of Psychopharmacology, 2nd Edition. Edited by Schatzberg AF, Nemeroff CB. Washington, DC, American Psychiatric Press, 1998, pp 901–916

Waldinger RJ, Frank AF: Clinicians' experiences in combining medication and psychotherapy in the treatment of borderline patients. Hospital and Community Psychiatry 40(7):712–718, 1989a

Waldinger RH, Frank AF: Transference and the vicissitudes of medication use by borderline patients. Psychiatry 52(4):416–427, 1989b

Wilcox JA: Divalproex sodium as a treatment for borderline personality disorder. Ann Clin Psychiatry 7(1):33–37, 1995

Zanarini MC, Frankenburg FR, Dubo ED, et al: Axis I comorbidity of borderline personality disorder. Am J Psychiatry 155(12):1733–1739, 1998

8

Cognitive-Behavioral Therapies

Dialectical Behavior Therapy, Cognitive Therapies, and Psychoeducation

Overview

A cognitive-behavioral (CB) concept of personality disorder involves pervasive and inflexible patterns of thought (cognitions), feeling (emotions), and behavior that are self-perpetuating (i.e., governed by the principles of operant conditioning) and self-reinforcing (i.e., governed by classical conditioning). It does not involve intrapsychic structures, an unconscious, or paradigmatic self-other units, as does a psychodynamic concept for personality disorders. In this chapter I review the clinical applications of CB therapies for borderline patients through the lens of a clinician who, though enthusiastic, is not sufficiently trained to claim expertise. Thus inadvertently in this chapter I try to bridge a gap that may also help others who similarly lack CB training.

The interest of cognitive-behavioral therapists in treating BPD has been quite limited until recently. As described below, the reasons for this are found within the history of changing treatment paradigms generally and in clinical considerations that are specific to BPD.

Historical Context

Schizophrenia offers a precedent illustrating the evolution of treatment strategies for BPD. The emergence of CB therapies for BPD in the 1990s parallels the development of structured cognitive and behavioral therapies for schizophrenia in the 1980s. An earlier emphasis on psychoanalytic therapies for schizophrenia began to give way in the 1970s, when empirical evidence established the value of medications. This change also occurred a decade later for BPD, although to a less dramatic extent (Chapter 6, this book).

What happened after medications gained acceptance with schizophrenic patients was that research showed that educational and directive sociotherapies enhanced social skills and diminished family hostilities in ways that greatly reduced hospital usage. Cognitive-behavioral therapies and the psychoeducational approach to patients, described in this chapter, and to families, described in Chapter 9 of this book, are conceptually similar to the social rehabilitative modalities that were found to help schizophrenic patients.

Because schizophrenic patients who had successfully benefited from medication, social skills training, and psychoeducational family interventions were still not fundamentally better in their ability to relate to others or to feel self-satisfaction, interest in the practical value of individual therapy has been revived. At this time, individual cognitive psychotherapies for schizophrenia are being developed and showing promise (Beck, in press; Hogarty et al. 1997). Borderline patients will benefit if the mental health field learns from that precedent. As noted in Chapter 3 of this book, sociotherapies are primarily designed to address observable social and behavioral signs of impairment. Cognitive-behavioral strategies are particularly suited to these problems. Interpersonal and intrapsychic impairments occur later and are the primary targets of other (interpersonal and psychoanalytic) modalities of treatment.

Clinical Cautions

Central to this book is the thesis that borderline patients require specialized modifications of any standardized or usual way of providing traditional institutional or outpatient therapies. Some related cautions about CB therapy are discussed in this section.

Inherent in the traditional application of CB forms of intervention is the assumption—much like the assumption behind medication prescription—that after an explicit, rational agreement about targets for change has been arrived at, patients will pursue these goals to the best of their abilities. As detailed by Young (1990), CB therapies have traditionally assumed that patients have access to feelings, thoughts, and discrete problems and a willingness to do homework. This approach no doubt arose because CB therapies developed as quasi-experimental services within academic psychology—not within hospital settings, where more severe, unselected, and unmotivated patients were found. Traditional cognitive-behavioral training sites have not provided guides for managing the intense interpersonal relationship (including the transference) or the hostile misattributions (e.g., malevolent control or abandonment) that characterize borderline patients.[1]

An assumption by CB therapists that patients will form rational working alliances to treat discrete problems can, in my experience and that of others (see Chapter 3 of this book), be harmful without modifications that take into account the special problems inherent in borderline psychopathology. CB therapies that fail to make these special provisions for BPD are doomed to fail, either from dropouts (Coker et al. 1993) or from adverse reactions (Friedman and Chernen 1994). Beck and Freeman (1990) and Young (1990) took a step toward avoiding the pitfall of covert resistance to change by emphasizing that before work on change is possible, the primary task is to establish a working alliance—a collaborative empirical approach.

As noted in Chapters 3, 4, and 6 of this book, this approach mirrors the emphasis given to the need to build an alliance within other types of therapy for borderline patients, except that within psychoanalytic therapies the *working* alliance is seen as an advanced form that is a goal of the therapy itself (Chapter 12 of this book). Beck and Freeman cited mistrust, rejection sensitivity, and the struggles over control as typical resistances to establishing such an alliance. They noted, however, that the rather active task-oriented and businesslike manner that characterizes most cognitive-behavioral therapists can dispel some of the relational problems, such as transference elaborations, that are found in dynamic therapies. Moreover, the collaborative empirical approach that characterizes CB theories is a useful model to guide primary clinicians and psychopharmacologists (as noted in Chapters 4 and 6 of this book, respectively).

CB therapists often are taught to appreciate the secondary gains (positive reinforcers) that can make patients' dysfunction desirable and thus resistant to

---

[1] Having said this, it also bears mentioning that doctors prescribing medication are often similarly naive (Chapter 6). Moreover, it is not clear that clinicians trained to do standard psychodynamic therapies handle these issues much better. Despite familiarity with the concepts of transference and projection, dynamic therapists who lack special training and experience working with borderline patients also are often ineffective (Chapter 11).

change. Yet these reinforcers may not be evident with borderline patients who resist therapist communications with other informants. Even if the CB therapist suspects that these reinforcers exist, he or she may find the subject difficult to address when the borderline patient carries a psychiatric diagnosis as an explanation for his/her disability. Moreover, although borderline patients might agree to work on making seemingly desirable changes (e.g., to stop purging or to attend classes), progress will be impeded if the CB therapist does not understand the meanings (in CB terminology, *underlying assumptions* or *learned associations*) attached to these changes—meanings that can make changes feel dangerous or undesirable to borderline patients.

Growth in the Use of Cognitive-Behavioral Therapy With BPD

There has been a notable surge of interest in CB approaches to BPD in recent years, generated in part by larger trends toward empiricism (cognitive-behavioral therapies are less inferential and more easily assessed than dynamic therapies) and the pressures of a managed care environment to define discrete goals and discrete time frameworks. Moreover, the pioneering contribution of a manual-guided BPD-specific behavioral treatment (discussed below) by Marsha Linehan (see Sidebar 11–3) has dramatically energized a whole new generation of cognitive-behavioral therapists.

Basic Operant Conditioning Applications for All Treatment Settings

All clinicians who work with BPD need to understand and apply basic operant and classical conditioning principles. This includes the recognition that much of what seems transparently maladaptive (e.g., withdrawal, rage, or self-destructive behavior) actually serves adaptive functions by virtue of the responses (reinforcing) that it evokes. Robbins (1988) was the first analyst to recognize this "functional" analytic understanding of self-destructive behaviors. For example, people with BPD act rather than talk about feelings because they have learned that actions evoke reinforcing responses such as attention, whereas talking about feelings evokes negative responses such as anger.

Therefore clinicians need to convey by word, and, even more important, by behavior, that the patients' behavioral adaptations are not useful in the present stage of their lives. This can mean pointing out (a verbal example) how the excessive demands for attention or reassurance that typify most relationships of borderline patients actually alienate the very people whose love and care they most hope to gain. This is called *contingency clarification*. Further, clinicians must always be conscious of how their reactions and behaviors reinforce or diminish patients' pathological behaviors. For example, a patient may demand attention (a dynamic interpretation) by staying beyond a session's contracted time. He/she should be responded to both with appreciation for the historically adaptive function of such behaviors and with negative consequences—for example, disapproval (an aversive interpersonal response intended to extinguish the behavior) or, if need be, by shortening the next appointment (an action to extinguish the behavior). If it is an option, I leave the office myself. (As an addendum to this example, the very effective aversive response I make is to begin working on other tasks when a patient is silent or otherwise disregarding the tasks of therapy.)

Here are two particularly important examples of how a consciousness about reinforcements should affect a clinician's reactions to borderline patients: 1) seeing them less frequently when they are more dysfunctional (e.g., in the hospital) and 2) consistently noting that suicidal acts or threats are reasons to doubt a therapy's value, not reasons for its continuation or intensification. In a larger sense, families, clinical settings, and psychotherapists should all consciously make efforts to offer less attention to negative (maladaptive) behaviors and more attention to positive (adaptive) behaviors. This means that patients who are getting better in therapy can expect to have it continued and that those who are failing to get better should get less of the current types of therapy than they have been receiving. One of the important guidelines for families is that they should always react to (never ignore) self-destructiveness or other crises, but they should not overreact (see Chapter 9 of this book). This principle exists basically to prevent patients' sense of being ignored or neglected but not to gratify (reinforce) the patients' expectation that crises or self-destructiveness can successfully be used to obtain power or sadistic control or to revive affection (all dynamic interpretations).

Of critical importance is that when responses by therapists or others that have reinforced negative behaviors are discontinued, the discontinuation be sustained, because they will initially evoke what behaviorists know as an *extinction burst*—that is, the unwanted behavior will increase before it decreases. A common example is that when a therapist changes his/her policy about accepting telephone calls between therapy sessions, a burst of phone calls will occur before the new policy is accepted. Another example: when a parent who has been an enabler (e.g., buying cigarettes for his/her child) says that he or she is going to stop, a redoubled burst of pleas, demands, and dramatic "withdrawal symptoms" is a predictable consequence. The occurrence of such extinction bursts is evidence that the recently initiated change is potentially powerful—if sustained.

Dialectical Behavior Therapy (DBT)

Since 1987, the single most remarkable entry in therapeutic strategies for borderline patients is a package of cognitive-behavioral strategies called *dialectical behavior therapy* (DBT; Linehan 1987a, 1987b). Basic DBT is a form of intensive outpatient program (IOP, level II; see Chapter 5 of this book) that has been the subject of 25 articles or books by its developer, Marsha Linehan, a behavioral psychologist (Scheel 2000). Workshops involving 10 days of training in DBT are oversubscribed in the United States, Europe, Australia, and Asia. Some U.S. state departments of mental health and managed care companies have endorsed DBT as a treatment of BPD, and some even protest payment for practitioners who offer non-DBT therapies. Clinical programs devoted to providing DBT are springing up throughout the United States and Europe. Major clinical trials that test its application in a variety of settings have been initiated here and abroad.

Swenson (2000) has suggested that the widespread dissemination of DBT reflects the hunger of the mental health community for a treatment that is clear, understandable, and seemingly learnable. This coincides with the hunger of funding agencies to invest in therapies with scientifically supported effectiveness. Beyond this, Swenson cites the undeniable value of DBT's capacity to invigorate and sustain enthusiasm for treating a group of patients who have often demoralized prior generations of clinicians.

DBT Theory

Linehan (1993a) proposed that the core psychopathology of borderline patients involves a biologically based failure of *emotional regulation* that has interacted with what she perceives as a socially pervasive *invalidating environment*. The biological side of Linehan's biosocial theory echoes theories that have been prominent in the psychiatric literature since the middle 1970s (Akiskal 1981; Klein 1977; Stone 1980) and subsequently given scientific substantiation by Siever and Davis (1991) as a type of psychobiological disposition to BPD (see Chapter 1 of this book). Linehan differs, however, by positing that the emotional problems are not anchored in or reflective of what psychiatrists call mood disorders. The social side of her theory picks up on a theme that is part of the clinical and research literature about BPD families. *Invalidation* reflects 1) the emphasis given to the marked discrepancies between the borderline patients' perceptions of themselves and their parents' perceptions and 2) the lack of communication about these differences (Feldman and Guttman 1984; Gunderson and Lyoo 1997; Gunderson et al. 1980; Shapiro 1982; Young and Gunderson 1995).

The emphasis in Linehan's biosocial theory on emotional dysregulation as the core BPD psychopathology is consistent with the DBT focus on maladaptive behavioral symptoms (e.g., impulsive and inappropriate expressions of emotions). This focus accords with the use of DBT for actively self-injurious patients whose maladaptive behaviors are believed to function as escapes from or expressions of negative emotions.

The Basic DBT Services

Although DBT is a set of behaviorally based treatment principles of direct relevance to BPD that can be implemented via a range of formats (e.g., groups, milieus, families), the basic DBT package described in this section is the one that has had empirical support. The package has three components: 1) once-weekly psychotherapy with a trained primary clinician-therapist whose work is coordinated with 2) a weekly 2½-hour skills training group led by trained co-leaders; both of these services are backed up by 3) telephone consultations with the primary therapist, or, if the therapist is unavailable, by arranged coverage. The point of phone contact is to *prevent* emergencies by providing skills coaching and/or relationship repair. Only as a last resort does the therapist use phone contact for assessing and managing emergencies. Of note is that a fourth nonoptional component of DBT does not include the patients. A weekly consultation meeting of the three members of the team is held to ensure adherence to the procedures and to diminish countertransference problems. Thus, each patient is receiving 3½ or more hours of direct contact (6 hours of therapist time) and an additional 3 hours of indirect therapist time each week. Together, these components offer a very structured, coordinated type of IOP program (see Chapter 5 of this book) that is intended to be comprehensive. Patients treated within Linehan's published research protocols are actively discouraged from using or relying on other therapies, such as hospitals or medications.

The group therapy component consists of a weekly 2½-hour social skills training. The course is composed of four social skills modules: mindfulness, emotion regulation, distress tolerance, and interpersonal effectiveness. A clearly written accompanying manual guides therapist interventions for each of these modules and provides text (with homework) for patients. Much of what DBT groups include has been offered by preexisting cognitive-behavioral therapies (e.g., contingency management, exposure, training in assertiveness or social skills, cognitive schemas as triggers). In DBT, these components are packaged in an integrated, learnable way, and they nicely connect with the agenda in the individual therapy. In my experience, many borderline patients find the structured educative format more useful and less stressful than the more expressive goals of interpersonal groups (see Chapter 9 of this book).

The individual psychotherapy component of DBT addresses a hierarchy of target problems, giving priority to self-destructive behaviors, "therapy-interfering behaviors" (Linehan's term), and problems of daily living (see Table 8–1 for first-stage targets).

TABLE 8–1. Hierarchy of first-stage targets in dialectical behavior therapy

1. Decreasing suicidal behaviors
2. Therapy-interfering behaviors
    - Nonattendance
    - Noncollaboration
    - Noncompliance
3. Quality-of-life-improving behaviors
    - Increasing behavioral skills
    - Mindfulness skills
    - Interpersonal effectiveness
    - Emotion regulation
    - Distress tolerance
    - Self-management

Source. Adapted from Linehan 1993a.

In accordance with DBT theory that invalidating environments are pathogenic, the therapist is actively supportive and specifically emphasizes validation of the patient's feelings, much as advocated by Adler (1986) and by others (e.g., Stevenson and Meares 1992) who deploy Kohut's self-psychology (see Chapter 12 of this book). The contract involving contingencies (see Chapter 10 of this book) recognizes the therapeutic necessity for protecting the limits and boundaries of the therapist, echoing a theme within the more general psychiatric literature (Chapters 3 and 4 of this book) and psychoanalytic literature (Chapters 11 and 12 of this book). In other respects, such as the structuring of the format and content of sessions and the unapologetic use of directive and educative techniques, this therapy is very different from traditional individual dynamic therapies. The dialectical tension between acceptance strategies such as validation and change strategies such as contingencies and homework is akin to the admixture of support and frustration found in dynamic therapies. Of interest is that in a small process study (Shearin and Linehan 1992) the advantage of having both acceptance and change techniques was confirmed.

The following vignette illustrates ways in which DBT's individual therapy can be distinguished from traditional dynamic therapies.

Vignette

Clinician (after greeting patient warmly): Let's start by looking at your diary card. [Therapist reviews the patient's daily diary reviewing suicidality, self-care, and periods of misery.]
Patient: It's been a good week—uh, two weeks actually.
Clinician: That's good. So tell me the reason you weren't here last week. [Inquiring about the second priority, therapy-interfering behavior.]
Patient: I overslept—had been unable to get to sleep, so finally I took a sleeping pill. I didn't want to, and I felt terrible when I woke up.
Clinician: That's a tough spot to be in. [Validates patient's dilemma.] Did you remember that you had an appointment?
Patient: Not until after I woke up. Then I knew I wouldn't be able to get here.
Clinician: How late did you sleep? [Assessing feasibility of her attending.]
Patient (irritated): I don't remember.
Therapist: You sound irritated.
Patient (calmer): Well, you make it seem as if I didn't want to come.
Therapist: Well, I'm sorry you missed. [Placating self-disclosure] It's good that you got the sleep you needed. Now let's discuss ways to see what we can do to prevent this from happening again. [Invites collaboration on problem solving.]

This brief and seemingly unremarkable interaction shows six ways in which DBT is distinguished from a dynamic therapy:

1. The DBT therapist structures the start of the session by asking to review the patient's diary card, reviewing suicidality (priority 1) and extreme emotional experiences. A dynamic therapist more typically would wait for the patient to identify what she wants to talk about.

2. The DBT therapist then inquires about therapy-interfering behavior (priority 2): the missed appointment. This might, and should, be pursued in a dynamic therapy too, but not as a standardized priority. Moreover, a dynamic therapist would probably make either a more open ended inquiry like "What's been going on?" or a negative transference inquiry, "Did your absence relate to our past session?"
3. In response to the patient's saying she had taken a sleeping pill to sleep and then had felt "terrible" when she awoke, the DBT therapist offers an empathic and validating response. Although some dynamic therapists might do this instinctively, common responses would be to make further inquiries about the insomnia (e.g., "What was on your mind?") or the medications (e.g., "Were you reluctant to use the sleeping pills?"), or the feeling bad (e.g., "What did you feel bad about?"). All of these inquiries would be based on the goal of adding meanings to the patient's understanding of these events.
4. When the patient gets irritated, the DBT therapist inquires about the in-the-moment interaction, with the rationale that the irritation could, if unattended to, become a problem interfering with therapy (priority 2). A good dynamic therapist would also inquire about the irritability, but would view it as potential material for a transference/countertransference analysis.
5. When the DBT therapist discloses that she is sorry the patient missed the appointment, she reveals that she wants the patient to come, and, by inference, that their sessions have value. The DBT therapist can be presumed to have assessed the risk that the response would reinforce the patient's absences and to have concluded that it would not. A dynamic therapist might be hesitant to make the response because it forecloses an opportunity to explore how the patient expected the therapist to feel—that is, to examine transference, or at least the therapeutic relationship.
6. The DBT therapist engages the patient in developing alternative ways of coping with the problem. The target problem is defined behaviorally as the missed appointment, and a functional analysis—the function served by missing, for example, a good night's sleep—is underscored. This validates the patient's need for self-care. A dynamic therapist would be hesitant to adopt a proactive, "what can be done" approach, fearing it would enact a parental transference, and the therapist would not define the problem behaviorally but would see it as an issue of conflict and motivation. Moreover, an analysis of the missed appointment would be less

likely to begin by the therapist's identifying that it served useful functions.

Empirical Support

Basic DBT (the combination of weekly individual and weekly group sessions) has established its ability to diminish patients' self-destructiveness and both emergency room and hospital usage significantly more than was observed in similar BPD patients who received treatment as usual (TAU) (Linehan et al. 1991, 1993). TAU consisted of whatever types of care the BPD patients were able to obtain. Though all were initially referred for individual therapy, TAU largely consisted of medication management, intermittent counseling, and hospital emergency services. All BPD patients received the treatment for 1 year and were followed up a year later. All were outpatients who were actively parasuicidal (meaning engaged in self-endangering behaviors that may or may not have been intentionally suicidal).

The diminution in self-destructive (parasuicidal) acts occurred even though DBT was no better than TAU at improving self-reports of hopelessness, suicidal ideation, or reasons for living. Patients in DBT had fewer psychiatric hospitalizations and fewer hospital days (8.5 days compared to 39 days) than those in TAU. This of course has obvious cost benefits. These evidences of efficacy are unquestionably tied to DBT's capacity to engage and sustain borderline patients in therapy: the 84% retention rate over the course of a year is significantly higher than the 50% for patients in TAU and significantly greater than can be expected in other nonspecialized outpatient psychotherapies (Gunderson et al. 1989; Skodol et al. 1983). On the other hand, the specialized Adlerian/Kohutian psychodynamic therapy empirically examined by Stevenson and Meares (1992) (see Chapter 12 of this book) had the same high retention rate. At the end of the study, the basic differences in outcome could be summarized thus: the DBT patients behaved better but still felt as miserable as those in TAU (Linehan et al. 1994). (This outcome departs from the usual generic sequence of changes described in Chapter 3 of this book, which might be due to the relative absence of medication use in this DBT sample.)

In this study, the comparative superiority of DBT in terms of patient participation, engagement, and remaining in DBT was doubtlessly strongly related to the conditions of the alternative treatment: treatment was of far less intensity and was provided by clinicians not selected for their particular skill or enthusiasm with borderline patients. This alternative treatment has important implications, since many clinicians are neither skilled in nor enthusiastic about working with borderline patients (B. Pfohl, K. Silk, C. Robins, M. Zimmerman, and J. Gunderson, unpublished data, May 1999) (see Chapter 11 of this book). In recognition of the weakness of the control condition, Linehan has subsequently been conducting a study comparing DBT to individual therapy that, although less intensive than the 3½ hours/week offered by DBT, is conducted by experienced and enthusiastic therapists. Results of that study remain unpublished at this time.

Within the health care system, basic DBT represents a particularly coherent form of level II, intensive outpatient care. As noted in Chapter 5 of this book, this level of care offers the minimal and therefore optimal level of care for actively self-destructive borderline patients. DBT has made one very important contribution, in my view, by documenting the advantages of mandatory combinations of individual and group therapies (split treatment) in "holding" patients and in diminishing the therapist burden (see Chapters 3 and 5 of this book). A second contribution of DBT is a valuable attitude: that borderline patients are in therapy for the purpose of changing (although, dialectically, the need to change is counterbalanced by acceptance of the reasons why they resist change). It is a very simple message, but no one before Linehan has previously been as direct and insistent in offering this challenge and this hope. It follows that goals need to be established and that the failure to make progress reflects poorly on the treatment.

Because empirical support for DBT elevates it above other outpatient psychosocial treatment approaches, I believe borderline patients should be advised to participate in this treatment if good-quality DBT therapists are available. Still, this endorsement must be qualified by a thoughtful recognition of the limitations of what is known about this new treatment (see Sidebar 8–1).

Sidebar 8–1: DBT's Limitations: Checking the Flood

So widespread is the enthusiasm for DBT, and in my view so generally well justified, that it seems hostile or cynical to introduce a skeptical viewpoint. Yet the twin risks of DBT's becoming prematurely reified (it is, after all, still being developed) and of its advocates' becoming a cult organized around special knowledge (as opposed to an advance within a clinical culture) impel a review of the limitations of our knowledge.

First, it is important to remember that empirically supported DBT is an outpatient package. The application of its principles within hospital (Springer and Silk 1996), residential (Simpson et al. 1998), or day treatment settings seems likely to enhance care, but this probability has not yet been established. Second, what has been empirically shown to be effective is the 1-year *combination* of the individual and skills group treatment components, nothing more or less. Many practitioners offer either the individual or the group component separately. Third, as impressive and distinctive as DBT's claims of efficacy are, they are based on only one relatively small (N = 44; DBT condition subjects = 23), unreplicated study. Fourth, DBT's efficacy is established in the behavioral realm; other therapies may have added advantages in the potentially more central realms of subjective distress and interpersonal function (Benjamin 1997). Results from Bateman and Fonagy's (1999) day hospital treatment (Chapter 5 of this book) or from Stevenson and Meares' (1992) dynamic therapy (Chapter 11 of this book) suggest more effectiveness in these other realms.

Other limitations derive from the difference between efficacy research (randomized controlled trials; RCTs) and effectiveness research (outcomes of treatment for samples that are not preselected) (R. E. Hoffman 1993; Seligman 1995; Wells 1999). This difference involves the following three DBT-specific considerations:

1. It is not known how well or in what ways basic DBT benefits will compare to effects from a therapy of another type (or types) offered at the same level of intensity by trained and enthusiastic therapists, which is in effect another type of coordinated intensive outpatient service.
2. It is not known what fraction of outpatients with BPD are willing or able to undertake DBT. Patient suitability depends on acceptance of the BPD diagnosis or on recognition that the emotional, behavioral, interpersonal, and self-awareness issues to which DBT is specifically addressed are problems that they want to change in themselves—for example, agreeing to the requisite contract. Agreeing to undertake DBT is especially difficult if it threatens ongoing contacts with preexisting and valued therapists or psychopharmacologists. Suitability for the group component also requires that patients be able to tolerate sharing attention and listening to others speak of their problems without getting so disturbed that they leave or become disruptive.
3. It remains unclear how exportable DBT is. The training considered to be necessary to provide DBT (two 5-day workshops) can be obtained only through Linehan herself and a few, albeit growing, number of other trainers (Linehan 1997). Still, Linehan (rightly, I think) does not feel confident that many therapists, even on completion of these workshops, can administer high-quality DBT, and she hopes to develop true credentialing criteria. In this respect, DBT is no different from other forms of treatment and is, I believe, easier than becoming psychody-

namically capable (see Chapter 11 of this book). One study indicated that 109 clinicians with diverse experience and training and roles trained by a state department of mental health could acquire reasonable *intellectual* mastering of DBT (Hawkins and Sinha 1998). I suspect that clinicians who have trouble being active, directive problem solvers and those who are deeply wedded to psychodynamic explorations find it hardest to adhere to or become competent in DBT. On the other hand, it is my impression that well-trained cognitive-behavioral therapists who are experienced in working with BPD patients and temperamentally comfortable being active and directive can learn to administer the individual therapy component of the DBT manual capably, even without the intensive workshops.

DBT's place in the therapeutic armamentarium for BPD is secure and can be expected to grow. It is worthwhile to discuss its limits to ensure that its growth is empirically rather than "epidemically" based. In the process of its growth, its uniqueness will be diminished, and referrals to it will become more discerning. It is hoped that Linehan and other DBT experts will help connect DBT with traditional biological and psychodynamic treatments and theories, just as some who are part of those traditions (e.g., Swenson 1989; Westen 1991) are doing.

Many BPD patients will not persevere in a DBT skills group (Linehan 1993b) (just as they will leave other groups; see Chapter 10 of this book) unless the primary clinician-therapist makes their attendance mandatory. Therapists thus often need to take the position that the skills learned in DBT group are necessary. Beyond therapists' being insistent and supportive, it is unclear what level of knowledge and coordination is required: in particular, it is unclear whether primary clinician-therapists need to have had DBT training themselves. In an unpublished study in which half of a sample of borderline patients who were receiving ongoing, non-DBT types of individual therapy were randomly assigned to receive the skills-training-group component of DBT, the skills group seemed to add little (study cited in Linehan and Heard 1993). Swenson (1989) had predicted that DBT groups without DBT individual therapists would diminish the group's potency, but its complete ineffectiveness surprised him. This finding surprises me too, because I have been impressed by the effectiveness of the skills training group when I've been the individual therapist (since I am not DBT trained) and because groups based on social learning theory have been reported by others (Goodpastor et al. 1983) to be effective for borderline patients.

The skills group component seems to be the most specific and discriminating aspect of DBT (i.e., the individual therapy's relationship components include many supportive relational elements found in dynamic therapies). I suspect that this failure of the skills group without a DBT individual therapist occurred because the group had a mandate that participants do assignments, complete homework, and make changes and this mandate was not taken seriously without active reinforcement by an individual therapist, including perhaps the contingency of the potential loss of that therapist. Moreover, the combination of the group with an actively supportive individual therapist may be essential for holding patient projections (see Chapter 4 of this book, section "Splits, Splitting, and the Principle of Split Treatment") and thereby greatly reducing dropouts. An alternate explanation for the failure of the DBT skills group to show benefits when provided in conjunction with a non-DBT therapist is that the individual therapy component of DBT accounts for most of the DBT package's benefits.

Patients can comfortably use DBT while participating in other therapies, such as the medication, family, and rehabilitation modalities. I agree with Swenson (1989), however, that combining the DBT skills group with dynamically based psychotherapy, especially intensive therapies (more than twice weekly), should be undertaken with caution. The supportive, validating aspect of the DBT approach—like that encouraged by the Stone Center's "relational therapy" (see Jordan et al. 1991 and Chapter 1 of this book)—will clearly invite an idealized split when combined with the unstructured, nondirective, and often frustrating approach of transference-based therapies. Another type of split may also occur. The expectation arising in DBT of learning and then applying new skills in living may become devalued when contrasted with a patient's work with a dynamic therapist, who can become idealized by virtue of his or her patient listening without explicit expectations of behavioral change. Whereas a dynamic therapist sees self destructive acts as generated by interpersonal stressors, the DBT therapist sees it as responsive to intense emotions (Kehrer and Linehan 1996). Such messages are not incompatible, but without thoughtful consideration, such differences can seed harmful splitting. The success of this combination depends on whether the therapists have goals in common, mutual respect, and frequent communication.

Vignette

A patient called her psychodynamic therapist on a Friday evening because she didn't "know whether to continue living is worthwhile." Her therapist listened empathically, but upon noting the patient's improved mood and her

> turn to more cheerful and prosaic topics, he then indicated that he needed to go. The patient said, "Oh, I'm sorry. I should have guessed you'd be busy." About 15 minutes later, she called her DBT therapist with the same concerns, and this therapist coached her to use self-soothing skills.
>
> The following week the patient and her two therapists met to clarify their roles. The dynamic therapist proposed that, since the patient seemed to feel better after being listened to by him, she would benefit from trying to understand why this was so. The patient agreed that being listened to helped, but she added that being coached by the DBT-trained therapist was actually more useful. The DBT therapist believed that the improved coping skills that derive from DBT offered more hope for change. The patient agreed with the DBT therapist, and they all agreed that the DBT therapist would have the role of responding to the patient's safety concerns in the future.

This vignette illustrates the very distinctive theories and responses of a DBT therapist and a psychodynamic therapist. The DBT therapist believed that by virtue of the specific coaching DBT can offer, he should assume the primary clinician's role. Discussion with the patient supported that. The dynamic therapist, however, continued to believe that the patient's relief came from caring attention and had little to do with skills the DBT therapist was coaching. Although the prospect of fewer phone calls was welcome to the dynamic therapist, he believed that the new plan would 1) make it less likely that the patient would become aware of what motivated her calls for help, 2) make the patient less insightful about her need for a dependent, secure attachment, and perhaps 3) make it less likely that this form of corrective relationship would evolve. The DBT therapist believed that the patient would learn to generalize the use of new coping skills and that that would allow her to need others' help less frequently.

DBT and dynamic therapies can be complementary but that relationship seems to rely on time-consuming efforts at collaboration. Basic DBT (group and individual components combined) appear to be highly useful in preparing patients for subsequent psychodynamic therapies by increasing patients' ability to recognize and tolerate emotions without action, a possibility recognized by Linehan (1997). DBT may make possible the emotional expression, interpersonal confrontations, and transference analysis that intensive dynamic therapies traditionally involve. It may also be that, when the patient has mastered the social skills modules in the group component of DBT, the advanced forms of individual DBT currently being developed can offer further opportunities for personal growth; the designated targets are the effects of trauma and improving the quality of life. A study under way in Sweden is examining 1) whether, in a second year of DBT, the individual therapy component can offer continued personal growth, and, if so, 2) whether or to what extent the added benefits derive from elements specific to the DBT interventions or from the nonspecific corrective aspects of the therapeutic relationship (R. Weinryb, personal communication, April 1999; see also Chapter 12 of this book).

PERSPECTIVE ON DBT

DBT treatment has rapidly become widely used and is sometimes advocated as a standard of care by Linehan and increasingly (as noted earlier) by others, including managed care companies and state departments of mental health. As noted in the preceding discussion, such a policy seems dangerously premature. Perspective will require time and more data.

DBT-trained therapists are developing applications for families (P. Hoffman 1999; P. Hoffman and Hooley 1998) and adolescents (Miller et al. 1997) and for inpatient (level IV) (Springer and Silk 1996; Bohus et al., in press) and partial hospital (level III) services (Simpson et al. 1998). All these applications and others that are in progress (Koerner and Dimeff 2000) require modifications of the basic DBT package. Insofar as outcome is measured by behavioral change, I expect that DBT will prove widely applicable when compared to usual nonspecialized services. I would also predict that its advantages will dramatically diminish when compared to alternative therapies offered with equal competence and intensity. I would hope, however, that findings on various types of BPD therapies would reveal some specificity of effects among the various therapies, such as added benefits in impulsive behaviors with DBT, as opposed to added benefits in interpersonal relationships with dynamic therapies. Although a committed empiricist like Linehan would say these are empirical questions, I think they are unlikely to be answered by RCTs because of the required length of treatment, the diversity of clinical settings and types of BPD patient, and the probable power of still unrecognized demographic factors like age, intelligence, and access to treatments.

COGNITIVE THERAPIES

Cognitive therapy clinicians postulate that borderline patients have disturbed cognitions that 1) develop early in their lives, 2) have maladaptive consequences, 3) are self-perpetuating, and 4) are, although difficult to change, the targets for cognitive therapies. The chief difference from behavioral therapies is that, whereas behavioral therapies focus on behaviors, cognitive therapies focus on changing dysfunctional cognitive schemata about oneself and one's environment. Although the distinction between cognitive approaches and behavioral approaches seems to disappear when applications are described, in principle cognitive therapies rest on the idea that behavioral (including interpersonal) problems are mediated by disturbed thinking. For example, a purposely self-destructive action would be seen as an outgrowth of a disturbed cognitive schema, such as the view of oneself as bad (Layden et al. 1993). The patient would be taught to recognize how this schema triggers self-destructive acts. The act itself would be identified as a decision, and the patient would be encouraged to consider options. The act might also warrant directives (e.g., "Stop. Consider that it's not good for you and doesn't get you what you want"). At this point, of course, the cognitive approach deploys behavioral techniques.

Specific maladaptive cognitive schema for BPD proposed by Young (1990) are: abandonment and loss, unlovability, dependence, subjugation, lack of identification, mistrust, inadequate self-discipline, fear of losing emotional control, guilt and punishment, and emotional deprivation. These are evaluated by a questionnaire and then examined to see what triggers the schema, how it is maintained, how it is avoided, and what would be an adaptive alternative way of behaving.

Beck and Freeman (1990) offer a different, but overlapping, dissection of the borderline patient's disturbed cognitions. Beck stresses three basic assumptions held by borderline patients: 1) The world is dangerous and malevolent. 2) I am powerless and vulnerable. 3) I am inherently unacceptable (Beck and Freeman 1990).

Beck also feels that dichotomous thinking is particularly common and problematic in borderline patients, who tend to perceive people, feelings, or issues in terms of mutually exclusive categories rather than seeing them as part of a continuum. He believes that the extreme (i.e., dichotomous) evaluation of situations is a cognitive handicap that leads borderline individuals to their extreme emotional responses and actions (in contrast to positing these individuals' basic failure of emotional or impulse regulation)—responses and actions that are then accompanied by rapid shifts to the opposite view. Beck postulates that the basic assumptions, the dichotomous thinking, and an unstable sense of identity are the particularly problematic cognitive features of borderline patients. Beck suggests that reducing and eliminating dichotomous thinking is an early goal of therapy. Still, he notes that the cognitive problems are so "encrusted" that a year is more likely to be needed than the 12 to 24 sessions that can affect other diagnostic types.

At this point, Beck, Freeman, and others (Perris 1994) have developed a thoughtful conceptual framework from which manual-guided treatments can be developed. As a result, in the next decade, empirical methods will probably be used to assess the benefits of cognitive therapies with borderline patients. This has already begun in short-term interventions, with promising results (see Sidebar 8–2). I have no doubt that benefits will be shown and that as a result cognitive therapies will take their place in the overall treatment of BPD.

Of note, Young (1990) and both Aaron and Judith Beck, as reported in *Clinical Psychiatry News* (Sherman 1999), recognize that borderline patients' transference offers a way to identify cognitive schema that can control their relationships (e.g., "My therapist wants to control me") or can be the triggers for their reactions within relationships (e.g., a therapist's lateness triggers abandonment fears). Judith Beck (Sherman 1999) even suggested that cognitive therapists may need to do work (cognitive therapy) on themselves because of their countertransferences. All the pioneering cognitive therapists give attention to the therapist's need to invest energy in establishing a trusting and collaborative working relationship.

Sidebar 8–2: Makes Sense, But Does it Work? Part 1–Preliminary Findings on Brief Cognitive Therapy

Tyrer and Davidson (2000) reported that a randomized controlled trial is under way in a large multicenter project in England and Scotland to study the effects of manual assisted cognitive therapy (MACT). MACT is a brief six-session intervention, using treatment booklets (bibliotherapy) and some skill training components of DBT, that is intended to diminish deliberate self-harm behaviors. Thirty-two patients with personality disorders who had at least two episodes of deliberate self-harm in the prior year were randomly assigned to receive MACT ($n = 18$) or treatment as usual ($n = 14$) and were then followed for 6 months. The data indicated that receiving MACT lowered the frequency of such acts (0.17 per month for MACT, 0.37 per month for TAU) and extended the median time until the next parasuicidal act (142 days for MACT, 114 days for TAU). There was also evidence of less depression and less cost of care among those in MACT. These intriguing results suggest an easily exportable intervention for use in the early phase of treating an important behavioral aspect of most borderline patients' presenting problems.

Westen (1991) has helped to bridge the conceptual and clinical gaps between the cognitive-behavioral and psychoanalytic approaches. Joining Beck and Freeman, he reconceptualized the borderline patient's defenses (e.g., splitting and projection) as disturbed cognitive patterns. Whereas Beck and Freeman (1990) refer to splitting as "dichotomous thinking," Westen identifies it as a misattributional style involving global or polarized judgments about self or others. In this scheme, projection is seen as misattributing one's own motives to others. Westen then describes how cognitive-behavioral techniques can be used within psychoanalytic therapy to diminish the borderline patient's overelaboration of affects and impulsive behaviors. Essentially, Westen advocates a cognitive technique of labeling (i.e., highlighting or setting apart) affect states (e.g., anger), words (e.g., "horrible" or "perfect"), or cognitions (e.g., "He distrusts me") that can subsequently be referred to as signals or red flags that will help that patient stop and think before reacting.

Psychoeducation for Patients

Although Brightman (1992) introduced a psychoeducational approach for borderline patients nearly a decade ago, such approaches remain relatively new (Ruiz-Sancho et al., in press). These services are based on the hope that patients diagnosed as having BPD will benefit from learning about their disorder (see Table 8–2). For psychoanalysts, this could seem to be reinforcing the patient's defenses. If one accepts Vaillant's or the Stone Center's assignment of pejorative connotations to the borderline diagnosis (see Chapter 1 of this book), one might think that psychoeducation is sadistically inviting the poor patients to "impale" themselves.

TABLE 8–2. Rationale for psychoeducation of BPD patients
Patient's right to know
Increases awareness of disorder—demystifies and destigmatizes
Diminishes sense of unique, unknown problems: knowledge that others have similar problems
Enrolls intellectual strengths and curiosity
Invites active participation in treatment planning
Establishes realistic hopes for change

Source. Adapted from Ruiz-Sancho et al., in press.

The psychoeducational approach rests heavily on the medical model of BPD as an illness. In this model, the behavioral problems associated with BPD are sequelae to disordered emotions and thinking. This message is usually welcome to patients. Certainly, psychoeducational therapists hope that these approaches will bring benefit to borderline patients by mobilizing their intelligence and curiosity. By informing patients about their disorder, this approach can make them more aware of how their feelings, behaviors, and thinking can cause problems. In a more general way, it helps to demystify and destigmatize the diagnosis. By informing patients about treatment options and the potential for change, psychoeducation helps establish realistic expectations for treatment. (It can be noted that this is done more commonly than is recognized during early sessions with case managers [Chapter 4 of this book] or with individual psychotherapy when a treatment plan or "contract" is being developed [see Chapter 11 of this book]). Certainly, the psychoeducational clinician's leadership, direction, and teacher-like role diminish heated, interpersonally focused transference; the danger, however, is that it can encourage a passive, tell-me-what-to-do-next approach to solving problems.

The use of psychoeducational methods within psychodynamically based interpersonal therapy was identified by Benjamin (1993). She actively informs borderline patients about the meanings and sources of their maladaptive relationship patterns. This method is very useful, in my experience (and I do it with increasing frequency and confidence), because it encourages intellectualization (a form of "mentalizing," as in Fonagy 1991) and with this, a type of valuable constraint on action. As noted elsewhere (Chapters 5 and 12 of this book), I am very explicit in making predictions about how BPD patients can expect to respond to forthcoming situations (e.g., a vacation or a step down in level of care). This is not to impress them with me; it's to impress upon them knowledge of who they are.

The simplest and most common psychoeducational intervention involves the diagnosis itself. Patients usually welcome reading the DSM-IV text (American Psychiatric Association 1994) and describing how the criteria do or don't apply to them (see Chapter 2 of this book). At the McLean Hospital outpatient clinic, we have a library of articles and a bibliography of books that patients are encouraged to read and then discuss with their primary clinicians (see the appendix at the end of Chapter 9 of this book).

The most ambitious psychoeducational approach, to my knowledge, was developed by Nancee Blum with help by Pfohl and St. John (Blum et al. 1999) at the University of Iowa Department of Psychiatry. It is called the Systems Training for Emotional Predictability and Problem Solving (STEPPS). This program offers a manual-guided series of about 15–20 classes (adapted from Bartels and Crotty 1992), designed to accommodate about 6–10 trainees at a time. The first section, entitled "Awareness of Illness," acquaints borderline patients and their significant others (the "reinforcement team") with the DSM-IV criteria and their applicability. The section also assesses early maladaptive cognitive schemas, using Young's questionnaire to help borderline patients recognize what types of thinking typify BPD (Young 1994). The second section of the course involves emotion management skills training. Following Bartels and Crotty (1992), the section conceptualizes BPD as a disorder of overly intense emotions, and the participating patients are taught specific regulatory skills. (Obviously, the formulation is very close to the one advanced by Linehan [see above], and both are derivative of the earlier literature citing affect dysregulation as core to this disorder [see Chapter 2 of this book]). The third section, "Behavioral Management," addresses social functioning impairments (e.g., eating, working), which are believed to result from the poor management of intense emotions.

Blum et al. (1999), in their abstract, reported that attendance at this course results in fewer hospitalizations, less need for more intensive services, and decreases in depression, negative feelings, and impulsive or self-destructive behaviors. Whereas some patients need to repeat the STEPPS program, graduates are invited to move on to a less intensive (twice-monthly), year-long follow-up program. The developers of this approach claim that it diminishes a borderline patient's need for individual therapy and that within therapies it diminishes the intensely dysfunctional relationships that patients form with therapists. The practical benefits of this approach are clearly measurable; when they have been demonstrated, the approach will no doubt undergo the same expansion that has been seen for DBT and may be foreseen for MACT (described above) and psychoeducational multiple-family groups (PE/MFGs) (to be discussed in Chapter 9 of this book).

Summary

Cognitive-behavioral approaches to the care of borderline patients have moved from the rear guard of modalities into the prominent foreground. The remarkable achievement of empirical substantiation for DBT has excited a new cadre of enthusiastic clinicians and a new intellectual ferment about mechanisms of therapeutic action within therapies. This chapter attempts to place this modality into its context alongside other modalities and within the history of treatment developments for BPD. Cognitive therapies are still in early stages of development. Less ambitious, but more easily exportable, are promising psychoeducational approaches. Even in modest form—telling patients their diagnosis and encouraging their learning about it—this intervention sets the stage for more respectful collaboration with patients in all modalities.

REFERENCES

Adler G: Borderline Psychopathology and Its Treatment. New York, Jason Aronson, 1986

Akiskal HS: Subaffective disorders: dysthymic, cyclothymic and bipolar II disorders in the "borderline" realm. Psychiatr Clin North Am 4(1):25–46, 1981

American Psychiatric Association: Diagnostic and Statistical Manual of Mental Disorders, 4th Edition. Washington, DC, American Psychiatric Association, 1994

Bartels N, Crotty M: The Borderline Personality Disorder Skill Training Manual. Winfield, IL, EID Treatment Systems, 1992

Bateman A, Fonagy P: The effectiveness of partial hospitalization in the treatment of BPD: a randomized controlled trial. Am J Psychiatry 156:1563–1569, 1999

Beck AT, Freeman AM: Cognitive Therapy of Personality Disorders, New York, Guilford Press, 1990

Benjamin LS: Interpersonal Diagnosis and Treatment of Personality Disorders. New York, Guilford, 1993

Benjamin LS: Models for treating borderline personality. J Personal Disord 11(4): 310–325, 1997

Blum N, Pfohl B, St. John D: Stairways: the next step in borderline personality disorder skills training. Paper presented at the International Society for the Study of Personality Disorders conference, Geneva, Switzerland, September 16, 1999

Bohus M, Haaf B, Stiglmayr C: Evaluation of inpatient DBT for borderline personality disorder: a prospective study. Behav Res Ther (in press)

Brightman BK: Peer support and education in the comprehensive care of patients with borderline personality disorder. Psychiatric Hospital 23(2):55–59, 1992

Coker S, Vize C, Wade T, et al: Patients with bulimia nervosa who fail to engage in cognitive behavior therapy. Int J Eat Disord 13(1):35–40, 1993

Feldman RB, Guttman HA: Families of borderline patients: literal-minded parents, borderline parents, and parental protectiveness. Am J Psychiatry 141(11):1392–1396, 1984

Friedman S, Chernen L: Discriminating the panic disorder patient from patients with borderline personality disorder. J Anxiety Disord 8(1):49–61, 1994

Fonagy P: Thinking about thinking: some clinical and theoretical considerations in the treatment of a borderline patient. Int J Psychoanal 72(4):639–656, 1991

Goodpastor WA, Pitts WM, Snyder S, et al: A social learning approach to group psychotherapy for hospitalized DSM–III borderline patients. Journal of Psychiatric Treatment and Evaluation 5(4):331–335, 1983

Gunderson JG, Lyoo IK: Family problems and relationships for adults with borderline personality disorder. Harv Rev Psychiatry 4(5):272–278, 1997

Gunderson JG, Kerr J, Englund DW: The families of borderlines: a comparative study. Arch Gen Psychiatry 37(1):27–33, 1980

Gunderson JG, Frank AF, Ronningstam EF, et al: Early discontinuance of borderline patients from psychotherapy. J Nerv Ment Dis 177(1):38–42, 1989

Hawkins KA, Sinha R: Can line clinicians master the conceptual complexities of dialectical behavior therapy? an evaluation of a State Department of Mental Health training program. J Psychiatr Res 32(6):379–384, 1998

Hoffman P: Family intervention: DBT family skills training. Presented at the Sixth International Congress on Disorders of Personality, Geneva Switzerland, September 1999

Hoffman P, Hooley JM: Expressed emotion and the treatment of BPD. In Session 4(3):39–54, 1998

Hoffman RE: Impact of treatment accessibility on clinical course of parasuicidal patients (letter). Arch Gen Psychiatry 50(2):157, 1993

Hogarty GE, Kornblith SJ, Greenwald D, et al: Three-year trials of personal therapy among schizophrenic patients living with or independent of family, I: description of study and effects on relapse rates. Am J Psychiatry 154:1504–1513, 1997

Hogarty GE, Kornblith SJ, Greenwald D, et al: Three-year trials of personal therapy among schizophrenic patients living with or independent of family, I: description of study and effects on relapse rates. Am J Psychiatry 154:1504–1513, 1997

Jordan J, Kaplan A, Miller J, et al: Women's Growth in Connection: Writings From the Stone Center. New York, Guilford, 1991

Kehrer C, Linehan MM: Interpersonal and emotional problem solving skills and parasuicide among women with borderline personality disorder. J Personal Disord 10:153–163, 1996

Klein D: Psychopharmacological treatment and delineation of borderline disorders, in Borderline Personality Disorders: The Concept, the Syndrome, the Patient. Edited by Hartocollis P. New York, International Universities Press, 1977, pp 365–384

Koerner K, Dimeff LA: Further data o dialectical behavior therapy. Clinical Psychology Science and Practice 7(1):104–112, 2000

Layden MA, Newman CF, Freeman A, et al: Cognitive Therapy of Borderline Personality Disorder. Boston, Allyn & Bacon, 1993

Linehan MM: Dialectical behavior therapy for borderline personality disorder: theory and method. Bull Menninger Clin 51(3):261–276, 1987a

Linehan MM: Dialectical behavioral therapy: a cognitive behavioral approach to parasuicide. J Personal Disord 1:328–333, 1987b

Linehan MM: Cognitive behavioral therapy of borderline personality disorder. New York, Guilford, 1993a

Linehan MM: Skills training manual for treating borderline personality disorder. New York, Guilford, 1993b

Linehan MM: Theory and treatment development and evaluation: reflections on Benjamin's "models" for treatment. J Personal Disord 11(4):325–335, 1997

Linehan MM, Heard HL: Impact of treatment accessibility on clinical course of parasuicidal patients (letter). Arch Gen Psychiatry 50(2):157–158, 1993

Linehan MM, Armstrong HE, Suarez A, et al: Cognitive-behavioral treatment of chronically parasuicidal borderline patients. Arch Gen Psychiatry 48(12):1060–1064, 1991

Linehan MM, Heard HL, Armstrong HE: Naturalistic follow-up of a behavioral treatment for chronically parasuicidal borderline patients. Arch Gen Psychiatry 50(12):971–974, 1993

Linehan MM, Tutek DA, Heard HL, et al: Interpersonal outcome of cognitive behavioral treatment for chronically suicidal borderline patients. Am J Psychiatry 151(12):1771–1776, 1994

Miller AL, Rathaus JH, Linehan M, et al: DBT for suicidal adolescents. Journal of Practical Psychiatry and Mental Health 3:78–86, 1997

Perris C: Cognitive therapy in the treatment of patients with borderline personality disorders. Acta Psychiatr Scand 89(379, suppl):69–72, 1994

Robbins M: The adaptive significance of destructiveness in primitive personalities. J Am Psychoanal Assoc 36(3):627–652, 1988

Ruiz-Sancho AM, Smith GW, Gunderson JG: Psychoeducational approaches, in Handbook of Personality Disorders. Edited by Livesley WJ. New York, Guilford, in press

Scheel KR: The empirical basis of dialectical behavior therapy: summary, critique, and implications. Clinical Psychology Science and Practice 7(1):68–86, 2000

Seligman MEP: The effectiveness of psychotherapy: the Consumer Reports study. Am Psychol 50:965–974, 1995

Shapiro ER: On curiosity: intrapsychic and interpersonal boundary formation in family life. International Journal of Family Psychiatry 3:69–89, 1982

Shearin EN, Linehan MM: Patient therapist ratings and relationship to progress in dialectical behavior therapy for borderline personality disorder. Behavior Therapy 23(4):730–741, 1992

Sherman C: Cognitive therapy's reach extends to Axis II. Clinical Psychiatry News, October 1999, pp 24–25

Siever LJ, Davis KL: A psychobiologic perspective on the personality disorders. Am J Psychiatry 148:1647–1658, 1991

Simpson EB, Pistorello J, Begin A, et al: Use of dialectical behavior therapy in a partial hospital program for women with borderline personality disorder. Psychiatr Serv 49(5):669–673, 1998

Skodol AE, Buckley P, Charles E: Is there a characteristic pattern to the treatment history of clinic outpatients with borderline personality? J Nerv Ment Dis 171(7): 405–410, 1983

Springer T, Silk KR: A review of inpatient group therapy for borderline personality disorder. Harv Rev Psychiatry 3(5):268–378, 1996

Stevenson J, Meares R: An outcome study of psychotherapy for patients with borderline personality disorder. Am J Psychiatry 149(3):358–362, 1992

Stone M: The Borderline Syndromes. New York, McGraw-Hill, 1980

Swenson C: Kernberg and Linehan: two approaches to the borderline patient. J Personal Disord 3(1):26–35, 1989

Swenson C: How can we account for DBT's popularity? Commentary re: article by Scheel. Clinical Psychology Science and Practice 7(1):87–91, 2000

Tyrer P, Davidson K: Cognitive therapy of personality disorders, in Psychotherapy for Personality Disorders. Edited by Gunderson JG, Gabbard GO (Review of Psychiatry Series, Vol 19; Oldham JO, Riba MB, series eds.). Washington, DC, American Psychiatric Press, 2000

Wells KB: Treatment research at the crossroads: the scientific interface of clinical trials and effectiveness research. Am J Psychiatry 156:5–10, 1999

Westen D: Cognitive-behavioral interventions in the psychoanalytic psychotherapy of borderline personality disorders. Clin Psychol Rev 11:211–230, 1991

Young JE: Cognitive Therapy for Personality Disorders. Sarasota, FL, Professional Resource Exchange, 1990

9

Family Therapies

Introduction

Family interventions of any type are sociotherapeutic (Chapter 5 of this book)—that is, they primarily affect the borderline patient's social adaptation. As is described in this chapter, family interventions for borderline patients are often initiated during crises, require education, and often require directives. Such interventions usually occur after the diagnosis is established and when the borderline patient is in more restricted levels of care (IV, hospital care, or III, residential or partial hospital care). These initial family interventions can make the interactions less stressful both for borderline family members and for others in a family. More sustained family interventions are usually needed to change a family's ways of communicating or relating. In the process of making such changes, families can become allies in proactively helping patients change. These changes will primarily take place when the patient is in level I (outpatient) or II (intensive outpatient) care.

In this chapter, an overall approach to families is described that integrates contributions from both psychoeducational and psychodynamic therapies. Indeed, as with group and individual therapies, these therapies are complementary but sequential. This family approach was developed after recognizing that traditional dynamically based family therapies usually end quickly—and badly. Borderline offspring can batter the parents into alienated flight, or the borderline individuals themselves can leave feeling betrayed and ganged up on. Yet the failure to involve families of borderline patients as supports for their treatment often makes the patients' own involvement in therapy either superficial or so fraught with fears of abandonment (often by ostensibly villainous parents) that using therapies to change themselves is impossible—a major reason for premature dropouts (Gunderson et al. 1989).

HISTORY

Efforts to intervene with families of borderline patients were first reported in the 1970s. These seminal reports came from a group of committed, analytically oriented family therapists. Their approach was based on psychodynamic and systems theories—theories that are linked in viewing psychopathology as resulting from conflictual forces within the designated patients' social systems. At its extreme, and consistent with the influential work by Masterson and Rinsley (1975), this meant that borderline psychopathology could not be expected to be meaningfully corrected without changing the borderline person's primary social milieu, which for many is the family. The initial reports were based on work done with adolescent samples on specialized, relatively long-term inpatient units at the National Institute of Mental Health (Shapiro et al. 1974; Zinner and Shapiro 1975) and subsequently McLean (Shapiro 1978a, 1978b, 1982). These therapists developed the theory that pathological forms of parental overinvolvement fostered the borderline offspring's dependency and abandonment fears. They also encouraged hopes that intensive long-term family therapy could bring about curative changes.

When such theory-based, intensive family therapy was immersed within containing inpatient services and was closely integrated with other modalities, it was, in my experience, a powerful approach that could be very useful. Its confrontational, authoritarian approach was, however, often resented even by the families who could benefit from it. They were, in any event, self-selected families who sought out and contracted to undertake this type of treatment program. It was, moreover, an approach that was not feasible in most settings and was not desirable to most families if they felt they could avoid it. Certainly, the approach was never considered appropriate for fragmented, abused, and nonverbal families or for those whose interactions with their borderline offspring were sparse—for example, those living elsewhere.

When studies of families with BPD members moved from the province of clinical observations to that of empirical studies in the 1980s, radical revisions in our understanding about the prototypical family occurred (Gunderson and Zanarini 1989; Links 1990). Our early work demonstrated that it was not true that most of these families were overinvolved and separation-resistant, as suggested by Masterson's theory (see Chapter 1 of this book) and by the pioneering family therapists noted above. Rather, we found, most families of borderline patients were insufficiently involved with the patients during their early development (Frank and Paris 1981; Gunderson et al. 1980; Soloff and Millward 1983a), and these families either perpetrated or were unavailable to help with traumatic experiences (Gunderson and Sabo 1993; Links and van Reekum 1993; Links et al. 1990; Millon 1987; Paris et al. 1994a, 1994b). Neglect and trauma were prototypical (Gunderson and Zanarini 1989; Zanarini 1997). Another series of studies showed that borderline patients' parents themselves had serious psychiatric problems, including substance abuse, depressions, and even borderline personality disorder itself (Akiskal et al. 1985; Goldman et al. 1993; Links et al. 1988; Loranger et al. 1982; Pope et al. 1983; Schachnow et al. 1997; Silverman et al. 1991; Soloff and Millward 1983b; Zanarini et al. 1990). All these studies combined to paint a very bleak and very critical picture of the health, function, and motivation of borderline patients' families. This perception is reflected in the virtual absence of any new papers about family therapies during the 1980s or 1990s.

The emergence during this last decade of a deficit model for BPD (Chapter 1 of this book) that is now superimposed upon the conflict model found in the early literature on families has quietly encouraged changes in the approach to families (Ruiz-Sancho et al., in press). While these changes in understanding the family environments of borderline patients were occurring, relevant research on treating families with another disorder was under way. Research on families with a member having schizophrenia showed that schizophrenic individuals in families who were high in expressed emotion (EE)—meaning hostile, critical, and overinvolved—had far higher relapse rates (50% versus 14%) over the course of 9 to 12 months and that a psychoeducational approach could reduce EE (i.e., the putative stressor) and thereby greatly reduce relapse rates (Goldstein 1995; Leff 1989; McFarlane and Dunne 1991; McFarlane et al. 1995). Indeed, the effect of these family interventions on relapse rates exceeded the effects resulting from the introduction of neuroleptics (Gabbard et al. 1997).

A review of the effectiveness of all types of psychosocial therapies for schizophrenia noted that these psychoeducational family interventions demonstrated the most powerful effects of any that have been tested (Gabbard et al. 1997). The basic principles of the psychoeducational family treatments (see Table 9–1) used in these studies with families who have schizophrenic offspring is radically different from the principles that guided the earlier family treatments based on psychodynamic system theory. Yet the rationale and the efficacy of these psychoeducational family treatments offered a model that could not be ignored by a new generation of clinicians with a more deficit-based construct of BPD.

TABLE 9–1. Principles of psychoeducation for families

Mental illness is a problem within the person, not a symptom of a problem family.
Family support is needed for treatment of mental illness.
Requires being informed about therapy, prognosis, and course.
Can diminish harmful anger, criticism.
Families often do not recognize the cost of the illness: family alienation and social isolation.
"Bad" parents are uninformed or ill, not malevolent.
Families are burdened; new management strategies can reduce this burden.

THERAPISTS AND COUNTERTRANSFERENCES

Families, specifically parents, do not see themselves as patients. They are consumers who clinicians can assume will be somewhat wary and defensive. Therefore clinicians should encourage them to carefully appraise treatment recommendations for their offspring or themselves. Anyone wanting to help families with a borderline relative needs to respect families' reservations. It helps to have firsthand knowledge about the hardships of parenting. Clinicians who believe that they themselves could never have a disturbed offspring or who believe they could readily manage the problems that borderline patients present to their families bring to therapy critical, intolerant attitudes that aggravate a family's guilt, anger, defensiveness, and isolation. Ideally, clinicians who do family interventions combine compassion for the family's plight with enough experience and confidence to inspire a family's trust.

Basic introductory family interventions (what will be described as phases 1 and 2) can often be done by the patient's primary clinician. More sustained family interventions (phases 3 and 4) profit by having an experienced family therapist who can comfortably coordinate his or her work with the patient's therapist. Whether a borderline patient's individual psychotherapist is suited for doing family therapy depends on that particular therapist's aptitude and the meaning of family therapy for the psychotherapeutic relationship. As long as the borderline patient is practicing self-endangering behaviors or is severely vocationally impaired (i.e., usually during the first 2 years of treatment), it is helpful for the individual therapist to periodically join family therapies when they are being coordinated by others. As discussed below, this helps family therapies become a stronger container (holding force) than when families fail to witness firsthand the individual therapist's respectful involvement with them.

GETTING STARTED: OVERCOMING RESISTANCE

Family interventions are indicated whenever a BPD patient has significant involvement with, or financial dependence on, his or her family. Hence, adolescents or young adult borderline patients are prime candidates. Unfortunately, it is in the nature of many borderline patients to emphatically resist involvement of their relatives by clinicians. Such disapproval or even prohibitions should not be accepted; this resistance requires a serious and sometimes extended working through (see Sidebar 9–1). It should be seen as symptomatic of the typically borderline pattern of devaluing prior caretakers out of hurt and out of a wish to invoke hope for a more idealized protective and exclusive relationship with a potential new caretaker. This pattern of being devaluative at intake, documented by Perry et al. (1990), has created a significant bias in the literature, because most of the research that has characterized families of borderline patients has relied on their accounts during intake evaluations (Gunderson and Lyoo 1997).

Vignette

Ms. F was a 23-year-old woman diagnosed with BPD who came for consultation at the recommendation of her psychopharmacologist. When I greeted her in the waiting room, she introduced me to her mother, who was sitting quietly a few seats away. During the course of the consultation, it became clear that Ms. F had remained very dependent on her parents, never having sustained a job ("I get too anxious and walk out") and having had boyfriends who at times have cohabited with her in her family's house.

After I invited the mother to join us, I began by reviewing the reasons for the referral and why the borderline diagnosis had been confirmed. The mother seemed to be familiar with the diagnosis and readily agreed that it described her daughter "perfectly." She went on to talk about how resistant her daughter had proved to a long train of therapies since the mother had begun taking her for help when Ms. F was age 13. I said that Ms. F would seem to be a good candidate for a DBT group, and we discussed the feasibility of that. Then I gave them reading materials ("What You Need to Know About BPD" and "Overview of Treatments") (see the appendix at the end of this chapter for these and other materials) and invited them to come back, with the patient's father if possible, in a week. The mother quietly, without explanation, said that it wouldn't be possible. I was a bit surprised, but agreed to meet in 2 weeks. Suddenly, I was aware that this therapy was unlikely to go smoothly. But why?

In the meeting 2 weeks later, it became clear that the mother had doubts about the likelihood that any therapy would change her daughter and that the patient's father, a silent man who drank heavily, believed that everything about the mental health field is a waste of money.

In this example, it became apparent that between her mother's codependency and her father's hostility, Ms. F would endanger her needed supports at home by being involved in therapy. Parental resistance therefore needed to be addressed first. A clinician wishing to treat Ms. F would not have any success unless Ms. F could believe that her involvement would not threaten her with the loss of her needed parental support. Her treatment would require her parents' being allied with her involvement in therapy and with its goals.

The initial phases of the family approach described here (phase 1, initial meeting, and phase 2, alliance building) are directed at calming the family's anxieties and establishing an alliance, rather than trying to treat the family per se. In this process, they are helped. Later phases (phase 3, psychoeducation, and phase 4, psychodynamic), identifiable as therapies, are explicitly intended to change the families. Special attention is given to the potential role of multiple-family groups (MFGs), because they have definite clinical and cost-benefit advantages over single-family interventions and because they are the only type of family intervention that has been examined empirically.

Sidebar 9–1: "You Can't Talk to My Parents"

Borderline patients frequently impose on their clinicians prohibitions about talking to their parents. Clinicians, eager to avoid conflict or build an alliance, can find it tempting to accept such prohibitions. Yet failure to enlist the support of a borderline patient's family is one of the major reasons for subsequently dropping out of psychotherapy (Gunderson et al. 1989). It helps to take a firm stance that, although the patient's objections are important, they fly in the face of the value you place on knowing firsthand about the important people in their lives. Persistence in examining and reality-testing the patient's fears (e.g., you'll betray confidences, you'll take the family's side, you'll "like them better," they will get too upset) and in explaining the possible benefits (e.g., this can help your family understand you better; this will help your parents be less suspicious, more supportive of your therapy) is often sufficient to gain permission.

When borderline patients are in a hospital setting, the usual evidence of possible dangerousness to self is almost always sufficient to provide legal justification for overriding the patients' prohibitions. Even if a clinician has questions about actual suicidal intention, this justification should be used to seize the opportunity it offers. When borderline patients are not in a hospital, there are still some occasions when they need to be told that the clinician cannot treat them (i.e., they cannot expect to improve) without enlisting their parents' support. This is the case when either 1) the families' responses to the patients are life endangering, or 2) the patients' involvement in therapy is experienced as a betrayal of their parents.

When the patients' therapy is paid for by their families, it is essential that this reality become an acknowledged part of establishing a realistic frame for the therapy (see Chapter 11 of this book). Patients may need to be reminded that their reliance on parental support for treatment means that excluding the parents jeopardizes its feasibility. Parents may need clinicians to remind them that, much like paying for a child's college education, they should help decide whether their investment in therapy is worthwhile. Therapists have a responsibility to inform parents who pay for a treatment about such issues as their child's attendance at, or motivation for, and apparent benefit from therapy. What remains confidential is what is being talked about.

Family interventions are often best begun during the crises that lead to hospitalizations. These crises are times when families often feel most in need of help—especially during the first few hospitalizations. Efforts to involve families whose borderline member has already been through many hospitalizations are less likely to be successful, since families have already established adaptations, often ones that are not helpful, such as giving up hope or having convictions about psychiatry's uselessness.

PHASE 1: INITIAL FAMILY MEETINGS

Problem identification, psychoeducation, and support are essential first steps in recruiting the borderline patient's significant others as allies. To begin an alliance requires that the clinician convey by word and attitude that he or she is sympathetic to the problems that significant others are struggling with and knows they have been doing the best they can. (Actually, the clinician should assume this last point.) The first meeting starts with unequivocal identification of the patient as having a serious disorder, or illness, and needing special support because of it. Not just parents, but spouses or children of married borderline patients can also benefit from the same initial contacts, but thereafter they pose special problems (see Sidebar 9-2).

Sidebar 9-2: Families of Married Borderline Patients

When the borderline patient is married, a clinician should inform the spouse about the borderline illness, in the hope that supportive allowance will be made for the spouse's handicaps. The clinician should simultaneously convey a need to respect and support that borderline partner's ongoing strengths. Psychoeducation for the spouse or even very structured skills enhancement instructions for both partners (Waldo and Harman 1998) can be helpful.

The clinician-therapist does not want to unnecessarily consign the marriage to a future in which caretaker-dependent roles are permanent. On the other hand, when such roles are already stably complementary, couples therapy is contraindicated (Paris and Braverman 1995). Couples therapy, like conjoint family therapy, sessions should await both members' being able to listen to what originally each partner could only say about the other in private–and being able to listen without getting enraged, terrified, or despairing (Seeman and Edwards-Evans 1979). For practical purposes, this means that significant change must have occurred in the borderline spouse before marital therapy is likely to be of value.

When the borderline patient is a mother, clinicians should recognize that the children are at high risk for psychiatric problems, including conduct disorders and attentional dysfunction (Links et al. 1990; Weiss et al. 1996). The patient (and spouse) should be educated about this risk, with compassionate efforts to ease undue guilt. Most borderline patients are grateful for evaluations of their children and for any recommendations for assistance.

Problem Identification

Clinicians should actively ask relatives to identify the problems that the borderline family member has created for them. In our initial survey of 40 families, the most common problems were (in order): 1) communication, 2) dealing with the hostile or rageful reactions, and 3) fears about suicide (Gunderson and Lyoo 1997). Once the problems are identified, clinicians can usually offer assurances that the burden created by these problems is familiar to mental health staff and can be significantly reduced, to everyone's benefit.

Psychoeducation

Psychoeducation (see Chapters 1 and 8 of this book) involves acquainting relatives with the borderline diagnosis by going through the diagnostic criteria together and making sure they are understood. This step is followed by evaluating how these criteria apply or are reflected in their borderline relative. When a clinician is asked whether someone has borderline personality disorder, it is useful to be able to describe it in a way that is relatively jargon free, allowing laypersons to reach their own conclusions about whether the diagnosis fits (see Chapter 1 of this book, the section titled "Misuses of the Borderline Diagnosis"). I make only modest revisions when talking to parents as opposed to the patients themselves, as shown here:

"People with a borderline personality disorder have grown up feeling that they were unfairly treated, that they didn't get the attention or care they needed. They are angry about that, and as young adults, they set out in search of someone who can make up to them for what they feel is missing. Hence, they set in motion intense, exclusive relationships, which then fail because they place unrealistic expectations on the other person. Upon failing, they feel rejected or abandoned, and they can either become enraged again about its unfairness (as they did when growing up), or they can feel they are bad and unlovable, in which case they become suicidal or self-destructive.

"Either their anger at being mistreated or their feeling bad and being self-destructive can cause others—especially parents—to feel guilty and try to make it up to them; it naturally evokes wishes to protect or rescue. Such responses from others, especially parents, unfortunately validate borderline persons' unrealistically high expectations of having their needs met, and the cycle is apt to repeat itself."

Central to the psychoeducation process is emphasizing that borderline patients have deficits or handicaps, which can, albeit slowly, be overcome. (Some patients don't want to hear the "slowly" aspect of this, whereas others find it reassuring to know that there is no short-term solution. This second group have often been confused or disillusioned by hearing unrealistically optimistic predictions or by being fundamentally aware that the problems are long-standing and deep-seated.) Encouraging relatives to read or view educative materials is often instructive. (See the appendix at the end of this chapter for psychoeducational materials.) Assigned reading (bibliotherapy) as homework to be discussed at the next meeting is a good idea. Equally important is to convey a message of respect: that to you the parents are important allies, not bad people and not rivals with you for their children's loyalties.

Support

A first point to be noted is that borderline patients are very difficult people to form helpful relationships with—for clinicians as well as for their families. Equally important is to empathize with how burdensome such patients are for a family. In a study that anticipated shifts in the borderline construct toward a model based more on medical deficits, Schulz et al. (1985) compared the burden of having a BPD family member to that of having someone with a chronic medical illness. Both conditions involve the burdens caused by dependency and unemployment; and in addition, BPD creates the burden of the borderline individual's behavioral problems (e.g., drunkenness, promiscuity) and the burden of families' feeling blamed, directly or by inference, by both the patients and the clinicians, who have typically excluded families. Clinicians can offer families an extremely important support by diminishing the families' feeling that they have been responsible for causing the illness—or their fear that clinicians hold them responsible (see Sidebar 9–3). Still, the psychoeducation used for other disorders that has given the reassuring impression that family environment has nothing to do with their offspring's illness is misleading (see Sidebar 13–1).

Sidebar 9-3: Finessing the Guilt Issue

Reiss et al. (1995) describe how families enter the mental health orbit with defensiveness and fear of blame. The very fact that they have a mentally ill offspring evokes in parents, regardless of the nature of their child's psychiatric problem, an immediate fear that they must have done something wrong and a defensiveness toward expected accusations. Certainly that defensiveness is exaggerated when the offspring has borderline personality disorder and thus is particularly angry and devaluative, and the child's hostilities cannot easily be discounted, because they are not psychotic (Baker et al. 1992). The stress of having an offspring who is clearly devaluative (Perry et al. 1990) and who often says about the family to anybody and everybody that "they did it; they're the ones" makes parents particularly fearful of what mental health professionals will say.

To reduce family guilt, it helps to emphasize to parents that they have a very disturbed and disturbing offspring–and that you are sympathetic to the problems that such an offspring creates for them. Say to them that there are many factors (inborn, developmental, and familial) that put children at risk for the development of BPD, that early attachment issues involve "goodness of fit" between a child's temperament and that of the caregivers (Thomas and Chess 1984), and that it takes complex interactions among multiple factors to develop this disorder. When families make more specific inquiries about their own responsibility for the disorder, note that it is a reasonable question but that unfortunately not enough is known to give a very meaningful answer. At this point, directly tell patients that because issues of causality are usually so heavily loaded with feelings of anger and guilt, these issues are rarely constructive for dealing with the present situation and recurrent crises. Actively move parents away from concerns about their possible causal role, and emphasize that the most constructive issues they can attend to is how to cope with the ongoing problems they face with this very troubled offspring. The causal issue is to some extent irrelevant; they have work to do right now.

This approach also sets a tone for their approach to their offspring's blaming: that it is not very relevant. Their son or daughter has problems and is going to have to learn how to cope better than at present. It is a very proactive, future-oriented approach.

PHASE 2: ESTABLISHING AN ALLIANCE

Establishing a satisfactory working alliance with a family may require only a few initial meetings, but often it requires more. One reason involves the guilt and defensiveness identified above. Conjoint meetings with the borderline offspring may be necessary if the patient is very dependent on the parents; in that situation, failure to have such meetings aggravates separation fears. Otherwise, however, conjoint meetings remain relatively contraindicated until both the family and the patient have first independently established a treatment alliance and have found the requisite perspective or strength to withstand the predictably powerful conflicts that occur in meeting together.

Two other issues—resistances that can delay forming an alliance—involve 1) the diagnosis itself and 2) the prospect of greater involvement in treatment.

Resistance to the Borderline Diagnosis

Some relatives greet the borderline diagnosis with skepticism, being relatively insistent that the problems are better understood as developmental (adolescence, authority issues, etc.) or are due to one of the more obvious (or pharmacologically responsive) symptom disorders (Axis I)—that is, depression, eating disorders, or substance abuse. Occasionally a family resists the BPD label because they have seen it applied to patients whom their offspring or the nursing staff have identified as offensive. In rare cases, families protest the diagnosis because they *know* something is wrong with their offspring's brain functioning. None of these causes for diagnostic resistance is inconsistent with the BPD diagnosis.

It is best to sidestep open disagreements about diagnostic questions. Clinicians can note how the BPD diagnosis has "added value": it offers families a way to understand why the patients' developmental problems, their symptoms, even their offensive behaviors, have proved resistant to treatment (or are unlikely to remit as rapidly as they hope). The clinician can help by persisting in efforts to address the relatives' skepticism about the diagnosis by offering more reading and didactic information about problematic issues such as rages, all-or-none thinking, and irresponsible role functioning. Patience and education will gradually lower resistance, enlist family collaboration, and allow families to accept the borderline diagnosis.

Resistance to Being Involved in Treatment

It is often difficult to involve parents who have been abusive or who are at present abusing substances. In both of these circumstances, involvement threatens their wish to preserve denial or to avoid shame. Such parents are often ill themselves—most often alcoholic—or have otherwise parented so irresponsibly (e.g., been abusive) that they have good reason, consciously or unconsciously, to fear vilification. Most of the time, when the parental marriage is intact, it is one parent-partner who is extremely hostile about mental health involvement, whereas the other is interested though hesitant. Occasionally, persistence by the interested parent can succeed in getting the hostile, resistant parent involved, but usually it is a standoff. Obviously, meetings with the interested parent should be offered, but when that parent gets involved, it can catalyze a separation or divorce within a dysfunctional marriage. Because the available parent rarely wants to jeopardize the marriage on account of this issue, he or she usually drops out or is too conflicted to gain much from family interventions. When parental separations occur, they can mobilize one or both parents to get more involved or otherwise become more attentive to their borderline offspring's care.

End of Phase 2: Transition From Treatment to Therapy

When the phase of alliance building is complete, the family is "ready" for therapy per se (i.e., ready to try to change). Readiness for involvement in family therapy is noted by three indications: 1) acceptance of the borderline diagnosis, or at least the possibility; 2) being reconciled to a long-term course of illness; and 3) wanting help in the way they relate to the borderline relative. At this point they are ready for interventions that will help them to change their ways of communicating and relating. Workshops in which 10–20 families meet for a half day to learn about the diagnosis, share experiences, and hear some hopeful messages offer an excellent vehicle for consolidating this phase (Berkowitz and Gunderson, in press).

PHASE 3: PSYCHOEDUCATIONAL FAMILY THERAPY

The goals of the psychoeducational approach in this phase are to improve family communication, diminish hostilities, and diminish burden. Table 9-2 outlines the range of issues with which psychoeducation can help. To accomplish these goals, families are taught how to create a more cool, calm, and predictable home environment. The therapist functions more as a teacher or leader than as an explorer, confidant, or transference object. Psychoeducational family therapies can be done with individual families or with a multiple-family group (MFG).

TABLE 9–2. Issues for psychoeducational family therapy

1. Lack of parental consensus building: predictable "good cop, bad cop" roles
2. "Parentifying" the child (Shane and Kovel 1988)
3. Misattributions of offspring
   - Independence (actually still dependent) (Young and Gunderson 1995)
   - Demandingness/hostility (actually often fearful) (Fonagy 1991)
   - Sociability (actually lacks close friends) (Young and Gunderson 1995)
4. Reducing emotionality (coping skills)
   - "Walk away"
   - Listen

Single-Family Interventions

Single-family interventions are usually more feasible for clinicians and more comfortable for parents. It should be emphasized that, as with the first two phases, conjoint meetings are not yet recommended. Parent management training (PMT), developed by Patterson (1982, 1992) for treatment of conduct disorder, offers a valuable model. This training is based on the idea that parent-child interactions may inadvertently promote angry and self-destructive behaviors by poorly thought through reinforcements and ineffectual or inconsistent punishments. Parents who stay up late to reprimand their borderline offspring for disregarding curfew may in fact be reinforcing this behavior. Parents are coached about alternative responses (e.g., stop staying awake and reprimanding; rather, cut back on your financial support). Parents then field-test their new learning with their offspring, returning to review what happened. Unfortunately, manuals for this coaching model have not yet been written, and it has not been tested with borderline patients.

Adaptations for a Multiple Family Group (MFG)

Psychoeducational multiple family groups (PE/MFGs) were independently begun at McLean Hospital in 1994 (Gunderson et al. 1997) and at Westchester Division of the New York Hospital in 1995 (Hoffman and Hooley 1998). These initiatives came after McFarlane had demonstrated advantages of MFGs over single-family interventions with families having a member with schizophrenia (McFarlane and Dunne 1991, McFarlane et al. 1995). Our experience and that of Hoffman (1999) has confirmed that MFGs are more satisfactory to consumers as well as more cost effective. The main problem with MFGs is logistical: they require clinical sites with a sufficient flow of borderline patients with suitable families to constitute a group. Hence the format is better suited to hospitals or clinics than to most office practices.

The format used in the McLean outpatient program follows a manual-guided book (Berkowitz and Gunderson, in press) that initially borrowed heavily from the one used by McFarlane for families with a member who has schizophrenia (McFarlane and Dunne 1990; McFarlane et al. 1995). Undertaking the psychoeducational approach by having multiple families meet together has advantages. By discussing their problems with similarly beleaguered—and often similarly isolated—families, participants gain a strong social support system.

Meetings are 1½ hours every 2 weeks. Four to six families is ideal to allow adequate attention to be paid to everyone. Socializing times at the start and end of meetings make them informal and reinforce the idea that there is more to life than problems. The structured agendas for the meetings help keep the meetings cool and task oriented. The groups can begin to effect changes after 3 months. Many families can leave after 1 year, although for some, 18 months seems preferable. Three stages of the PE/MFG are outlined below. (A variation on this format is offered by Hoffman, who uses larger groups with more frequent sessions and more didactic DBT-based exercises [Hoffman 1997; Hoffman and Hooley 1998]).

Three Stages of Psychoeducational Family Therapies

These stages (early, middle, late) apply to either single-family or multiple-family psychoeducational interventions.

The Early Stage

The early stage involves a more intensive schedule (weekly, if possible, for about 2 months) and more active direction and didactics by the family therapist–teacher. The leader's active structuring of sessions deliberately decreases the emotionality of meetings. It is especially important to recognize how upsetting it can be for some parents to hear about others' problems. A disproportionate number of the families who enter therapy are hypersensitive, rather than callous, to being exposed to feelings of sadness and anger or signs of conflict. Fonagy (1995) and Fonagy et al. (1995) have suggested that parental difficulty in recognizing, tolerating, or expressing feeling is one of the situations that can lead to children's developing borderline deficits. The ongoing process of didactic psychoeducation exercises can also ease common anxieties about self-disclosure or help seeking.

Family guidelines are given (Table 9–3), and leaders actively promote adherence to them, advising families to keep them on the refrigerator door or under their pillows. In virtually every group session, leaders make frequent reference to them during discussions. The effect, beyond the literal application of guidelines, is to cause parents to stop and think before reacting.

One guideline referred to often during the early phase concerns self-harm (guideline 7). This guideline can lead to immediate changes in a family's response, which will bring its members relief and diminish both the opportunities and the need for splitting or secondary gain and for their sequelae,

TABLE 9–3. Family guidelines in relationships with a borderline member

Goals: go slowly

1. ***Remember that change is difficult to achieve and fraught with fears.*** Be cautious about suggesting that "great progress" has been made and about giving "you can do it" reassurances. **"Progress" evokes fears of abandonment.**
2. ***Lower your expectations.*** Set realistic goals that are attainable. **Solve big problems in small steps.** Work on one thing at a time. Big goals or long-term goals lead to discouragement and failure.

Family environment: keep things cool

3. ***Keep things cool and calm.*** Appreciation is normal. Tone it down. Disagreement is normal. Tone it down too.
4. ***Maintain family routines as much as possible.*** Stay in touch with family and friends. There's more to life than problems, so don't give up the good times.
5. ***Find time to talk.*** Chats about light or neutral matters are helpful. Schedule times for this if you need to.

Managing crises: pay attention but stay calm

6. ***Don't get defensive in the face of accusations and criticisms.*** However unfair, say little and don't fight. **Allow yourself to be hurt.** Admit to whatever is true in the criticisms.
7. ***Self-destructive acts or threats require attention.*** **Don't ignore. Don't panic.** It's good to know. **Do not keep secrets about this area.** Talk about it openly with your family member and make sure professionals know.
8. ***Listen. People need to have their feelings heard***. Don't say "It isn't so." Don't try to make the feelings go away. Using words to express fear, loneliness, inadequacy, anger, or needs is good. **It's better to use words than to act out on feelings.**

Addressing problems: collaborate and be consistent

9. ***When solving a family member's problems, always:***

   Involve the family member in identifying what needs to be done.

   Ask whether the person can "do" what's needed in the solution.

   Ask whether he or she wants you to "do" what's needed.
10. ***Family members need to act in concert with one another.*** Parental inconsistencies fuel severe family conflicts. Develop strategies that everyone can stick to.
11. ***If you have concerns about medications or therapist interventions, make sure that both your family member and his or her therapist or doctor know.*** If you have financial responsibility, you have the right to address your concerns to the therapist or doctor.

Limit setting: be direct but careful

12. ***Set limits by stating the limits of your tolerance.*** Let your expectations be known in clear, simple language. **Everyone needs to know what is expected of them.**
13. ***Do not protect family members from the natural consequences of their actions.*** Allow them to learn about reality. Bumping into a few walls is usually necessary.

TABLE 9–3. Family guidelines in relationships with a borderline member *(continued)*

14. ***Do not tolerate abusive treatment such as tantrums, threats, hitting, and spitting.*** Walk away and return to discuss the issue later.
15. ***Be cautious about using threats and ultimatums. They are a last resort.*** Do not use threats and ultimatums as a means of convincing others to change. Give them only when you can and will carry through. Let others—including professionals—help you decide when to give them.

emergency room or hospital services. Another guideline that may provide immediate benefits involves severely split parental roles (guideline 10) (see Sidebar 9–4).

Sidebar 9–4: "Good Cop/Bad Cop": A Parental Problem

It is not unusual for parents to divide the roles that they play, by common agreement, for their children. The most common example is that one parent, the "good cop," provides an abundance of the caretaking and protection (usually the mother), whereas the other parent, the "bad cop," embodies the needed disciplinary and authoritarian roles (usually the father). Under ordinary circumstances this works satisfactorily, but for an offspring with borderline personality disorder, such a division invites trouble. The nurturing parent's attitudes help consolidate the borderline offspring's desires into entitlements, and the disciplinary parent allows the borderline offspring to translate his or her own disappointments into parental cruelties.

In such circumstances, parents who recognize their pattern of splitting can benefit from guideline 10. They are told to conscientiously correct splitting by 1) always communicating with each other and only then deciding on mutually acceptable responses to problems and 2) having the bad cop offer a favorable parental response and having the good cop offer a response that the offspring does not want. This directive has immediate benefits. Parents working collaboratively diminish their alienation from each other; both feel more supported and confident. The borderline offspring feels less responsible for parental conflict and more truly held by the family.

During the early phase, a variety of exercises can begin to modify habitual patterns of interaction with the borderline offspring:

1. The book *Don't Shoot the Dog: The New Art of Teaching and Training* (Pryor 1999) can be used to teach parents basic skills in behavioral conditioning.
2. *Communications and Confrontations exercise.* Family members are asked to role-play the how-to of doing confrontations in prescribed ways. There are three components: "I feel...."; "You did...."; and "I want...." Hoffman (1999) uses the DBT-based "Dear Man" exercise for similar purposes.
3. *Managing Criticism exercise.* This exercise relates to guideline 6. It uses some standard behavioral therapy techniques and is reinforced by instructive imagery, e.g., using a sponge as a metaphor for patience and resiliency during confrontations.
4. *Attributions exercises.* This exercise borrows from Fonagy's (1991, 1995) description of how interactional patterns in childhood have led to some typical ways in which borderline patients misattribute feelings or motives to parents and others. Adapted from Fonagy's concept of "mentalizing," this guideline teaches parents to "speak Borderlinese" (i.e., to develop an awareness of the thoughts, fears, and needs underlying their borderline offspring's words and behaviors). For example, when people with BPD say they "hate" someone, it usually means that they feel rejected; when they say they "don't need anyone," it means that they believe being needy is unacceptable. By this means, parents learn how to more accurately understand and respond to such typically all-or-none borderline statements.

The Middle Stage

The frequency of meetings now diminishes to every 2 weeks. It is at this point that conjoint meetings with the borderline offspring can begin, based on the premise that the parents have enough distance, support, humility, and new understanding not to respond to the inevitable opportunities to get into heated struggles. Good indicators of the borderline patients' ability to use the conjoint meetings successfully are that the patients have an alliance with a primary clinician-therapist or are within a more intensive treatment setting (levels II–IV) where they can process the feelings evoked by meeting with their parents.

The format in the meetings now deals more exclusively with problem solving. Families are expected to describe a current situation with the expectation that other family members and the therapist will offer suggestions about how to respond. The family of the borderline patient are aware that they will be encouraged to change patterns of response to the patient. Again, during this stage, the therapist often encourages the family to make reference to the guidelines and often underscores the message that change is not easy—for anyone. Within MFGs, this is the stage when the group "comes together"—develops a cohesion based, in part, on a good working knowledge of one another's shared problems.

The Late Stage

Existing evidence shows that the family functions better now (see Sidebar 9–5). Conjoint meetings with the borderline member have become more comfortable; open hostilities are usually bypassed. The problem-solving format is predictable; family members feel bolder, more confident in giving feedback to each other. Some have made changes that they take pride in; others have persisting difficult-to-solve problems that everyone is familiar with. It helps when the borderline offspring knows that a parent is trying to change, even if he or she fails.

The therapist's role now is seldom directive; rather, the therapist facilitates efforts to understand or communicate that family members can increasingly undertake themselves. Gains made by this time (approximately 1 year) may lead to termination. Sometimes this is a time when particularly emotional statements about guilt or angry feelings toward the borderline family member are voiced. Within the MFG, this usually evokes much support from others.

The psychoeducational therapist encourages families to make ongoing use of the new skills, move on to psychodynamic therapy if it is indicated, return for added psychoeducational meetings as needed, or join self-help groups and become proactive advocates for other families with problems like themselves (Chapter 13 of this book).

Sidebar 9–5: Makes Sense, But Does it Work?–Part 2: Preliminary Findings of the PE/MFG

The goals of psychoeducational therapies are to effect changes in the borderline patient's family that will secondarily effect positive changes in the patient's course of illness. More specific goals involve improving communications, diminishing hostilities, and diminishing struggles over control and independence. One of the central vehicles by which this is accomplished is making families better informed. Two of the expected benefits from the changes are decreased family burden and decreased feelings of alienation.

Up to the present, there has been only one empirical investigation of PE therapies: a pilot study using PE/MFGs (Gunderson et al. 1997). Results are shown (Table 9–4) from 11 families who participated in two PE/MFG groups that were 1 year in duration.

The BPD subjects made changes in desirable ways during the year: diminished hospitalizations and self-destructive acts. Of course, it is not possible to infer that the family changes were responsible. What is very clear is that the consumers felt very pleased with what they learned.

TABLE 9–4. Preliminary results of pilot study using psychoeducational multiple-family groups (N = 11)

Area assessed	Degree of change[a]
Communication	++
Hostilities/conflict	+
Criticism	+
Independence/control	++
Conflict about	+
Separation anxiety	+
Feeling overcontrolled	+
Emotional overinvolvement	±
Knowledge	++
Burden	++

[a]Level of change: ++ = > 1 SD in desired direction; + = .5 to 1 SD in desired direction; ± = mixed results.

Phase 4: Psychodynamic Family Therapy

Psychodynamic family therapy requires the borderline patient's active participation. It should be used selectively, where family readiness has been established by the family's completing less-demanding interventions of the types described in the earlier phases. The readiness to communicate, the ability to recognize (and not act on) feelings, and the use of validation are indications. Without such preparation, this phase is contraindicated: it often results in alienating either the patient or the family members to such a degree that treatment of any sort may be unfeasible. Therapy of a psychodynamic kind is not focused on crisis management and on learning to talk and listen to each other better.

Usually, the duration of psychodynamically based family therapies is open ended. The therapy with families having a borderline member involves an effort to 1) enhance family closeness through the expression of feelings toward each other and 2) enhance understanding of one another through personal self-disclosures and the recognition and acceptance of individual differences.

What distinguishes these goals from any other good-quality, standard psychodynamic family therapy can be found in the particular significance of certain types of family dynamics in families with a borderline member (see Table 9–5). Earlier accounts of dynamically based therapies with families having a borderline member—beyond noting inconsistencies and role problems, with which the educational-behavioral-managerial approach described above can help—were largely concerned with the recognition of projections and projective identifications and with repossessing ("owning") what rightly belongs to each family member's own self (Shapiro 1992).

TABLE 9–5. Issues for psychodynamic family therapy in families with a borderline member

Hostile or withdrawing responses to separation initiatives (Masterson 1972)
Marital bonding that promotes distance, projection, and invalidation of the borderline offspring (Feldman and Guttman 1984; Gunderson et al. 1980; Shane and Kovel 1988)
Projective identification: projections evoking confirmatory (but unrepresentative) responses from others (Feldman and Guttman 1984; Shapiro et al. 1975)
Lack of curiosity about offspring combined with pathological certainty (Shapiro 1982)

Note. These issues can be two-way: the borderline offspring can behave toward the parents in the same ways that parents behave toward the offspring.

SUMMARY

The introduction of structured psychoeducational approaches to families with a borderline member has been welcomed. Such an approach actively allies families with treatment goals, builds skills, and, if done well, improves communication and reduces hostilities with the borderline family member. Whereas the format presented in this chapter seems to work well, other formats are feasible and can be expected to evolve along with the growth of clinical experience and of scientifically based knowledge about the pathogenic—or ameliorative—role of the family. What is clearly evident already is that such interventions require only modest training, are readily exportable, and are very cost effective. The role of traditional expressive psychodynamic therapies may still be important, but these therapies should be initiated selectively, often only after families have already benefited from more educational approaches.

References

Akiskal HS: The nosologic status of borderline personality: clinical and polysomnographic study. Am J Psychiatry 142(2):192–198, 1985

Akiskal HS, Chen SE, Davis GC, et al: Borderline: an adjective in search of a noun. J Clin Psychiatry 46(2):41–48, 1985

Baker L, Silk KR, Westen D, et al: Malevolence, splitting, and parental ratings by borderlines. J Nerv Ment Dis 180(4):258–264, 1992

Berkowitz CB, Gunderson JG: Multifamily psychoeducational treatment of borderline personalty disorder, in The Multifamily Group. Edited by McFarlane WR. London, Oxford University Press, pp 593–613 (in press)

Feldman RB, Guttman HA: Families of borderline patients: literal-minded parents, borderline parents, and parental protectiveness. Am J Psychiatry 141(11):1392–1396, 1984

Fonagy P: Thinking about thinking: some clinical and theoretical considerations in the treatment of a borderline patient. Int J Psychoanal 72:639–656, 1991

Fonagy P: Playing with reality: the development of psychic reality and its malfunction in borderline personalities. International Journal of Psycho-Analysis 76(Pt 1): 39–44, 1995

Fonagy P, Steele M, Steele H, et al: Attachment, the reflective self, and borderline states: the predictive specificity of the Adult Attachment Interview and pathological emotional development, in Attachment Theory: Social, Developmental, and Clinical Perspective. Edited by Goldberg S, Muir R, et al. Hillsdale, NJ, Analytic Press, 1995, pp 223–278

Frank H, Paris J: Recollections of family experience in borderline patients. Arch Gen Psychiatry 38:1031–1034, 1981

Gabbard GO, Lazar SG, Hornberger J, et al: The economic impact of psychotherapy: a review. Am J Psychiatry 154(2):147–155, 1997

Goldman SJ, D'Angelo EJ, DeMaso DR: Psychopathology in the families of children and adolescents with borderline personality disorder. Am J Psychiatry 150:1832–1835, 1993

Goldstein MJ: Psychoeducation and relapse prevention. Int Clin Psychopharmacol 9(5):59–69, 1995

Gunderson JG, Lyoo IK: Family problems and relationships for adults with borderline personality disorder. Harv Rev Psychiatry 4(5):272–278, 1997

Gunderson JG, Sabo AN: The phenomenological and conceptual interface between borderline personality disorder and PTSD. Am J Psychiatry 150(1):19–27, 1993

Gunderson JG, Zanarini MC: Pathogenesis of borderline personality disorder, in American Psychiatric Press Review of Psychiatry, Vol 8. Edited by Tasman A, Hales RE, Frances AJ. Washington, DC, American Psychiatric Press, 1989, pp 25–48

Gunderson JG, Kerr J, Englund DW: The families of borderlines: a comparative study. Arch Gen Psychiatry 37(1):27–33, 1980

Gunderson JG, Frank AF, Ronningstam EF, et al: Early discontinuance of borderline patients from psychotherapy. J Nerv Ment Dis 177(1):38–42, 1989

Gunderson JG, Berkowitz C, Ruiz-Sancho A: Families of borderline patients: a psychoeducational approach. Bull Menninger Clin 61(4):446–457, 1997

Hoffman PD: A family partnership. Journal of the California Alliance for the Mentally Ill 8:52–53, 1997

Hoffman P: Family intervention: DBT family skills training. Presented at the Sixth International Congress on Disorders of Personality, Geneva Switzerland, September 1999

Hoffman PD, Hooley JM: Expressed emotion and the treatment of borderline personality disorder. In Session 4(3):39–54, 1998

Leff J: Controversial issues and growing points in research on relatives' expressed emotions. Int J Soc Psychiatry 35:133–145, 1989

Links PS (ed): Family Environment and Borderline Personality Disorder. Washington, DC, American Psychiatric Press, 1990

Links PS, van Reekum R: Childhood sexual abuse, parental impairment and the development of borderline personality disorder. Can J Psychiatry 38:472–474, 1993

Links PS, Steiner M, Huxley G: The occurrence of borderline personality disorder in the families of borderline patients. J Personal Disord 2:14–20, 1988

Links P, Boiago I, Huxley G: Sexual abuse and biparental failure as etiologic models in BPD, in Family Environment and Borderline Personality Disorder. Edited by Links PS. Washington, DC, American Psychiatric Press, 1990, pp 105–120

Loranger AW, Oldham JM, Tulis EH: Familial transmission of DSM-III borderline personality disorder. Arch Gen Psychiatry 39(7):795–799, 1982

Masterson J: Treatment of the Borderline Adolescent: A Developmental Approach. New York, Wiley, 1972

Masterson JF, Rinsley DB: The borderline syndrome: the role of the mother in the genesis and psychic structure of the borderline personality. Int J Psychoanal 56(2):163–177, 1975

McFarlane WR, Dunne E: Family psychoeducation and multi-family groups in the treatment of schizophrenia. Directions in Psychiatry 11(20):2–7, 1991

McFarlane WR, Lukens E, Link B, et al: Multiple-family groups and psychoeducation in the treatment of schizophrenia. Arch Gen Psychiatry 52:679–687, 1995

Millon T: On the genesis and prevalence of the borderline personality disorder: a social learning thesis. J Personal Disord 1(4):354–372, 1987

Paris J, Braverman S: Successful and unsuccessful marriages in borderline patients. J Am Acad Psychoanal 23(1):153–166, 1995

Paris J, Zweig-Frank H, Guzder J: Psychological risk factors for borderline personality disorder in female patients. Compr Psychiatry 35:301–305, 1994a

Paris J, Zweig-Frank H, Guzder J: Risk factors for borderline personality in male outpatients. J Nerv Ment Dis 182:375–380, 1994b

Patterson GR: Coercive Family Process. Eugene, OR, Castalia Publishing, 1982

Patterson GR, Reid JB, Dishion TJ: Antisocial Boys. Eugene, OR, Castalia Publishing, 1992

Perry JC, Herman JL, van der Kolk BA, et al: Psychotherapy and psychological trauma in borderline personality disorder. Psychiatric Annals 20(1):33–43, 1990

Pope HG Jr, Jonas JM, Hudson JI, et al: The validity of DSM-III borderline personality disorder: a phenomenologic, family history, treatment response, and long-term follow-up study. Arch Gen Psychiatry 40(1):23–30, 1983

Pryor K: Don't Shoot the Dog: The New Art of Teaching and Training, Revised Edition. New York, Bantam Doubleday Dell, 1999

Reiss D, Hetherington EM, Plomin R, et al: Genetic questions for environmental studies: differential parenting and psychopathology in adolescence. Arch Gen Psychiatry 52:925–936, 1995

Ruiz-Sancho AM, Smith GW, Gunderson JG: Psychoeducational approaches, in Handbook of Personality Disorders. Edited by Livesley WJ. New York, Guilford (in press)

Schachnow J, ClarkinJ, DePalma CS, et al: Biparental psychopathology and borderline personality disorder. Psychiatry 60:171–181, 1997

Schulz PM, Schulz SCH, Hamer R, et al: The impact of borderline and schizotypal personality disorders on patients and their families. Hospital and Community Psychiatry 36:879–881, 1985

Seeman MV, Edwards-Evans B: Marital therapy with borderline patients: is it beneficial? J Clin Psychiatry 40(7):308–312, 1979

Shane M, Kovel V: Family therapy in severe personality disorders. International Journal of Family Psychiatry 9:241–258, 1988

Shapiro ER: The psychodynamics and developmental psychology of the borderline patient: a review of the literature. Am J Psychiatry 135:1305–1315, 1978a

Shapiro ER: Research on family dynamics: indications for family and individual treatment in adolescence. Adolescent Psychiatry 6:360–376, 1978b

Shapiro ER: On curiosity: intrapsychic and interpersonal boundary formation in family life. International Journal of Family Psychiatry 3:69–89, 1982

Shapiro ER: Family dynamics and borderline personality disorder, in Handbook of Borderline Disorders. Edited by Silver D, Rosenbluth M. Madison, CT, International Universities Press, 1992, pp 471–493

Shapiro RL, Zinner J, Shapiro ER: Concurrent family treatment of narcissistic disorders in adolescents. Int J Psychoanal Psychother 4:379–396, 1974

Shapiro ER, Zinner J, Shapiro RL, et al: The influence of family experience on borderline personality development. International Review of Psychoanalysis 2(4): 399–411, 1975

Silverman JM, Pinkham L, Horvath TB, et al: Affective and impulsive personality traits in relatives of borderline patients. Am J Psychiatry 148:1378–1385, 1991

Soloff PH, Millward JW: Developmental histories of borderline patients. Compr Psychiatry 24:574–588, 1983a

Soloff PH, Millward JW: Psychiatric disorders in the families of borderline patients. Arch Gen Psychiatry 40:37–44, 1983b

Thomas A, Chess S: Genesis and evolution of behavioral disorders: from infancy to early adult life. Am J Psychiatry 141:1–9, 1984

Waldo M, Harman MJ: Borderline personality disorder and relationship enhancement martial therapy, in The Disordered Couple. Edited by Carlson J, Sperry L, et al. Bristol, PA, Brunner/Mazel, 1998, pp 285–297

Weiss M, Zelkowitz P, Feldman RB: Psychopathology in offspring of mothers with borderline personality disorder: a pilot study. Can J Psychiatry 41(5):285–290, 1996

Young DW, Gunderson JG: Family images of borderline adolescents. Psychiatry 58(2):164–172, 1995

Zanarini MC (ed): Evolving perspectives on the etiology of borderline personality disorder, in Role of Sexual Abuse in the Etiology of Borderline Personality Disorder. Washington, DC, American Psychiatric Press, 1997, pp 1–14

Zanarini MC, Gunderson JG, Marino MF, et al: Psychiatric disorders in the families of borderline outpatients, in Family Environment and Borderline Personality Disorder. Edited by Links PS. Washington, DC, American Psychiatric Press, 1990, pp 67–84

Zinner J, Shapiro ER: Splitting in families of borderline adolescents, in Borderline States in Psychiatry. Edited by Mack J. New York, Grune & Stratton, 1975

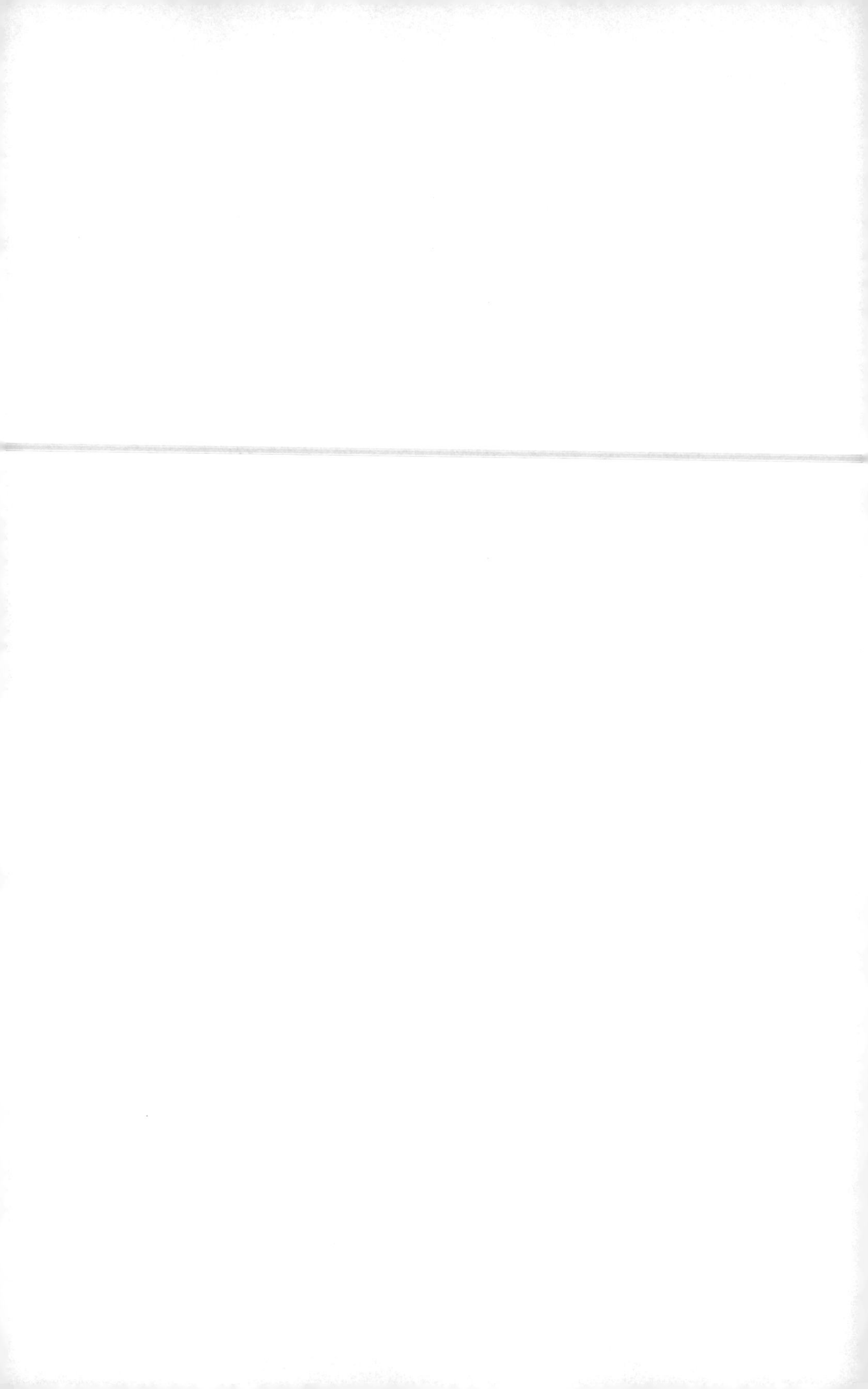

APPENDIX

Suggested Psychoeducational Printed Materials, Videos, Films, and Web Sites

PRINTED MATERIALS

Overviews

"Borderline Personality Disorder." *Journal of the California Alliance for the Mentally Ill*, Vol. 8, No. 1, 1997.

Wide-ranging and very readable comments from experts, families, and persons with BPD.

Borderline Personality Disorder: What You Need to Know, by J. Gunderson, Psychosocial Research, McLean Hospital, Belmont, MA.

A concise, informative summary.

I Hate You, Don't Leave Me, by J. Kreisman and A. Strauss. Los Angeles, CA, The Body Press, 1989.

Readable and instructive.

Imbroglio, by J. Cauwels. New York, W. W. Norton, 1992.

Scholarly and understandable.

"The Pain of Being Borderline," by M. Zanarini, F. Frankenburg, J. Gunderson, and others. *Harvard Review of Psychiatry*, Vol. 6 (Nov.–Dec. 1998), pp. 201–207.

Scientific description of negative thoughts and feelings in individuals with BPD.

Family Issues

"Walking on Eggshells," pamphlet, by P. Mason and R. Krieger. BPD Central, 1996. Web site address, http://www.BPDCentral.com

Useful description of problems for families or others.

"Family Problems and Relationships For Adults With Borderline Personality Disorder," by J. Gunderson and I. K. Lyoo, Psychosocial Research, McLean Hospital, Belmont, MA. *Harvard Review of Psychiatry,* Vol. 4, pp. 272–278, 1997.

Scientific description.

The Family Crucible, by C. Whitaker and A. Napier. New York, Bantam Books, 1978.

How one family member can bring covert family issues to light.

Instructive Books

Search For the Real Self, by J. Masterson, New York, Free Press, 1988.

Readable psychodynamic approach.

Girl, Interrupted, by S. Kaysen. New York, Turtle Bay Books, 1993.

A best-seller. Highlights treatment impasses, black-and-white thinking.

Lost in the Mirror, by R. Moskovitz. Dallas, TX, Taylor Publications, 1993.

Borderline patients can recognize themselves. Vivid and compassionate.

Marilyn: A Biography, by N. Mailer. New York, Grosset and Dunlap, 1973.

History's most celebrated exemplar of borderline personality disorder.

Eclipses: Behind the Borderline Personality Disorder, by M. F. Thornton, E. W. Peterson, and W. D. Barley. Madison, AL, Monte Sano Publishing, 1997.

Effective Psychotherapy with Borderline Patients, by R. Waldinger and J. Gunderson. Washington, DC, American Psychiatric Press, 1989.

Case reports of successful long-term therapies.

Diana: In Search of Herself (1999), by S. B. Smith. New York, Times Books, 1999.

Readable, insightful glimpse of the distinction between public persona and internal strife.

Personality Self-Portrait, by J. M. Oldham and C. B. Morris. New York, Bantam Books, 1990.

Makes personality disorders understandable. Instructive chapter on BPD.

A Bright Red Scream: Self-Mutilation and the Language of Pain, by M. Strong. New York, Penguin Books, 1998.

Newsletters

NEDPA News. From New England Personality Disorders Association (NEDPA), McLean Hospital, Belmont, MA 02478.

Valuable personal accounts.

TARA Times. From TARA, 23 Greene St., New York, NY 10013

Good account of public advocacy initiatives and opportunities.

VIDEOS

"The Borderline Syndrome," PBS, 1988. Albany, NY, Olive Tree Productions.

An instructive introduction.

Companion to "The Borderline Syndrome," PBS, 1988. Albany, NY, Olive Tree Productions.

FILMS

Looking for Mr. Goodbar (with Diane Keaton). Paramount Pictures, 1977.

Captures emptiness, thrill seeking, and good/bad split self.

Fatal Attraction (with Glenn Close). Paramount Pictures, 1987.

Frightening portrait of abandonment rage.

Lethal Weapon (with Mel Gibson). Warner Bros., 1987.

Captures identity disturbance.

Taxi Driver (with Robert De Niro and Jodie Foster). Columbia Pictures, 1976.

Play Misty for Me (with Clint Eastwood). Universal Studios, 1971.

Torment by others who resist being possessed.

Girl, Interrupted (with Winona Ryder and Angelina Jolie). Columbia, 2000.

More vivid than the book (see above for book listing).

Bliss (with Craig Sheffer and Sheryl Lee). Triumph Films/Stewart Pictures, 1997.

A poignant look at a lost soul with a history of childhood sexual abuse.

World Wide Web

BPD Central
http://www.bpdcentral.com
By Krieger and Mason (authors of *Walking on Eggshells*; see above in "Family Issues").

Balances facts and compassion.

Mental Health Net (link from CMHC Systems home page)
http://www.cmhc.com

Well organized and frequently updated.

National Alliance for the Mentally Ill (NAMI) home page
http://www.nami.org

DBT Network
http://www.dbt-seattle.com

Up-to-date developments of dialectical behavior therapy–related research and services.

The Borderline Sanctuary
http://www.mhsanctuary.com/borderline

Supportive and hopeful testimony by/for borderline patients.

Soul's Self-Help Central
http://www.soulselfhelp.on.ca (On the opening screen, click on "Borderline Personality Disorder" in the list of topics at the left.)

Supportive and hopeful testimonials and e-mail support group.

10

Interpersonal Group Therapy

Introduction

Group therapies are one of the psychosocial modalities that target the borderline patient's socially maladaptive behaviors (Chapter 4 of this book). Many clinicians have noted that the interpersonal and social deficits characterizing BPD are ideal targets for the goals served by interpersonal group therapies (IPGs) (Finn and Shakir 1990; Flapan 1983; Target and Fonagy 1996). These groups combine involvement with support (see Chapter 3 of this book) and have obvious relevance to borderline patients. In addition, the large number of reasonably qualified interpersonal group therapists and the available evidence of efficacy and cost benefits (discussed below) make it incumbent on any outpatient clinic purporting to treat borderline patients to offer interpersonal groups. In my experience, referral to an IPG should always be considered as a potential split-treatment partner (Chapter 4 of this book) for outpatient care by primary clinicians, psychopharmacologists, and psychotherapists.

Marziali and Munroe-Blum (1994) pointed out that an IPG is considerably more cost effective—even with the use of cotherapists—than individual psychotherapy. Over the course of a year, an IPG group with 7 patients would consume 150 hours of therapist time (2 therapists × 50 sessions × 1½ hours/session), whereas 7 patients in individual therapy would require 350 hours of therapist time (7 patients × 50 sessions × 1 hour/session). If, say, the group cost $45/session and individual therapy cost $50/session, for seven patients the group would cost $6,750 and the individual therapy $40,500—six times the cost.

Still, neither the relatively low cost of IPGs nor the growth in multimodal treatments for BPD seem to have appreciably changed the level of research on IPGs or use of the groups. Even though, in my experience, the value of IPG therapy is modestly more widely recognized than in the past, there remains a reluctance by many psychotherapists, case managers, and outpatient clinics to rely on this modality. In principle, the use of IPGs should be expanded by two current phenomena: 1) the growth in demand for intensified outpatient therapies, mandated by the lack of long-term hospital or residential services, and 2) the growth in demand for cost-beneficial alternatives mandated by managed care (Segal and Weideman 1995). Underuse is clearly related to borderline patients' typical resistance to this modality. Still, it will be in the interest of the patients if appropriately more, and more enthusiastic, referrals to IPGs occur, either through cost containment pressures or through more enlightened clinicians.

Indications

Although IPGs are indicated for many patients, it is important to exercise judgment and be selective about who is referred. Interpersonal groups may be initiated when patients are in level III (residential or partial hospital) or level II (intensive outpatient) programs. Indeed, the use of such groups at the Ulleval Hospital in Norway as a step-down from day hospitals has been described, with good supporting evidence, by Wilberg et al. (1998). That study showed that the 12 patients who attended IPGs had fewer hospitalizations and suicide attempts and were better off symptomatically and in overall health on follow-up nearly 3 years later than the 31 patients who did not go to an IPG.

IPGs are not suitable for borderline patients with seriously life-endangering behaviors. This modality is primarily suited for the many borderline patients who do not require hospital or partial hospital care and whose level I outpatient care might otherwise consist of only medications and psychotherapy. Piper and Josie (1998) believe that group therapy is particularly welcome to patients who are threatened by the intimacy required in individual therapy or the authority often seen in medical intervention. As described in Chapter 5 of this book, in my experience this modality takes its place as an alternative or sequel to the social-skills groups of dialectical behavior therapy (DBT).

Vignette

Ms. G was a 28-year-old woman who had had four hospitalizations in the previous year, the year in which she relocated to a distant city for a work opportunity. When she returned to live with her mother, her suicidal impulses

> diminished, but she remained troubled by "unrealistically negative thinking," meaning that she expected to be rejected, and by recurrent anger—especially toward her mother–that she did not express and that caused her to "feel bad." She had had several boyfriends but no one recently, because she had become too upset ("I lose my identity") and had cut herself when relationships ended.

This vignette underscores two general guidelines involving motivation and aptitude for referring borderline patients to an IPG: 1) patients should recognize problems in their interpersonal relations that they would like to work on. (It is insufficient for a clinician or anyone else other than the patient to recognize such problems.) 2) Patients should be sufficiently in control of impulses (and suicidality) that they can be expected (and be able) to sit through and participate in emotionally wrought discussions.

Ms. G's suitability for an IPG were evident, because her issues were so patently interpersonal, notably a hostile-dependent relationship with her mother, rejection sensitivity and withdrawal in heterosexual relations, and her relative absence of a social network (especially girlfriends). In addition, because her behavioral problems were quite minor—she had no patterns of self-destructive acts and was capable of sustained role functioning within school and work settings—she was an ideal candidate for an IPG. Although her relatively poor skills in affect recognition and expression might be helped by cognitive-behavioral interventions, the potential bonus of better peer relations that derive from IPGs seemed in her case to be an overriding consideration.

IPG STRUCTURE, DURATION, AND LEADERS

Structure: Group Size and Meeting Schedule

Four members is the minimal size and a useful minimum to keep in mind for getting started. Having four members translates into the likelihood of having three in attendance, and although starting with only three attendees may be hard to justify in cost-benefit terms, it has advantages over a long delay while waiting for enough members ready to join. Borderline patients are always ambivalent about joining groups, and delay can easily flip the balance toward not starting. Six to eight members is optimal. A larger size does not permit enough individual activity to keep everyone engaged.

Meetings are once or twice weekly and last for 1–1½ hours. Twice a week offers the group more of a holding function, but this frequency is rarely feasible because of the ambivalence that typifies most borderline patients. Groups should meet in early evenings to diminish conflicts with vocational activities.

Duration

Given that the IPG primary goals are social and interpersonal, the benefits can be expected to require a minimum of 4 months but will usually accrue for 1½–2 years (see Chapter 3 of this book). After 2 years, the rate of added benefit often diminishes. Because of the socializing function that IPGs can serve for borderline patients, it is best not to limit continued involvement, even if it seems to involve little new learning. The group therapy aftercare given at Ulleval Hospital had a mean duration of 1 year, but as experience with this modality grew, this duration seemed "rather short" (Wilberg et al. 1998, p. 218). The duration suggested here (1½–2 years) extends that suggested by Marziali and Munroe-Blum (1994). At the start of their project, they, like Piper and Josie (1998), believed that having a preestablished time limit (they thought 30 sessions) for the IPG would "accelerate the achievement of important changes" (p. 689). But after their project, they concluded that a longer period in IPG (at least a year) might offer further advantages—especially for a subgroup they termed "pseudocompetent patients," meaning the borderline patients who were intellectually well defended.

Group Therapists

Most experienced group therapists can effectively lead IPGs for borderline patients. This, as pointed out by Marziali and Munroe-Blum (1994), is one of the really significant assets of this modality. Second only to dynamic psychotherapy, it is a standard treatment of which many psychologists, social workers, and even psychiatrists have a working knowledge. Still, the ability of the IPG group leaders to establish a positive relational alliance with the borderline members turns out to be a very important prediction of outcome (Marziali et al. 1997). Horwitz (1987) recommended having the same therapist conduct both individual and group therapies, since observations made in the group can offer valuable material for working through in the individual therapy. In my experience, however, the problems usually outweigh the advantages. These problems involve the imbalance and consequent rivalry experienced by IPG members who do not have the leader as an individual therapist and the intensification of "special patient" expectations by those who do.

Moreover, having BPD group members involves special considerations for leaders. Because the risks of impulsive, self-destructive, or inappropriate (boundary-violating) relationships are greater with borderline group members, prior clinical experience and especially experience with clinical administration are valuable assets. Often, conducting groups in either inpatient or residential settings teaches clinicians about limit setting, safety assessments, communication with other team members, and other administrative roles needed for work with borderline patients. Having acquired these skills, clinicians can combine them comfortably with the usual supportive, interpretive, and other facilitative functions needed for good outpatient interpersonal group leadership. (Such learning is also needed to be able to function as a borderline patient's primary clinician-therapist; see Chapters 5 and 11 of this book.)

Coleaders are often beneficial. Here too the principle of split treatment is at work: the patient who is angry at one therapist can preserve a "good" image for the other, which makes flight less likely. Cotherapists help to check each other's countertransference reactions, maintain continuity of treatment during absences, and otherwise decrease the burden of running groups (Greenbaum and Pinney 1982). In the absence of a cotherapist, IPG group leaders, like DBT skills training groups (Chapter 7 of this book), will benefit from having supervision or peer group discussion.

GETTING THE GROUP STARTED

Membership

The warning offered in earlier literature about having too many borderline patients in a group (Horwitz 1987; Pines 1990; Roth 1990a; Wong 1980) now seems, on the basis of experience at McLean and elsewhere, to be unjustified (Marziali and Monroe-Blum 1994; O'Leary et al. 1991). It is critically important for IPGs to provide BPD patients with the benefit of feedback from others with the same issues. These issues include the phenomena of intense affects and unstable relationships, but also, as Koseff (1990) noted, similarities in developmental experiences and defenses. I therefore think it is desirable to have at least three borderline members; otherwise, a selective diagnostic mix is fine. Dependent, schizoid, chronically depressed, and narcissistic patients mix well. Although the preponderance of BPD patients are female, it is desirable to have male members in IPG groups. Patients who are so exploitative or otherwise antisocial that they are unlikely to seek change and are likely to affect others harmfully should be excluded. Patients with active, serious substance abuse should not enter IPGs without concurrent active involvement in substance abuse treatment. Neither patients who are significantly healthier nor patients who have chronic psychoses will find BPD groups useful or comfortable.

Engagement

Borderline patients do not select IPG (or any group therapy) as their treatment of choice. Indeed, their resistance is so severe that coercive pressures often need to be used: the primary clinician-therapist must insist on their participation as part of a larger treatment plan that includes one-to-one contacts with them, which, invariably, is what borderline patients prefer. In the only randomized controlled study of IPGs for borderline patients, Marziali and Munroe-Blum (1994) reported that 31 of the 110 borderline patients dropped out after being assigned to the IPG condition. Of the 79 patients who began treatment, another 13 dropped out in the first 3 sessions. Thus, 40% dropped out. Many of the remaining 66 patients dropped out before 9 sessions. These data highlight the very significant problem of getting BPD patients engaged. A recent analysis suggested that patients in IPGs are slower to develop a treatment alliance than those in individual therapy (Marziali et al. 1999).

To get borderline patients engaged, I tell them, "You need to join a group. You can learn things there that you can't learn in individual psychotherapy. Specifically, you can learn how others cope with the same problems and how you unknowingly impede making the close relationships that you want. Moreover, you can learn some things faster in groups than you can in individual therapy. For example, you can learn to listen when people express feelings you usually can't stand, and you can learn to understand why people have those feelings." Patients are usually receptive to the idea that it is easier to understand or recognize a problem when it is observed in others, and that this awareness may help them understand or recognize their own problems.

I also tell patients that "my own experience shows that participation in a group makes it more likely that your psychotherapy will succeed. I (or any individual therapist) can easily underestimate the stressful effects of things I say or do; thus, there will probably be times you will want to leave therapy. Groups offer a useful way to process such stress. And conversely, the group will undoubtedly prove stressful at times, and when that occurs, I (or another individual therapist) can help you learn from that experience."

Sidebar 10-1: Makes Sense, But Does It Work?—Part 3: Preliminary Findings on Efficacy of IPG

Research on the efficacy of IPGs is very limited. Nehls (1991) pioneered this area with a report that borderline patients who attended groups showed improved Global Assessment Scale (GAS) and symptom outcomes. But it is Marziali and Munroe-Blum (1994) who have really advanced empirical examination of whether IPGs can benefit borderline patients. Their study offered thirty 1½-hour sessions of an IPG led by trained, multidisciplinary cotherapists. Their manual-guided IPG, modeled after Dawson's (Dawson 1988, Dawson and MacMillan 1993) management style (see Chapter 4 of this book, section titled "Relationship Management"), emphasized empathy and deemphasized interpretation. The 38 borderline outpatients randomly assigned to IPG were compared to 41 others assigned to weekly individual psychodynamic therapy that, insofar as it was modeled after that described by Kernberg (1968, 1975, 1986; see Chapter 12 of this book), emphasized interpretations. The psychodynamic therapy (the control condition) was conducted by therapists with training and experience equal to that of those providing the IPG (Marziali and Munroe-Blum 1995).

Outcome variables emphasizing problematic behaviors, depressive symptoms, and social adjustment were assessed during the 1 year when patients received therapy and on follow-up a year later. Both groups showed clinically significant but similar levels of improvement at 1 year, and both groups sustained those improvements during the follow-up. Improvements were most dramatic in behaviors (e.g., hospitalization, suicidal acts, impulsivity), to a lesser degree in depression, and least for social adjustment. The investigators did not believe that the patients' overall "character pathology" was much affected.

Encouraging results, but the study's conditions seriously limit what can be concluded. Notably, the investigators adopted a very generous definition for "treatment compliance": attendance at three or more sessions in the subject's assigned treatment. Of the 66 patients who were in their assigned treatment for 3 or more sessions, only about 67% provided outcome data. Many of the IPG subjects had only between 3 and 9 sessions—enough that this subgroup was compared to those who had had 10 or more. No differences were found. This disturbing finding was used by Marziali and Munroe-Blum (1994) to suggest that the benefits may occur rapidly. It may, however, have other explanations. For example, the improvements seen in the treatment group could be due to nonspecific or placebo effects—that is, it could be true that the benefits at 1 year and follow-up a year later for both the IPG sample and the psychodynamic therapy group reflect the natural course of the disorder. Another explanation may relate to the waiting time. The IPG patients often had to wait for several months before enough were present to start a group. During this period, they had frequent visits with a research assistant familiar with IPG interventions. The waiting patients may have benefited before they entered what frequently turned out to be a very short-term IPG intervention.

All in all, this study by itself does not offer a strong empirical endorsement for the value of an IPG for borderline patients. However, the endorsement of IPGs in this study is strengthened by the results from the study by Nehls (1991) and by the very impressive conclusions about IPGs found in Wilberg et al.'s (1998) naturalistic follow-along study of borderline patients leaving a day hospital (described earlier in this chapter). Munroe-Blum and Marziali (1995) concluded that the results show that IPGs offer a reasonable response to the market's demand for a low-cost therapy that can be offered by a wide range of providers. I agree; I would also conclude that the studies by Marziali and Munroe-Blum, as well as the other studies, provide a very strong rationale for conducting more definitive studies.

I would like to bolster these arguments for why borderline patients should join an IPG by citing research evidence, but the results (see Sidebar 10–1), although supportive, are not compelling. What really fosters my convictions about the role of IPG, therefore, is personal experience and the significance I attach to using a complementary second modality (i.e., the principle of split treatment discussed in Chapter 5 of this book).

Some borderline patients can become engaged in a group only if they have a highly idealized view of the leaders (Roth 1990b) or if they can establish a "twinship self-object" relationship with another member (Bacal 1990). Without these protective relationships, they feel too vulnerable or victimized to stay. Roth (1990b) noted that some borderline patients require emotional distance to stay in groups and that they are likely to flee when other members of an IPG make changes that call for more intimacy.

Establishing a Contract

In establishing a contract, it is useful to specify IPG goals and what the leader's and participants' roles will be. This activity is often facilitated by the group leaders' writing out a standardized guide for goals and roles (a "contract") that is given to prospective patients (see Table 10–1 for an example).

The contract is then reviewed before starting. Whereas the role of such formal contracts is controversial for setting the framework for treatment (Chapter 4 of this book) or for starting individual psychotherapy (Chapter 11 of this book), it seems more consistently useful for IPGs. It standardizes the development of a contractual alliance (Chapter 3 of this book), facilitates a sense of belonging, and, by establishing norms, diminishes the likelihood of regressions. It assumes that all members, though strangers, have arrived with some common understanding of what to expect from one another. Some therapists like to have the contract signed, formally indicating that patients understand and agree to these goals and roles.

TABLE 10–1. A contract for interpersonal group therapy

Goals

To understand how your interpersonal style affects others and how others, in turn, affect you. Participation in the group can be expected to improve your communication skills and help with appropriate expressions of feelings. It is also expected to enhance your capacity to understand feelings and motives in others and your comfort in close relationships.

Roles

Participants are expected to attend, to pay regularly, and to let the group leaders know if they are unable to do either. In sessions, members are expected to talk about issues in their lives and to listen and respond to those disclosed by others.

It is expected that leaders and all members will respect each other's confidentiality. If you think that you want to leave the group, it will be discussed in the group, with adequate time for others to respond.

Therapists are expected to encourage members to discuss personal problems and their responses to each other. Therapists will also comment on group process issues such as cohesion, avoidance, or trust, and they will help the group identify interactions whose interpersonal significance might otherwise be unnoticed—for example, competitiveness, exclusiveness, or covert hostility.

PROCESSES OF THERAPY

The processes described in this section have an overall containing function that can be powerfully beneficial for borderline patients and that can replace the more formal containment performed at higher levels of care.

Interpersonal Learning

Borrowing from Yalom's (1995) list of group processes, interpersonal learning (as opposed to, say, insight, skill training, or catharsis) is central to IPGs for borderline patients. The following four are particularly valuable examples (Yalom 1995):

1. *Learning that others have similar experiences—"I'm not alone."* Hearing others voice feelings or concerns that a patient has not articulated or has felt as shameful sets the stage for improved capacities for socializing.
2. *Being able to express feelings without being rejected.* Not only useful in their own right, such experiences lead to examining why such feelings are generated.
3. *Learning how one affects others.* Learning about oneself through others' reactions is a basic step toward being psychological-minded and gaining a sense of personal agency.
4. *Learning that disagreeing is different from invalidation.* Many borderline patients are so starved for validation that they experience any disagreement or confrontation as cruel and undermining.

Group leaders can facilitate such learning by underscoring these experiences when they occur and by actively inviting members to discuss their responses to each other. Over time, these experiences of having the freedom to speak and hear the truth can give an IPG a major holding or containing function.

Cohesion

Because the personal relationships of borderline patients are typically either intense, demanding, exclusive relationships that end badly or unfulfilling and superficial relationships, the IPG offers a powerful opportunity to develop different (less intense), more adaptive (task-sharing), and more satisfying ways of relating. The severe interpersonal impairment that characterizes borderline patients means that—borrowing again from Yalom's list of therapeutic procedures—*cohesion* of the group is a primary therapeutic process. *Cohesion* refers to the processes that tie participants to the group. Marziali et al. (1997) suggested that the development of strong group cohesion is facilitated by members' having established a strong alliance with the group leader. My experience, like that of Marziali and Munroe-Blum (1994), is that the process is also facilitated by similarities in age and background among group members, which enhance the ability of members to identify with each other. Using self-psychology to promote cohesion, Macaskill (1980) interprets the angry, self-contained, or devaluing behaviors as defenses against pain and a poor self-image. Cohesion is also helped by experiences of acceptance by each other and by leader interventions that focus on group processes, reinforcing the group's identity as an entity (e.g., "The group seemed disturbed by. . .]."). Borderline patients who feel valued by being a part of the group, rather than being either merged with or excluded from it, learn a very valuable capacity. Macaskill (1982) found that borderline patients particularly valued altruistic experiences within groups, and he noted that group members learn to comfort each other, following the example set by group leaders. Horwitz (1977, 1987) believes that the interpersonal learning experiences attained in IPGs are helpful in setting the stage for individual psychotherapy. I strongly agree and, as mentioned, would also note the complementary functions each serves for the other.

Owning and Expressing Hostilities

Borderline patients typically have easily awakened grievances that, when triggered, offend others with their expression—whether in the form of inappropriate anger, intimidating attitudes, or acting unrealistically entitled (e.g., "I'm owed special exemptions"). Thus they drive away the people to whom they might otherwise become attached. As Marziali and Munroe-Blum (1995) pointed out, this problem may become evident early in IPGs, when the borderline members begin to criticize the IPG leaders' skill ("You should have. . . .") or value ("We were doing fine until you said. . . ."). Marziali and Munroe-Blum advised leaders to tolerate the attacks and to acknowledge that the IPG or they themselves (the group leaders) may in fact not be helpful (as in Dawson 1988, Dawson and MacMillan 1993—see Chapter 4 of this book, section titled "Relationship Management"). Although I agree that this approach may disarm some borderline patients, it can have some negative effects. It may fuel fears that the leader(s) are not in charge, that they can be bullied, or that they also doubt whether the group therapy can help. I would encourage leaders' being more educative about the time course in which changes might occur and about the leaders' reasons for saying or not saying things. At the same time, such bitter expressions of hostility toward the group or the leader(s) offer opportunities to address how expressions of impatience or unrealistic expectations make it difficult to form good working relationships. Inviting other patients to describe their reactions to a member's expression of hostility is also very useful. IPGs are particularly useful in drawing attention to the maladaptiveness with which these feelings are managed.

Vignette

Leader: What's the matter, Sheila? You look dazed.
Sheila: I'm dissociating.
Leader: When did that start?
Sheila: I don't know. I guess right after we started.
Leader: Why was that? What happened?
Sheila: I don't know.
Henry: I'll bet you got upset by what I said about my wife fucking around.
Jane (sarcastically). There's nothing new about that, Henry. But what I remember is I got irritated right off the bat because as usual you arrived five minutes late. (Now with open hostility) And then you take over the group! It's rude.
Leader: Do other people share Jane's reaction?
Sheila: It's just that he does the same thing every week.
Leader: You mean you felt irritated too?
Sheila: (Subdued): Yes, I did.

This vignette highlights the many ways in which IPGs help borderline patients learn about owning and expressing angry feelings. IPGs can help patients own angry feelings that they would otherwise ignore or recognize but express in symptoms—which Sheila's "dissociating" seemed to be—or otherwise fail to communicate—as Sheila subsequently, although hesitantly, was enabled to do. This shift by Sheila was in part due to the modeling role served by the more outspoken Jane, by the manifest acceptance of such anger in the leader's response and further inquiries, and by the fact that other members subsequently also acknowledged Jane's anger at Henry. In the context of an IPG, it is likely that Jane will eventually learn that her sarcastic outspokenness intimidates others, even if they admire her, and that it helps account for her ongoing failure to have dates. Finally, Henry, with time, may learn that his recurrent lateness acts out, passively, his hostile resistance to compliance with any rules—one of many passive-aggressive ways that he unwittingly provokes his wife's affairs. Just as in individual therapy, the sequence involves helping patients 1) see their anger, 2) see it as others see it, 3) see its consequences, and then 4) support change.

Split Treatment: Communicating With Primary Clinicians and Other Therapists

It isn't always true that a group leader and individual therapist (or primary clinician) need to talk to each other about a shared patient, but this option must be open. Actual communication is needed when there are attendance problems, there are safety risks, or the patent's behavior otherwise endangers the usefulness of either therapy (e.g., drug use, an affair with another group member). Occasionally, a borderline patient is in an IPG with no other therapy, but this option has inherent problems for patients who practice dangerous self-destructive behaviors. The IPG therapist may be forced to take on a responsibility for that patient's safety that will be very disruptive to the group's function. (Marziali et al. [1997] did report, however, that sometimes the other members of an IPG take this responsibility on themselves.) Usually, borderline patients in an IPG will benefit from having a primary clinician who serves as the therapist. Here it is critical that the IPG leader and the primary clinician/therapist respect the value of each other's modality so that, when either party is told by the patient how stupid or insensitive the care in that other modality has been, the therapists are neither sympathetic nor protective. (See "Splits, Splitting, and the Principle of Split Treatment" in Chapter 4 of this book.) Actually, one of the potential misuses of communication between a therapist and group leader would be to report to each other when a borderline patient says anything critical or devaluative about the other. The clinicians need to be able to contain such charges and retain the separateness of the two modalities.

Outside-the-Group Contacts

The propensity for BPD patients to want to meet outside the group sessions invariably creates tension for IPG groups. In the worst case, borderline patients who meet outside the IPG develop covert alliances that then exclude others and create an intimidating team within sessions. In the best case, such outside-the-group socialization addresses the facts that BPD patients usually have few friends and that the experience of psychiatric care, especially hospitalization, has added to their alienation from community-based peers. Because of the potential value of social networking as an outgrowth of IPG and the potential harm from a control struggle, it is usually unwise for leaders explicitly to discourage outside contact. This principle is counter to established expectations for interpersonal or dynamically based group therapies, but it accommodates some of the unique aspects of borderline patients. Instead, it is best to identify explicitly how such outside contacts can create group problems (e.g., "It is very hard to say in the group anything someone doesn't want to hear if you risk a friendship because of it"). It is realistic and sufficient to expect that IPG group members will identify and be prepared to discuss any significant contacts they have outside groups.

Summary

Interpersonal group therapies for borderline patients are a greatly underused therapeutic modality. This is due partly to the apprehensiveness many therapists feel about the behavioral management problems expected and partly to the logistics that make it difficult to get such groups up and running. Still, the transparent cost-beneficial aspects of this modality and the available empirical evidence should impel far greater use of IPGs in the future.

This chapter has described ways in which IPGs nicely complement psychodynamic therapies as usual case management practices. IPGs offer a valuable holding function through their clarity of structure and expectations and by most of their critical therapeutic processes, which can provide much of what more intensive levels of care typically offer. In addition, IPGs offer unique learning experiences that are central to borderline patients' social rehabilitation. Much more knowledge is needed to improve the ability to retain borderline patients in this modality.

References

Bacal HA: Objective relations in the group from the perspective of self-psychology, in The Different Patient in Group. Edited by Roth B, Stone W, Kibel H. Madison, CT, International Universities Press, 1990, pp 157–174

Dawson D: Therapy of the borderline client, relationship management. Can J Psychiatry 33:370–374, 1988

Dawson D, MacMillan HL: Relationship Management and the Borderline Patient. New York, Brunner/Mazel, 1993

Finn B, Shakir SA: Intensive group psychotherapy of borderline patients. Group 14(2):99–110, 1990

Flapan D: The borderline patient in group psychotherapy. Issues in Ego Psychology 6(1–2):52–57, 1983

Greenbaum DN, Pinney EL: Some comments on the role of cotherapists in group psychotherapy with borderline patients. Group 6(1):41–47, 1982

Horwitz L: A group-centered approach to group psychotherapy. Int J Group Psychother 27:423–439, 1977

Horwitz L: Indications for group psychotherapy with borderline and narcissistic patients. Bull Menninger Clin 51:248–260, 1987

Kernberg O: The treatment of patients with borderline personality organization. Int J Psychoanal 49:600–619, 1968

Kernberg O: Borderline Conditions and Pathological Narcissism. New York, Jason Aronson, 1975

Kernberg O: Severe Personality Disorders: Psychotherapeutic Strategies. New Haven, CT, Yale University Press, 1986

Koseff JW: Anchoring the self through the group: congruences, play, and the potential for change, in The Different Patient in Group. Edited by Roth B, Stone W, Kibel H. Madison, CT, International Universities Press, 1990, pp 87–114

Macaskill ND: The narcissistic core as a focus in the group therapy of the borderline patient. Br J Med Psychol 53(2):137–143, 1980

Marziali E, Munroe-Blum H: Interpersonal Group Psychotherapy for Borderline Personality Disorder. New York, Basic Books, 1994

Marziali E, Munroe-Blum H: An interpersonal approach to group psychotherapy with borderline personality disorder. J Personal Disord 9(3):179–189, 1995

Marziali E, Munroe-Blum H, McCleary L: The contribution of group cohesion and group alliance to the outcome of group psychotherapy. Int J Group Psychother 47(4):475–479, 1997

Marziali E, Munroe-Blum H, McCleary L: The effects of therapeutic alliance on the outcomes of individual and group psychotherapy with BPD. Psychotherapy Research 9(4):424–436, 1999

Monroe-Blum H, Marziali E: A controlled trial of short-term group treatment for borderline personality disorder. J Personal Disord 9(3):190–198, 1995

Nehls N: Borderline personality disorder and group therapy. Arch Psychiatr Nurs 5(3):137–146, 1991

O'Leary KM, Turner ER, Gardner DL, et al: Homogeneous group therapy of borderline personality disorder. Group 15(1):56–64, 1991

Pines M: Group analytic psychotherapy of the borderline patient. Group Analysis 11:115–126, 1978

Piper WE, Josie JS: Group treatment of personality disorders: the power of the group in the intensive treatment of personality disorders. Psychotherapy in Practice 4(4):19–34, 1998

Roth BE: The group that would not relate to itself, in The Difficult Patient in Group. Edited by Roth B, Stone W, Kibel H. Madison, CT, International Universities Press, 1990a, pp 127–156

Roth BE: Countertransference and the group therapist's state of mind, in The Difficult Patient in Group. Edited by Roth BE, Stone WN, Kibel HD. Madison, CT, International Universities Press, 1990b, pp 287–294

Segal BM, Weideman R: Outpatient groups for patients with personality disorders, in Effective Use of Group Therapy in Managed Care. Edited by MacKenzie KR. Washington, DC, American Psychiatric Press, 1995, pp 147–164

Target M, Fonagy P: Playing with reality, II: the development of psychic reality from a theoretical perspective. Int J Psychoanal 77:459–479, 1996

Wilberg T, Friis S, Karterud S, et al: Outpatient group psychotherapy: a valuable continuation treatment for patients with borderline personality disorder treated in a day hospital? a 3-year follow-up study. Nordic Journal of Psychiatry 52(3):213–221, 1998

Wong N: Combined group and individual treatment of borderline and narcissistic patients: heterogeneous versus homogeneous groups. Int J Group Psychother 30(4):389–404, 1980

Yalom ID: The Theory and Practice of Group Psychotherapy, 4th Edition. New York, Basic Books, 1995

11

Individual Psychotherapies, Phase 1

Getting Started

Introduction

Without question, individual psychotherapies have been the cornerstone of treatments for borderline patients. A recent study shows that more than 90% of those who received any treatment had individual psychotherapy (Bender et al., in press). In that study, the mean length of time in their prior psychotherapy was 51 months. Although some of what these patients called psychotherapy doubtless included what in this book is referred to as primary clinician functions or case management (see Chapter 4 of this book), Bender and colleagues' finding is all the more remarkable for having occurred within a managed care environment, where such lengths of treatment are discouraged.

Psychotherapy, as used here, refers to a modality that is not primarily designed to "stop bad things"—that is, relieve symptoms or diminish self-destructive or otherwise maladaptive behaviors. Psychotherapy is designed to "do good things": to help patients change for the better—to develop new psychological capacities. As such, *therapies* differ from *treatments.* As noted in Chapter 3 of this book, treatments (e.g., medication, diet, hospitalization) are given to patients; a patient passively receives (or resists) but does not initiate. Therapies require shared goals and at least intermittent collaboration. These abilities—that is, readiness for psychotherapy (see Table 11–1) often develop out of work with someone who had a case manager/primary clinician role. Establishing sustained collaboration (a working alliance) is itself an achievement for borderline patients (Chapter 3 of this book), signifying a beneficial change resulting from psychotherapy (see Chapter 12 of this book) or, as described elsewhere, from involvement in any one of a number of other modalities (Chapters 6–10 of this book).

TABLE 11-1. Readiness for psychotherapy

Patient	Therapist
Sees problem in self	Trained in skills that facilitate change
Seeks change in self	Agrees with patient's goals
Patient (or others) in principle can assume primary responsibility for patient's safety	Can contain patient's emotions but does not assure patient's safety

I believe it is necessary and desirable to distinguish psychotherapy from case management, since many problems in treating borderline patients derive from misguided efforts to implement psychotherapies (i.e., from having mistakenly assumed patients' readiness, with shared goals and collaborative intentions) when borderline patients need more and other forms of treatment. Individual psychotherapies may begin while borderline patients are in hospital, residential, or intensive outpatient programs. However, in the context of these higher levels of care (Chapter 4 of this book), the role of individual psychotherapy is often adjunctive, and the specific goals of psychotherapy are secondary to case management goals, which are symptom relief and behavioral management.

In reference to the five therapeutic functions described in Chapter 3 of this book, all psychotherapies involve nonspecific forms of support (e.g., concerned attention and empathy). Psychotherapies vary in their level of structure. Because most borderline patients require more structure than do other patient types, psychotherapists need to be particularly attentive to developing agreed-upon roles and goals, boundaries, and the like. The considerable within-session structure (e.g., role playing, directives, education, homework, mental exercises) typically offered in cognitive therapies makes them antiregressive and anxiety relieving. In contrast, dynamic therapies, which traditionally depend heavily on the functions of involvement and validation, are typically anxiety provoking because they offer modest amounts of structure within sessions and impose implicit demands for close emotional engagement with an important other. As is described in Chapter 12, dynamic therapies with borderline patients differ from dynamic therapies with other diagnostic groups in that they cannot rely on the patient's initiatives and that therapists need to provide more than the usual levels of structure by being particularly active and interactive. The therapeutic processes of involvement and validation (as described in Chapter 3 of this book) are what distinguish individual psychotherapies from other modalities. The sustained involvement with a trustworthy and caring other offers a powerful corrective attachment experience (discussed in Chapter 12 of this book). The validation process is particularly critical to the subject of this chapter—helping borderline patients become engaged—although validation as a technique that helps them own (i.e., experience as part of who they are) feelings and motives is also a longer-term process in other effective psychotherapies.

GETTING STARTED

The Problem of Dropouts

A series of studies initiated in the 1980s documented a very high rate of dropout from individual psychotherapies by borderline patients. Skodol et al. (1983) found that 67% of borderline patients dropped out of individual psychotherapy in 3 months. Manual-guided transference focused psychotherapies (TFP), a type of therapy developed by Kernberg, have often ended prematurely. Yeomans et al. (1993) discovered that 9 of the first 14 therapies ended prematurely (within 12 months). The dropouts scored particularly high on narcissistic themes (Horner and Diamond 1996) and on impulsivity (Yeomans et al. 1994). A subsequent report indicating that 11 of 36 patients in TFP dropped out by 3 months (Smith et al. 1995) suggests that more skills in engaging patients may have developed. In the Treatment of Depression Study, 40% of the cluster B patients dropped out within 16 weeks (Shea et al. 1990).

Several other studies done by my McLean-based research program have underscored this problem. In a study of 60 borderline patients who were beginning individual psychotherapies at McLean Hospital (Gunderson et al. 1989), we found that 25 (42%) dropped out within six months. The most common reasons were: 1) too much frustration, 2) lack of family support, and 3) logistics (travel, time, costs). As Yeomans et al. (1993) noted, the rate of dropouts in our study is lower than can reasonably be expected in outpatient settings, since some of our sample were hospitalized for all or most of the initial 6 months. It is of note that our healthier BPD patients were more likely to stay in psychotherapy if it was started in outpatient settings (not overly controlled), whereas the more severe BPD patients were more likely to remain in psychotherapies that were started during inpatient stays. In another study (Waldinger and Gunderson 1984) we surveyed senior and expert therapists who had contributed to this literature. We discovered a similar pattern. This survey indicated that in office practice, even the experts have problems keeping borderline patients engaged in psychotherapies: of 790 borderline patients, 54% continued psychotherapy beyond 6 months and only one-third (33%) went on to complete their therapy satisfactorily. These studies have made it clear that engaging borderline patients in individual psychotherapy is a difficult task and that whatever role individual psychotherapies might be able to play, it is likely to be unfulfilled because roughly half of patients will leave before its benefits can be expected. A clear implication is that before initiating psychotherapy both a patient and a therapist should carefully consider their readiness (see Table 11–1).

Little is known about what characteristics distinguish borderline patients who are suitable candidates for psychodynamic psychotherapy. Kernberg (1982) warned against the use of this modality for those with serious antisocial traits, those for whom secondary gain was very extreme, or cases in which either extreme situational instability or impulsivity would preoccupy the treatment content. He cited capacity for introspection and psychological-mindedness as assets. In a retrospective review of 299 patients with borderline personality organization (see Chapter 1 of this book), of whom 206 had DSM-III BPD, who had all received intensive (≥3 sessions a week), psychoanalytically oriented therapies, Stone (personal communication, April 1999) considered 132 of the patients ideally amenable to this modality. A disproportionate number of the less amenable were among the 206 patients who met criteria for BPD. Stone would add serious substance abuse to Kernberg's list of poor amenability factors, and like me he would emphasize the issue of motivation cited in Table 11–1.

Contracting Roles

As described in Chapter 3 of this book, the earliest (i.e., contractual) form of alliance involves an agreement between the patient and the clinician about goals and their respective roles. In an effort to engage borderline patients in psychotherapy more successfully, Kernberg's transference focused psychotherapy (TFP) formalizes the process of creating a contract (Clarkin et al. 1999; Selzer et al. 1987; Yeomans et al. 1993). This approach involves the process by which a patient and a therapist develop an agreement about the therapy's goals and their respective roles (see Table 11–2). It includes agreeing about practical issues such as fees, payment scheduling, and frequency of visits (to be discussed separately in the next section of this chapter, "Structuring

TABLE 11–2. Contracting: possible patient/therapist pre-agreements

Practicalities

Fee, schedule for payments

Schedule of visits

Attendance, missed appointments

Vacations

Crisis management

Patient's goals

Insight: to understand yourself

Change: to modify maladaptive attitudes and behaviors or to resolve conflicts or to develop new ways to attain satisfaction

Relational: to establish new capacities for sharing, attachment, empathy

Mental: new capacities to think, conceptualize

Roles and responsibilities

Therapist	Patient
Listen, observe	Discuss self
Guide, direct	Discuss therapy
Respond informatively	
Recognize limits of responsibilities	

the Therapeutic Frame: External Boundaries"). Yeomans et al. (1994) found that their therapist activity in contracting was associated with retaining patients. Akhtar (1992), like Kernberg et al. (1989), uses contracting to create an agreed-upon frame, which he refers to when problems are encountered; thus the frame does not seem arbitrary, reactive, or punitive. Linehan (1993) also gives great significance to establishing a contract for borderline patients before starting dialectical behavior therapy (DBT)—for example, establishing clear goals (target behaviors) for change and making a specific commitment to those changes, as well as a commitment to attend regularly (see Chapter 8 of this book). These clinicians may use multiple sessions, almost always a minimum of two, to reach an agreement about roles and goals before therapy begins.

Spending time on developing such a contract is consistent with one of the overall theses of this book: individual psychotherapies that rely heavily on a borderline patient's ability to control impulses and that invite affect expression often require patients to have unusual strengths, or to have attained these strengths by other types of therapy. Indeed, in the absence of such strengths, other modalities, including for example DBT or case management, are preferable.

Yeomans et al. (1993) emphasized that the contract should be explicit about the limits of the therapist's role and responsibilities; for example, "it does *not* fall within the role of the therapist to get involved in the actions of the patient's life through phone calls, emergency room visits, etc." (p. 256). This limit, reflecting Kernberg's viewpoint (Kernberg et al. 1989), stems from a conviction that a therapist's involvement with the patient's life outside sessions is frequently the cause of treatment failures. Yeomans et al. (1993, 1994) noted that the contract begins with a statement by the therapist about the (minimal) conditions under which therapy can be conducted and that this statement is followed by a dialogue that invites the patient to respond. During the dialogue, again at the therapist's initiative, problems are anticipated (e.g., coming to sessions intoxicated, intercession crises, or the patient's not wanting to leave) that are based on the patient's prior history (see Sidebar 11–1).

Sidebar 11–1: Anticipating Problems in Psychotherapy

When a new patient is known to have posed serious behavioral problems in prior therapies, Kernberg (Kernberg et al. 1989) recommended that "preconditions and structure for their management must be established" (p. 29) before treatment can take place. He cited as an example a patient who repeatedly refused to leave a former therapist's office and then had spent much of each day in that therapist's waiting room hoping to talk to her between appointments. Kernberg recommended telling such a patient, "'You will leave my office and waiting room at the end of each session. Do you understand why I am saying this [presumably it has been explained], and is this something you feel you can do?'" Should the patient voice uncertainty, the therapist is advised to continue, "'If you do not leave, I will call for help in removing you. If I have to do that three times, the treatment will end. I shall inform your parents about this so that they, like you, will know in advance that this treatment could turn out to be brief'" (p. 29).

My own approach would be quite different. The initial assumption about the failure of a prior therapy would be that the failure involved misunderstanding by the therapist as well as misconduct by the patient. With respect to this patient's prior refusal to leave, I'd start by noting that such a habit would pose a difficult problem for any new therapy too. If asked, "What will you do?" I would respond by saying, "Do? I don't know. I know that I, as well as other patients who come here, would feel haunted by your lingering presence. You probably already know that, don't you? Would you wish for that? Once you knew your presence was disturbing, would you feel like staying anyway?" If the patient indicated he or she "just" wanted to talk or see the therapist between appointments, I would quickly note that such a desire is a good and important issue to talk about and just the sort of issue that would interest me. "But," I'd add, "I know that I would not want to talk with you–or even to be observed by you–under those particular circumstances. It's important for my welfare to use my time on other issues (e.g., to attend to myself, to prepare for what's next on my schedule, to take notes, etc.)." If the patient seemed unsympathetic to this statement, I'd say, "I know I would begin to resent your disregard for my wishes and needs." If pushed further about what I would do, I'd become more insistent about my earlier inquiries: "*Why you could want to do that*–especially when you would already know that it is unwelcome and could engender resentment–would really be the question. Possibly you have needs that go beyond what psychotherapy can offer. So tell me, what would cause you to do this? Is it my privacy you wish to share, or is it your isolation you wish to avoid?" In this way, I would expect to be able to avoid setting limits (see Chapter 4 of this book), if possible.

Although the idea of a contract is generally helpful, it has some significant downsides. The most important is that most borderline patients are neither reliable nor foresighted enough to broker a meaningful contract. Contracts offer advantages when patients are being recruited into a randomized controlled psychotherapy study, as was the case when Linehan developed her contracts, because it excludes the patients who are most unlikely to succeed. Randomized controlled trials are conducted only under ideal circumstances. It is estimated that only about 10% of the patients who meet diagnostic criteria for any diagnosis will pass all other inclusion criteria and then stay compliant with psychotherapy research protocols long enough to provide outcome data (Gunderson and Gabbard 1999). This was clearly true for the study of interpersonal group therapy (Chapter 10 of this book). (These finding are a major reason why the scientific community is now giving more credibility to *effectiveness* research than to *efficacy*—that is, controlled-outcome—research.) Therefore a major problem with contracting is that for clinicians with assigned responsibilities for a borderline patient and with limited access to other modalities, formalizing a contract will often be asking the patient to agree to a plan that will prove impossible.

What is the patient seeking therapy then to do? Does the patient say OK to an impossible contract, then either feel disdain for the clinicians' naivete or feel ashamed when the contract is broken? And what is that clinician to do should the patient say that he or she cannot fulfill the contract—for example, say that he or she cannot come regularly or stay sober? The clinician cannot send the patient elsewhere; therefor he or she needs to say that although *therapy* is impossible, *treatment* is not. Hopefully, that clinician has other ways to work with the patient, such as case management (Chapter 4 of this book), psychopharmacology (Chapter 6 of this book), or family education (Chapter 9 of this book).

Although I agree with Kernberg that anticipating problems on the basis of a patient's prior history in therapies can prevent later dropping out or impasses, my approach is somewhat different (see Sidebar 11–1). I prefer to limit "contracting" to an agreement about practical issues, usually behavioral or interpersonal, and a few simple statements about my role. For example, I will say, "I see my role as helping you understand yourself. I believe that will allow you to change." I will then cite issues that arose during the evaluation that seemed to have troubled the patient and that I foresee as amenable to change. I underscore, as does Linehan (Chapter 8 of this book), that change is expected—that change is the explicit measure by which I judge, and encourage patients to judge, whether therapy is a worthwhile investment of our time and their money.

I specifically do *not* tell a prospective or new borderline patient that I will not be available except for emergencies or how they can expect me to respond to boundary issues. When a patient has had specific behaviors that potentially endanger therapy or safety, they should of course be addressed, but I would prefer the style described in Sidebar 11–1. Otherwise, I think that for therapists to actively anticipate such behaviors sets an unnecessarily defensive and adversarial tone for the therapy. Having said this, I recognize that a more formal contracting process may have advantages for therapists who don't feel confident that they can responsibly respond to whatever crises arise.

Structuring the Therapeutic Frame (External Boundaries)

It is the therapist's responsibility to establish a framework for a therapy (Spruiell 1983). These frames are the obvious signs that the therapist is a professional at work, work that involves discipline, expectations, and restraints. Therefore these frames are the skeletal representation of the therapist's boundaries, boundaries that have obvious interpersonal counterparts (as discussed in Chapter 4 of this book and elsewhere in this chapter). Components of the external boundaries are billing, scheduling, and the seating arrangement.

Bills

Some clinicians in private practice see borderline patients only if they receive a high fee, justifying this requirement on the basis of the extra difficulties they expect. High fees may be justified for these patients, but fees should be based on expertise. The therapist who is apprehensive about the difficulties expected from borderline patients can justify the high fees only if he or she uses the money to pay for supervision. Otherwise, these patients should be referred.

Getting the bill paid consistently is often a problem with borderline patients. Therapists need to distinguish tardy or missing payments that are based on a patient's general lack of organization and conscientiousness from those that are based on anger, denial, or feelings of entitlement. When payment problems are due to a general lack of responsible functioning, skill building through education, reminders, and planning may be helpful. Problems that are an expression of acting out angry or entitled feelings about the therapy (or life) require interpretation and potentially limit setting. It is often a useful option to have patients who are delinquent about their bill pay at each session so that the issue is very hard to overlook. The following vignette looks at payment problems.

Vignette

Ms. H had been in therapy for 2–3 sessions a week at a reduced fee for several years. When her increasingly intrusive demands proved unresponsive to my efforts to set limits, it led to termination of the therapy. Ms. H had built up a significant unpaid bill, but she had contracted to pay it off gradually as a condition I required before I would agree to begin seeing her once weekly. I also told her that, though it was not my usual practice, I would want her to pay her bill each session. She did this quite satisfactorily at the end of her first few sessions. I treated this as an expected and unremarkable event until at the end of the third session, she neglected to pay her bill, whereupon I took it up actively on her fourth visit. She was duly apologetic and assured me that it wouldn't be an issue. That day, a few minutes after the end of the session, she returned. She inquired about the amount and then asked for a pen with which to make out her check. I was aware that by helping her pay the bill I was extending her session, but not to do so might have excused her negligence. I told her that I was sorry that this couldn't be discussed, but I was sure she could find a pen.

It is tempting to bypass borderline patients' involvement with their bill payments when payment can more reliably be taken care of by billing others (insurers or family). Most patients ask the clinician to do this, and although I try to keep the patient as the responsible intermediary, I confess that sometimes the game isn't worth the candle. Even when billing is taken care of by others, I underscore to the patient that the issue of being financially responsible inevitably must return—that to become the respectable person the patient wants to be will require the now liberated, but "not yet adult," patient to assume such burdens.

The issue of whether to bill for missed sessions can be of particular trouble to borderline patients. Therapists differ in their standards about this, but borderline patients periodically test the clinician's willingness to make exceptions for them. Therefore therapists will find it valuable to advise patients of their policy and be prepared to maintain it. I think it is useful for most borderline patients to agree that they are expected to pay for any missed session short of emergencies (which do not include hangovers, headaches, and unexpected guests).

Frequency

Figure 11–1 and Table 11–3 show the relationship of the frequency of visits to therapeutic goals. If the therapeutic relationship is to be sufficient for the correction of unstable introjects or remission of a pattern of insecure attachments, two or more psychotherapy sessions a week are probably required, although this principle is untested. Kernberg too (Kernberg et al. 1989) advocated a minimum of twice-weekly appointments for psychodynamic therapies to be capable of affecting structural change (although his emphasis is more on the requirements for transference analysis than on the requirements for the relationship to have corrective potential). Therapies with the mandate to help patients understand themselves, a mandate on which psychodynamic therapies rest, almost always require more than once-weekly sessions. The exception to this general rule is that dynamic therapy once a week is feasible when therapists see a patient who is being "held" by attending residential or intensive outpatient services (levels of care II–IV) three or more times a week.

If, however, the therapist sees the patient once weekly in the absence of other modalities, the therapist must provide the holding functions: must get involved in crisis management, emergency phone calls, medications, and other issues of the patient's current reality—activities by the therapist that carry great meaning to the patient but are inadequately understood. This type of

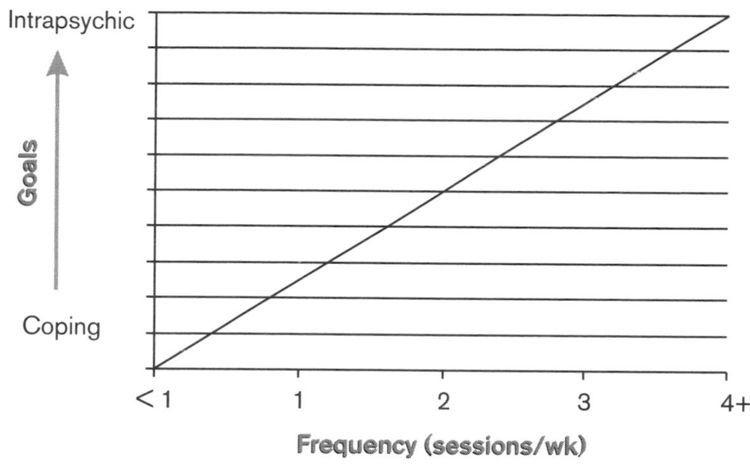

FIGURE 11–1. Relationship of frequency of sessions and treatment goals.

TABLE 11–3. Relationship between goals and frequency of sessions

Frequency (per week)	Goal
1	Management grows into support; this can be an anchor (a stabilizing influence) that helps the patient to learn and grow from life experiences.
2	Sufficient for management and "therapy": can foster change via insight, using either dynamic or cognitive strategies.
3	Optimal for dynamic therapies when examination of relationship is central. Personal growth can occur by virtue of therapy.
≥4	The patient's life is likely to revolve around therapy until growth occurs; frequency can be useful for patients who need an object but carries significant potential for being harmful.

"therapy" requires enough directives, advice, limits, and the like that the therapist's activities involve what is better labeled case management, and the therapist's role is what has been identified here (Chapter 4 of this book) as that of the primary clinician. It is misleading to think of this work as therapy, since although it has growth-enhancing potential it does not have purpose. Therefore the clinician might consider either reduced frequency or reduced duration of sessions.

For a twice-weekly outpatient psychodynamic therapy to succeed in the absence of a second modality, the patient will need to have good impulse control and low liability risks. Twice-weekly sessions are sufficient for the holding function, but this frequency often lends itself to more supportive, current-events–focused therapy for borderline patients who lack significant other supports. Three times a week is far more desirable with competent therapists for development of themes and for focusing on the therapeutic relationship. The corrective benefit of developing a trusting and secure attachment is far more likely than with twice-weekly therapies, no matter how skillfully delivered. Still, in addition to the problem of financial feasibility, such intensive therapies should be undertaken only when therapists are appropriately ready (see below). For patients, being ready for such therapy means having adequate social skills and impulse control.

Scheduling

Therapists generally try to do their best to accommodate the scheduling that patients request. Two caveats here relate to BPD. One is that sometimes borderline patients' ambivalence about assuming a responsible role combines with the idealization and dependency they feel toward their therapists to cause them too readily to schedule appointments at a therapist's convenience, at the expense of work, school, or other "get-a-life" activities. Therapists must recognize this tendency by patients and facilitate making appointments at times that are helpful to patients. A second caveat is that therapists may adopt too rigid a stance about appointments with borderline patients to avoid getting caught in control struggles or being manipulated. Both are possible, but it's better to discover and discuss such occurrences—then perhaps become firm—than to assume the worst.

Gutheil and Gabbard (1993) point out another issue, the "specialness" that patients can attribute to being the last patient in a therapist's day. Although the authors point out how this can be part of a slippery slope leading to boundary violations, what may be more generally useful in regard to borderline patients is that when a very intense transference develops, with marginal or erratic reality testing, it is best to schedule such patients during high-traffic times when there are evidences of other patients, other staff, and other interests by a therapist.

Seating

This discussion assumes that therapy appointments will take place within an office occupied by the therapist. The general principles about seating are to let the patient decide where he or she would like to sit but to retain a role as adviser. Of the three standard arrangements—across, convergent, and parallel—borderline patients may initially prefer to sit across to protect their distance. That is fine, but I encourage patients to see the convergent arrangement as a step forward in trust. (In this arrangement, the chairs are side by side, angled somewhat toward each other, so that when each person looks ahead, his or her vision converges separately from the other person's.) Psychoanalysis, where the parallel arrangement exists, is the only therapy where patients are disinvited to look at the therapist. Because of fearfulness (projections), few borderline patients would want or accept this, although counterphobic borderline patients will occasionally impulsively get on a couch if it is available (also see Sidebar 11–2).

Sidebar 11–2: What Is the Role of Psychoanalysis for BPD Patients?

Since 1968, at least 53 books have been written by psychoanalysts about treatment of borderline patients by psychoanalytic psychotherapies (data from Library of Congress database search). (There are, of course, a vastly larger number of additional journal articles and book chapters devoted to the subject.) In most instances, these books report on intensive (3 sessions a week or more) therapies conducted while sitting in the converging arrangement, with a focus on insights gained by examination of the relationship. In some instances, psychoanalysis proper (i.e., the parallel, lying-down arrangement) has been described (Abend et al. 1983; Volkan 1987). Some books have contained detailed case studies (Abend et al. 1983; Chessick 1977; Searles 1986; Volkan 1987). Of these 26 psychotherapeutic case studies, 18 patients did not meet criteria for BPD (Gunderson and Gabbard 1999), although they did have the primitive defenses and identity issues consistent with the broader concept of borderline personality organization (see Chapter 1 of this book). By DSM standards, the 18 non-BPD cases would meet criteria for other types of personality disorder, primarily narcissistic ($n = 6$) or schizoid ($n = 4$).

The psychopathology of BPD makes psychoanalysis proper relatively contraindicated. BPD patients need structure, supports, and a corrective relationship, all of which are difficult to achieve with the open-endedness of psychoanalysis. The Menninger Psychotherapy Research Project (MPRP) showed that all the borderline patients who were assigned to psychoanalysis alone got worse. (For discussion of the MPRP, see Horwitz 1982; Kernberg et al. 1972; Wallerstein 1986; and Chapter 12 of this book, including Table 12–1.) Still, borderline patients who have attained internal controls and stable role functioning may want to deepen their therapy and, in effect, expand their object relatedness by learning to examine the increased frustrations and projections that are invited by going on the couch. If they have achieved these capabilities, they are by then, arguably, no longer borderline. In my experience, such patients can then go on to achieve considerable further growth.

Fonagy (1995) referred to a borderline patient who sat on the floor of his office, paced back and forth, or lay on his couch facing him. His acceptance of these arrangements is no doubt encouraged by his training in child analysis. I view such tolerance with adult patients as dangerously regressive. It underestimates a borderline patient's expectable awareness of the behavior's inappropriateness and undermines the task orientation that therapists need to sustain. It is not that a limit needs to be set; it is that the meaning of any grossly inappropriate behavior needs to be the subject of an exploration, actively initiated by the therapist's inquiring about its meaning. I prefer to pursue such exploration, even if a patient is resistant, because of my concern for how the behavior (such as sitting on the floor) distracts from the task of understanding whether the behavior is serving useful or maladaptive functions. Limits are rarely needed (see Chapters 3 and 12 of this book).

THERAPISTS

Qualifications

This book is a testimonial to the complicating consequences of greater knowledge about treating borderline patients, specifically that the therapeutic tasks and modalities required for most patients at various points need to involve clinical staff who have differing experience, training, and personal qualities. Even within the relatively narrower group of therapeutic tasks that are needed for borderline patients who are ready to undertake individual psychodynamic therapy, the factors of experience, training, and personal qualities still need to be considered (see Fine 1989).

Regrettably, therapists vary considerably in their skill with borderline patients. Some psychiatrists, many social workers, and most nurses recognize that they "aren't good for borderline patients" and would happily avoid them (B. Pfohl, K. Silk, C. Robins, M. Zimmerman, and J. Gunderson, "Attitudes Towards Borderline PD: A Survey of 752 Clinicians," unpublished data, May 1999). However, there remain many mental health professionals who believe they are capable with borderline patients but are still not in fact good for them. This overestimation of oneself is usually based on naivete about oneself or about borderline patients, but it is sometimes based on the appeal (Main 1957) such patients can have for prospective therapists: the promise of being very helpful to someone for whom life has been unfair and whom others have failed. Being blind to one's limits can also be propelled by the very practical pressures to fill one's time, whether in private practice or in a clinic.

Pfohl et al.'s study also indicated that mental health professionals with more administrative experience in hospital or residential programs had less polarized ideas about the borderline patient's likely responsiveness to psychotherapies; and that psychologists proved distinctly, and quite uniformly, more optimistic.

Borderline patients are still likely to get into psychotherapies with clinicians whose training or experience are clearly inappropriate for the therapeutic goals (see Figure 11–2). One common example involves clinicians with experience and training only in short-term or nonintensive behavioral therapies who, often in response to borderline patients' requests, escalate the frequency of visits to three or even more times a week. Such intensity invites a regressive dependency, which then cannot be adequately used for personal growth because of the therapist's lack of training and of transference management skills. Rather, borderline patients' dependent hopes for direction, protection, or nurturance are likely to be enacted in a relationship with such therapists, who interpret these hopes as needs. Borderline patients welcome such therapies, but they conclude that being sick or otherwise victimized determines whether their hopes are fated to be fulfilled. The point here is that only psychodynamically trained therapists have a theory-based treatment that can convert intensive visits into a growth-facilitating experience. Linehan (Chapter 8 of this book) is developing a long-term individual therapy based on cognitive-behavioral principles that may prove useful. However, given the mutual problem solving orientation of cognitive-behavioral therapies, it seems unlikely that any longer-term therapy based on this approach can attain the same depth as can dynamic therapies, whose theory and technologies emphasize examination of the relationship to the therapist. Even Linehan, usually critical of analytic speculations, notes the potential role for such therapies after DBT (Linehan 1997).

Vignette

Ms. J was a 31-year-old woman with talent as a writer; she was the mother of a 3-year-old daughter. She entered therapy after the sec-

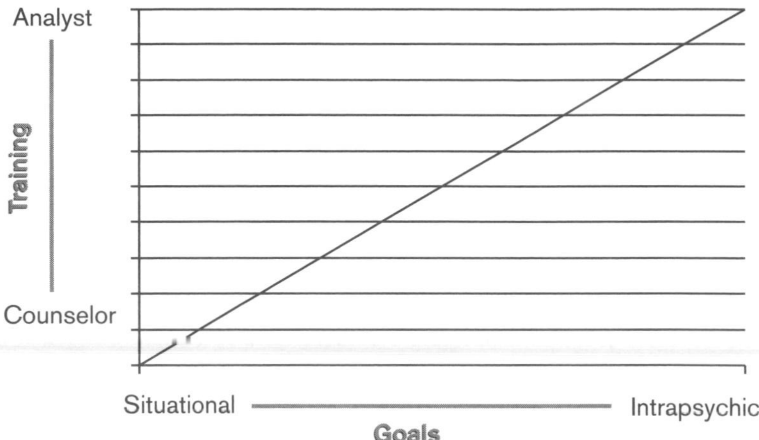

FIGURE 11–2. Relationship of therapist type and treatment goals.

ond of two hospitalizations for suicidality, during which it was uncovered that since being deserted by her husband, she had been drinking very heavily. She was assigned to begin therapy with a young female psychiatrist who had graduated from a dynamically oriented training program, where she had been recognized for her conscientiousness and supportive attitudes and where she had specialized in treatment of substance abusers. Within a few days after Ms. J's hospitalization, during meetings with her new therapist, Ms. J was without evidence of depression; indeed, she seemed outgoing and energetic.

Because of Ms. J's intellectual curiosity and her wish to get over her "habit" quickly (and because finances were not an issue), on discharge from the hospital the therapist agreed to meet with her twice weekly. Within the first week, Ms. J called twice with concerns about her depression (i.e., her sense of "badness") returning. On the second phone call, this problem gave way to talking about the patient's daughter's cough. In response to Ms. J's request, the therapist gave advice about medication, spelled out the names, and, in an attempt to be helpful, advised the patient about a pharmacy close to where she lived.

Within a few weeks, a pattern began whereby the patient came three times a week and called two or three evenings, often regarding the care of her child. The therapist, becoming resentful about the growing demands on her time, hesitantly suggested that she would charge for the phone time. When the patient got angry ("I thought you really cared," "If you want to quit, just say so," etc.), the therapist responded by dropping the issue. The therapist then felt even more resentful and sought supervision.

This vignette illustrates how neither psychiatric training nor a generally good set of skills in a related area can offer assurances to patients about selecting a qualified therapist. To become good with borderline patients requires experience and training; specifically, otherwise good therapists still need to have supervised experience with these patients. To develop the needed skills usually requires 2–3 years of fairly extensive, preferably multifaceted, contacts such as those derived from inpatient or residential settings. Psychiatrists who manage medications for many borderline outpatients usually learn the basics; such experiences make one comfortable with the management issues.

If an otherwise good therapist wants to develop psychotherapeutic skills for borderline patients but has not had case management experience, he or she will need good supervision while treating several patients over the course of the first year or two of treatment (when management issues are prominent). Only psychiatrists or psychologists who have already seen borderline patients nonintensively, with good psychodynamic supervision, and who then undertake advanced psychotherapeutic training (most often in psychoanalytic institutes, where students are immersed in dynamic thinking), are good candidates to do intensive psychoanalytic therapies with properly selected borderline patients, provided there is good supervision.

Even with intensive training or good supervision, high-frequency sessions with patients should be undertaken with caution, because personal qualities are also important. It isn't merely a matching issue: therapists who do well with one patient will do well with most. Therapists should not take on borderline patients without consideration of the issues about the patients and themselves listed in Table 11–4.

Note that important exceptions to these cautions about initiating individual psychotherapies involve clinicians in training. Many are (as I was) sufficiently apprehensive or offended by borderline patients that they will not voluntarily start psychotherapy with these patients if Table 11–4 is used as a measure of readiness. However, trainees who want to become good psychotherapists and who have good supervision available should embrace the opportunity to work with such patients, who offer exceptional learning experiences. Therapists who do not find interesting the issues that surround the treatment of borderline patients (action, dependency, anger) or who do not ac-

TABLE 11–4. Reasons for a therapist's taking a borderline patient

A therapist's readiness to take a borderline patient should involve the following considerations:
This patient is interesting (challenging, touching, confusing, attractive, needy, smart, etc.).
I believe the patient can change (for the better).
This is essential, not adjunctive, therapy—a serious responsibility for which I have time and energy.
The patient is suffering (hostilities, acting out, and symptoms are there for a reason).
I believe that I can help, but that cannot be assured (both beliefs are presumably based on experience).
I'm prepared to persevere despite the expectation of doing things I don't want, being criticized or hurt, possibly failing.
I know that if treatment doesn't seem helpful, I will seek consultation, and I can discontinue. (The therapy is not a lifetime contract for the patient or for me.)
My life is good. (Life outside my role as a therapist is reasonably fulfilling.)

tually like such patients will be unlikely to do well with them; these therapists are unlikely to find the exceptional borderline patients with whom they will be able to work well.

The vignette about Ms. J also illustrates the pressures that borderline patients bring to bear on inexperienced, naive, or untrained therapists. Borderline patients welcome anyone's attention and support, and they are willing to give up ego or social functions in the service of feeling taken care of (the issue of regression is discussed in Chapter 2 of this book and Sidebar 12–3). Patients cannot be relied on to make an informed selection of a therapist that is based on who can help them to change. As described in Chapter 13, the section titled "Development of Specialists and Special Services," I think specialists should be identified (also see Chapter 12 of this book).

Qualities

Some qualities cannot be taught, or untaught. This explains why therapists with very different training and theories can become excellent therapists (see Sidebar 11–3). One study (Rosenkrantz and Morrison 1992) concluded that therapists who are high on "anaclitic, depressive and fusion tendencies" do poorly, whereas those who are "high boundary" therapists function well. In my experience, therapists who do well are usually reliable, somewhat adventurous, action oriented, and good-humored. This translates into being active and responsive. Positively unworkable are therapists who are effete, genteel, or controlling.

Sidebar 11–3: Listening to Kernberg or Linehan: Can Charisma Cure BPD?

Listening to Kernberg, clinicians aspiring to treat borderline patients could feel convinced that clinicians' ability would depend on their comfort with aggression (their own and others') and their ability to identify and interpret unrecognized motivations or conflicts and might, in addition, be increased by completing psychoanalytic training.

Listening to Linehan, clinicians with the same hopes could conclude that to attain the same goal would depend on their identifying problems the patient wants to change and having mastered the comparatively clear DBT theory and skills; mastery in this instance would require attendance at several intensive weeks of workshops and would, in addition, be assisted by more extensive training in cognitive-behavioral therapy.

Still, both these renowned experts have had many otherwise capable students who, after receiving the training, still cannot treat borderline patients well. Many of the clinicians who have attended Linehan's rigorous training are still unable to conduct therapy with high levels of competence. Similarly, efforts to train therapists to do Kernberg's manual-guided transference focused psychotherapy (Kernberg et al. 1989) have also been frustrated by the discovery that most therapists fail to adhere to the prescribed practices (Yeomans et al. 1992). These difficulties within research settings confirm what I've observed over the course of my career: many therapists are not good with borderline patients. So maybe the success of both Kernberg and Linehan with borderline patients is not attributable to either their theories or their training.

Perhaps the secret lies in what has been disparagingly called the nonspecific components of what they offer. Both Kernberg and Linehan are charismatic. They are authoritative: they embody confidence, clarity, forcefulness, and certainty. Swenson (1989) noted that both meet "the patient's emotional intensity or lability head on with a steady emotional intensity of their own. Both therapists give the patient the feeling that they are present, engaged, and indestructible" (p. 32). No doubt patients are transported by the same impulse to accept what these therapists say that has led many professionals to try to do as they say. Moreover, both Kernberg and Linehan seem undaunted by controversy, perhaps even enjoying debate and challenge. Both welcome opportunities to demarcate their positions and to clarify how their views may be distinguished from the views of others. No doubt patients are impressed by these therapists' efforts to make themselves clear and by their attention to fine distinctions. And both are prepared to share their viewpoints, whether sought or not. Patients of either Kernberg or Linehan, I believe, feel confident that their opinions, judgments, or decisions will be heard and responded to–what Swenson summarized as feeling "emotionally held" (p. 32).

Attentive, challenging, and responsive: it is my impression these same qualities distinguish others who are excellent therapists with borderline patients. Certainly, these qualities seem valuable in getting borderline patients engaged, but the long-term processes by which it is possible for BPD to be cured (see Chapter 12 of this book) are no doubt where differences in theory and training can be critical.

Many borderline patients have strong preferences for one gender or the other, but their reasons bear exploration. It may be that they associate femininity with qualities of closeness and empathy—admittedly more common in females, but hardly unheard of in males, especially those who have chosen the helping professions. It may be that patients associate masculinity with protectiveness and directiveness—again, qualities more common in males, but hardly confined to them. As an approach to finding a therapist, gender is far less useful than the desired personal qualities.

So how does a borderline patient select a good therapist? It isn't easy (see Table 11–5). Patients should be cautious, since many therapists are neither qualified to treat them nor really interested in their issues. As discussed previously in the chapter, certain therapist qualities also seem almost universally desirable for borderline patients. For example, therapists need to like working with issues of action, anger, and dependency.

TABLE 11–5. How a borderline patient should choose a therapist

The patient should ask himself or herself these questions about the therapist:
Do I want to be involved with this person? (Do I like him or her?)
Does the therapist seem to want to get involved with me? (Does he or she seem interested in me?)
Can I learn something from the therapist? (Does he or she seem confident, ready to convey what he or she knows?)
Is the therapist able to help with what I want? (Does he or she have the needed training, skills, and experience?)
Is the therapist sufficiently reliable, conscientious, and durable? (Does he or she seem fragile, unpredictable, or restless?)

ENGAGEMENT

In the first phase of treatment with a borderline patient, the therapist's goal should be primarily to engage the patient. How a prospective therapist manages the issues discussed earlier about contracting and establishing a framework, as well as the therapist's personal qualities, are important determinants of whether a patient becomes engaged. Still, engagement per se involves moving the alliance from the contractual type described earlier to the relational type (to be discussed in Chapter 12 of this book). The earliest indications of patient engagement involve the perception that the therapist is likable or wants to be helpful (Alexander et al. 1993). Engagement is unlikely when the therapist is described as "no personality," "blah," "nothing to say." Research indicates that even by 6 weeks of therapy, patients should indicate an overall positive relationship with a new therapist and a hopefulness about benefiting from the therapy (Gunderson et al. 1997; Horwitz et al. 1996). Therapies that fail to get this type of start may warrant consultation.

The three components of helping the patient becoming engaged are

- Invoking the patient's attachment to the therapist
- Invoking the patient's hopes for change
- Invoking the patient's interest in the process of self-disclosure and self-examination (i.e., the learning process)

As noted in Chapter 6 of this book, a therapist who administers medications often can jump-start a borderline patient's hopes for change and his or her confidence in the therapist's intention to be helpful. During these initial few months, it is very useful for the therapist to be quite active in structuring the sessions, encouraging the patient with tasks such as writing an autobiography between sessions, and giving the patient encouragement to think about what they have discussed. Psychodynamic therapists who might otherwise expect the patient to take the lead can learn from cognitive-behavioral therapists, who have found that a directive, businesslike approach that purposely does not evoke intense transference is useful in alliance building (see Chapter 8 of this book). The therapist should convey an interest in the psychotherapeutic task and implicitly—sometimes explicitly—offer hope that the patient is capable of change and capable of having a more satisfactory future. With these supports, a borderline patient begins to develop both a realistic hope that change can occur, albeit slowly, and an appreciation of the therapist's commitment to him or her as well as to the task. Table 12–4 sets forth how these developments relate to and set the stage for later changes.

The basic axiom of dynamic therapies, to let positive transference alone but to be active about early signs of negative transference, applies to borderline patients. Still, when borderline patients begin treatment with extreme idealization and optimism about therapy or the therapist, these tendencies should not be mistaken for a sign either that they are committed to the treatment tasks or that their hopes are connected to the need for personal change. Indeed, whenever such idealization and optimism become evident, I conscientiously and good-naturedly demur in order to diminish the risk that the inevitable disillusionment will be too bitter. This is similar to Dawson and MacMillan's (1993) warning about being "too therapeutic" (see Chapter 4 of this book), but less extreme. Even the patients who begin their treatment with skepticism and devaluation should by 6 months have acquired some hope that "therapy might help," a hope that derives primarily from the experience of the therapist's involvement and borrows heavily on the therapist's convictions.

Borderline patients are very sensitive to whether a prospective therapist seems interested in them. For most borderline patients, lack of interest translates into rejection and being unwanted. The more fearful about lack of interest the patient is, the more sensitive to signals of inattention he or she will be; for the patient, signs of a therapist's lack of interest are worse even than signs of being misunderstood. At signs of inattention, some borderline patients will become silent and withdrawn. Others will become irritated and say "Pay attention," or "You're not listening, are you?" or demand, "What are you thinking about?" These protests are clear and meaningful requests that therapists should attend to by becoming more active and interactive. Therapists whom borderline patients want to return to (i.e., become engaged with) are those whose interest in them was manifest by being reactive and interactive: patients call them "all there," a "real person." These qualities are interpreted by borderline patients as a therapist's "likability" and "helpfulness," the qualities that best determine whether patients will want to become engaged (Alexander et al. 1993).

Likability is most closely related to a therapist's level of activity and interest. It is usually evident in the small, off-the-record exchanges at the start or end of sessions, during which patients and therapists often exchange comments on things like weather, clothing, transportation, or the news. Common values should become apparent through such informal comments as well as in relation to the patient's description of his or her life. It is useful for therapists to disclose common values, attitudes, and the like in the service of developing the relational alliance (Chapter 3 of this book).

In the early 1990s, leaders from McLean Hospital and Wellesley College's Stone Center (Jordan et al. 1991) developed a psychotherapeutic approach based on women's psychology that proved instructive about how to engage borderline patients in therapy. This encouraged many therapists, especially female psychologists, to bring an openly caring (empathic, validating, nonconfrontational) approach to borderline patients. This approach, as shown by Linehan, could effectively help patients become attached; and it diminished, I believe, the usual frequency of early dropouts. Unlike Linehan, the McLean–Stone Center therapists placed their contribution within the context of the earlier clinical theory by Kohut (1971) and its application to BPD by Adler (see Chapter 12 of this book). Unfortunately, the virtues of this approach by Stone Center therapists brought with it three problems: 1) many of the therapists were not trained in case management (i.e., primary clinician) tasks (as described in Chapter 4), 2) some unnecessarily vilified male therapists, and 3) in my opinion, they did not take advantage of what is useful from earlier contributions to theory and technique (most notably by Kernberg) that can help borderline patients own and use their aggression. What the empathic, validating approach does is ignite an idealizing transference, which will encourage engagement with therapists of either gender. But whether the therapy facilitates change (via a corrective attachment and new learning) depends on a therapist's other techniques.

Several characteristics of borderline patients, unrelated to a therapist's interventions or style, can affect whether they become engaged in therapy. Borderline patients who start within longer-term baseline hospitalizations or who have had more prior psychotherapy are more likely to become engaged in further psychotherapy (Gunderson et al. 1989). This observation may reflect the more general observation that psychotherapy patients with higher education and higher socioeconomic status are less likely to drop out (Garfield 1994); it may also mean that borderline patients learn from past experience to become more tolerant of the limits of therapy. In any event, the more general principle of split treatment (Chapter 4 of this book)—that is, the use of a second collaborating and complementary modality to help contain splits, projections, and flight—can greatly enhance the likelihood of engagement in psychotherapy.

SUMMARY

This chapter has discussed the conditions that can determine whether psychotherapy with a borderline patient should be initiated and, if so, what the conditions are that will allow it to succeed. Hopefully, readers will recognize that, although exceptions to every rule exist, it makes no sense to ignore probabilities. Clearly, not all borderline patients are candidates for psychotherapy. Capability and motivation need to be assessed. How the therapy framework is established is of critical importance, and therapists should have a good understanding of issues of scheduling, billing, and agreed-upon goals to give the venture the best chance of success. Of particular importance is to recognize how the framework should be fitted to the patient's needs and to the capabilities of both patient and therapist. It is also clear that not everyone can treat borderline patients well; therapists should consider their capabilities. Finally, intensive schedules of psychotherapy should be offered only by qualified professionals.

References

Abend SM, Porder MS, Willick MS: Borderline Patients: Psychoanalytic Perspectives. New York, International Universities Press, 1983

Akhtar S: Broken structures: Severe personality disorders and their treatment. Northvale, NJ, Jason Aronson, 1992

Alexander LB, Barber JP, Luborsky L, et al: On what bases do patients choose their therapists? Journal of Psychotherapy practice and Research 2(2):135–146, 1993

Bender DS, Dolan RT, Skodol AE, et al: Treatment utilization by patients with personality disorders. Am J Psychiatry (in press)

Chessick RD: Intensive Psychotherapy of the Borderline Patient. New York, Jason Aronson, 1977

Clarkin JF, Yeomans FE, Kernberg OF: Psychotherapy for Borderline Personality. New York, Wiley, 1999

Dawson D, MacMillan HL: Relationship Management and the Borderline Patient. New York, Brunner/Mazel, 1993

Fine R (ed): Current and Historical Perspectives on the Borderline Patient. New York, Brunner/Mazel, 1989

Fonagy P: Playing with reality: the development of psychic reality and its malfunction in borderline personalities. International Journal of Psycho-Analysis 76(Pt 1):39–44, 1995

Garfield SL: Research on client variables in psychotherapy, in Handbook of Psychotherapy and Behavior Change. Edited by Bergin AE, Garfield SL. New York, Wiley, 1994

Gunderson JG: The borderline patient's intolerance of aloneness: insecure attachments and therapist availability. Am J Psychiatry 153(6):752–758, 1996

Gunderson JG, Gabbard GO: Making the case for psychoanalytic therapies in the current psychiatric environment. J Am Psychoanal Assoc, 1999

Gunderson JG, Frank AF, Ronningstam EF, et al: Early discontinuance of borderline patients from psychotherapy. J Nerv Ment Dis 177(1):38–42, 1989

Gunderson JG, Najavits LM, Leonhard C, et al: Ontogeny of the therapeutic alliance in borderline patients. Psychotherapy Research 7(3):301–309, 1997

Gutheil TG, Gabbard GO: The concept of boundaries in clinical practice: theoretical and risk-management dimensions. Am J Psychiatry 150(2):188–196,1993

Horner MS, Diamond D: Object relations development and psychotherapy dropout in borderline outpatients. Psychoanalytic Psychology 13(2):205–223, 1996

Horwitz L: Clinical and projective assessments of borderline patients. Paper presented at a symposium, The Borderline Patient: A Multiaxial View, Department of Psychiatry, University of Miami School of Medicine, Key Biscayne, FL, 1982

Horwitz L, Gabbard GO, Allen JG, et al: Borderline Personality Disorder: Tailoring the Psychotherapy to the Patient. Washington, DC, American Psychiatric Press, 1996

Jordan J, Kaplan A, Miller J, et al: Women's Growth in Connection: Writings from the Stone Center. New York, Guilford, 1991

Kernberg OF: The psychotherapeutic treatment of borderline personalities, in Psychiatry 1982: Annual Review (Review of Psychiatry series, Vol 1. Grinspoon L, series ed.) Washington, DC, American Psychiatric Press, 1982, pp 470–486

Kernberg OF, Burstein ED, Coyne L, et al: Psychotherapy and psychoanalysis (final report of the Menninger Foundation's Psychotherapy Research Project). Bull Menninger Clin 36:1–275, 1972

Kernberg O, Selzer M, Koeningsberg HW, et al: Psychodynamic Psychotherapy of Borderline Patients. New York, Basic Books, 1989

Kohut H: The Analysis of the Self. New York, International Universities Press, 1971

Linehan MM: Cognitive-Behavioral Treatment of Borderline Personality Disorder. New York, Guilford, 1993

Linehan MM: Theory and treatment development and evaluation: reflections on Benjamin's "models" for treatment. J Personal Disord 11(4):325–335, 1997

Main T: The ailment. Br J Med Psychol 30:129–145, 1957

Rosenkrantz J, Morrison TL: Psychotherapist personality characteristics and the perception of self and patients in the treatment of borderline personality disorder. J Clin Psychol 48(4):544–553, 1992

Searles HF: My Work with Borderline Patients. Northvale, NJ, Jason Aronson, 1986

Selzer MA, Koenigsberg HW, Kernberg OF: The initial contract in the treatment of borderline patients. Am J Psychiatry 144(7):927–930, 1987

Shea MT, Pilkonis PA, Beckham E, et al: Personality disorders and treatment outcome in the NIMH Treatment of Depression Collaborative Research Program. Am J Psychiatry 147:711–718, 1990

Skodol AE, Buckley P, Charles E: Is there a characteristic pattern to the treatment history of clinic outpatients with borderline personality? J Nerv Ment Dis 171(7):405–410, 1983

Smith TE, Koenigsberg HW, Yeomans FE, et al: Predictors of dropout in psychodynamic psychotherapy of borderline personality disorder. Journal of Psychotherapy Practice and Research 4(3):205–213, 1995

Spruiell V: The rules and frames of the psychoanalytic situation. Psychoanal Q 52(1): 1–33, 1983

Swenson C: Kernberg and Linehan: two approaches to the borderline patient. J Personal Disord 3(1):26–35, 1989

Volkan VD: Six Steps in the Treatment of Borderline Personality Organization. New York, Jason Aronson, 1987

Waldinger RJ, Gunderson JG: Completed psychotherapies with borderline patients. Am J Psychother 38(2):190–202, 1984

Wallerstein R: Forty-Two Lives in Treatment. New York, Guilford, 1986

Yeomans F, Selzer M, Clarkin J: Studying the treatment contract in intensive psychotherapy with borderline patients. Psychiatry 56(3):254–263, 1993

Yeomans FE, Gutfreund J, Selzer MA, et al: Factors related to drop-outs by borderline patients: treatment contract and therapeutic alliance. Journal of Psychotherapy Practice and Research 3(1):16–24, 1994

12

Individual Psychotherapies, Phases 2, 3, and 4

Processes of Change

THE IDENTIFICATION OF BORDERLINE personality psychopathology arose out of observations from within psychoanalytically oriented treatment settings (Chapter 1 of this book), and the term *borderline* became widely used only after—I think because—Kernberg (1968) and Masterson (1971) promoted hopes that skilled, intensive, long-term psychodynamic psychotherapies could bring about curative, basic structural changes. In the ensuing 30 years the literature has been flooded with articles and books on the problems, processes, and potential for such therapies. Psychotherapies remain central to most treatment plans. As noted, during what was identified (Chapter 11 of this book) as the first phase, the therapist's early tasks usually involve case management activities. This chapter discusses the processes within long-term therapeutic relationships that allow internal psychological changes of a more basic, structural, and enduring nature to occur. Mirroring the changes that have occurred within psychoanalytic conceptions about processes of change (Stern et al. 1998), the psychoanalytic literature relevant to borderline patients has moved from ego-psychology or object relations theories and techniques into *relational* perspectives that have attached more significance to processes of engagement and attachment.

Therapies can start at basically any level of care, but as noted above (and in Chapters 3, 4, and 11 of this book), psychoanalytic therapies directed at growth should not be confused with case management. Psychotherapies intended to bring about psychological growth require readiness and motivation by patients, training and experience by therapists, and a frequency of two or more sessions per week (Chapter 11 of this book). Regardless of whether psychotherapy is initiated when a borderline patient is in level I or level II care, it is primarily an office practice modality whose distinguishing advantages rely on a duration of at least a year.

With respect to the framework of the five therapeutic functions described in Chapter 3 of this book, those that are most specific to psychoanalytic therapies are involvement and validation. Involvement refers to the process by which a level of closeness, trust, and intimacy develops that exceeds what patients have previously experienced and that gives patients new abilities to form such relationships with others. Validation refers to the process by which patients develop recognition and acceptance of themselves as unique. It develops out of increased awareness and understanding of oneself. This function has special significance for borderline patients, whose recognition of feelings or motives is impaired and whose sense of self is often confused or distorted.

In this chapter I review some aspects of the extensive literature on individual psychotherapies and then delineate two major processes of change: those related to relational experiences and those related to learning. These psychotherapeutic processes are sometimes referred to respectively as corrective attachment experiences and as insight (or as changes in cognitive schema). I then identify three phases of change that allow therapists and patients to recognize whether therapies are progressing or have reached an impasse. Common types of impasse in each phase are described.

Prior Literature

Outcome Studies

A series of naturalistic prospective follow-along studies have explored what benefits can be expected from long-term psychoanalytic therapies (see Table 12–1).

The first and most recognized by far of these studies is the Menninger Psychotherapy Research Project (Kernberg 1972; Wallerstein 1986). The majority of the 42 patients in this naturalistic prospective study suffered from severe personality disorders. In the study design, patients were assigned to receive psychoanalysis, expressive psychotherapy (meaning investigative, in-

TABLE 12–1. Summary of outcome studies

Study	Sample	Type of psychotherapy	Therapists
Menninger Psychotherapy Research Project (Horwitz 1982; Kernberg et al. 1972; Wallerstein 1986)	N = 16 who met criteria for BPO and were referred for long-term treatment with intermittent use of hospitalization	Assigned to receive either "expressive," i.e., psychoanalysis (n = 6) or psychoanalytic (n = 5) psychotherapy or "supportive" (n = 5) on basis of clinical judgment. Frequency = ≥3/wk for expressive and 1/wk for supportive.	MD and PhD with extensive experience
Northwestern University Department of Psychology (Howard et al. 1986)	N = 23 outpatient "borderline-psychotic" subjects from various study samples	Unstandardized, "generic"; most patients seen ≤ once weekly by trainees	Unstated, many
McLean Psychotherapy Engagement Project (Gunderson et al. 1989, 1997; Najavits and Gunderson 1995).	N = 60 hospitalized patients meeting DIB/DSM criteria for BPD; all were starting a new psychotherapy	"Psychodynamic" without standardization of technique, theory, or intensity; most were seen once weekly	MDs and PhDs of varying experience, including trainees
New South Wales (Stevenson and Meares 1992, 1999; Meares et al. 1999).	N = 30 outpatients meeting DSM-IV criteria for BPD	Standardized, "self-psychological" with intensive supervision; frequency was twice weekly	MD and PhD trainees

Note. DIB = Diagnostic Interview for Borderline Patients.

sight oriented, emotion generating), or supportive psychotherapy (meaning directive, defense-reinforcing, emotion inhibiting).

Hospitalization was a concurrent modality for most patients in the course of the treatments. Horwitz (1982) later attempted to draw more specific conclusions about the outcomes of a subgroup of 16 patients of the original 42 who might qualify for a diagnosis of borderline personality. This subgroup was identified by the presence of a poorly formed identity, nonspecific evidence of ego weakness, and intrusion of primary-process thinking in their psychological tests. Of these 16 patients, 5 were considered successes, 5 were considered unchanged, and 6 were thought to have become worse. The type of treatment the subgroup sample received was divided equally between psychoanalysis and psychotherapy. All 6 borderline patients who got worse had received psychoanalysis. The two others who received psychoanalysis did well, but they were considered to have higher levels of ego strength. All 5 of the successful outcomes occurred in patients who had received psychotherapy (presumably supportive-expressive). Nevertheless, 4 of these 5 still had evidence of primary-process thinking on psychological tests conducted at the follow-up evaluation.

A second set of studies, in which I participated, initiated at McLean Hospital in the 1980s, was prompted by the question whether it would be possible to evaluate the efficacy of psychoanalytic therapy through controlled outcome research. Drawing on lessons learned from a previous experience in conducting such a study with schizophrenic subjects (Gunderson et al. 1984; Stanton et al. 1984), we were determined as a first step to document that major structural benefits occur from psychoanalytic psychotherapy and to identify how often and how long such benefits take. As noted in Chapter 11 of this book, Waldinger and I found that even expert, published psychoanalytic therapists rarely (10%) judged their therapies with borderline patients to have ended successfully (Waldinger and Gunderson 1984). Success meant change from a moderately severe level of social impairment to modest impairment—that is, having become only minimally self-destructive and having taken on a functional role.

The second approach to this study took place at McLean, where many therapists, like those in the Menninger study, had been practicing intensive long-term therapies for many years. When those staff were invited to identify cases that they felt had gone on to curative changes, surprisingly few could do so. Five cases were subsequently detailed in case reports (Waldinger and Gunderson 1989). This study showed that borderline patients could undergo curative changes in long-term therapies (4–7 years). It was important to document that this was possible, although a strong causal connection could not be made. Still, the more instructive finding was to discover how rare such instances are.

The third part of this investigation was a naturalistic prospective study with unselected therapists of variable experience. This study documented a high frequency of dropouts from therapy (Gunderson et al. 1989), a decline in suicidality (Sabo et al. 1995), and an overall variability in outcomes (Najavits and Gunderson 1995). As a result of these studies, we concluded that even with senior, experienced therapists, major successes were unusual and took many years, and that, without pilot data that could identify what qualities of therapist and borderline patient made effectiveness possible, controlled outcome research on psychoanalytic therapy with borderline patients was not feasible.

A third outcome study was reported by Howard et al. (1986) as part of a meta-analysis in which an overall relationship between number of sessions and successful outcome was documented. A smaller sample at his own clinic, 23 patients grouped as "borderline-psychotic," required a significantly greater number of sessions to achieve improvement than did patients who were depressed or anxious. In what was usually once-weekly therapies, about half of the "borderline-psychotic" sample who remained in therapy had improved by 6 months, about 75% by 1 year, and nearly 90% by 2 years. Although encouraging, this study has a nonstandardized threshold for improvement and does not, of course, identify what percent of patients discontinued therapy because they were not improving.

The fourth and most important major outcome study came from New South Wales, Australia. Stevenson and Meares (1992) conducted a naturalistic prospective study of the effectiveness of psychodynamic psychotherapy that is decidedly more encouraging than what was observed in either the Menninger or the McLean study. The therapies were conducted twice weekly by young trainees who received extensive supervision from audiotapes. The 30 borderline patients were quite dysfunctional and had failed in prior therapies. After 12 months of therapy, there were follow-ups at 1 year and 5 years (Meares et al. 1999). Of note is that only 16% dropped out—the same rate as in Linehan's study of DBT—testifying to a very successful engagement process. At the 1-year follow-up there was a significant decline in the mean number of DSM-IV BPD criteria met by these patients (from 17.4 to 10.5), and 30% of treated patients no longer met the threshold for BPD diagnosis. There was a dramatic decrease in visits to medical professionals (from 3.50 to 0.47 per month), episodes of self-harm (from 3.77 per year to 0.83 per year), hospital admissions (from 1.77 to 0.73 per year), and the mean number of months spent as inpatients (from 3 to 1.47 months). It is of note that, unlike those treated with DBT (Chapter 7 of this book), the patients had significant and sustained reductions in anxiety and depressive symptoms. Improvements were maintained on follow-up to 5 years. The cost of treatment for the sample in the year prior to treatment was 16 times greater than in the year of therapy (Stevenson and Meares 1999).

This study was done without a control group, but the rather remarkable results held up when the outcomes were compared to those for another 30 BPD patients, who were on a waiting list for a year before receiving treatment as usual, consisting of supportive or cognitive therapy and crisis management (Meares et al. 1999). The low frequency of dropouts is far better than was found in the other research on outpatient psychotherapies (cited above and detailed in Chapter 10 of this book). Moreover, the high quality of the outcome is dramatic, consistent with or better than that observed in the widely cited DBT (see Chapter 7 of this book) and seemingly much better than observed in either the McLean study (Najavits and Gunderson 1995) or the Menninger study (Horwitz 1982). These results are even more notable considering the youth and inexperience of the therapists (contrasting with what is recommended in Chapter 11 of this book) and considering that the therapies were discontinued successfully at 1 year (contrasting with what I will recommend in this chapter). Replication with a control group is the much-awaited next stage.

Currently under way is research in psychodynamic or psychoanalytic therapies with borderline patients that will shed further light on the value and the role of these therapies. Of special note have been the impressive efforts to manualize Kernberg's particular transference focused psychotherapy (TFP). The effort began with the still theory-laden and clinically rich draft of a manual published by Kernberg and colleagues (1989).The draft then underwent considerable further development, giving way a decade later to a more pragmatic, specific, and operationalized version (Clarkin et al. 1999). This effort was led by Clarkin, a distinguished psychotherapy researcher. Perhaps pushed by the example set by Linehan for DBT (see Table 8–1), TFP has also now identified a hierarchy of treatment goals. As shown in Table 12–2, like DBT, TFP's hierarchy begins by addressing suicidal threats—also including violent behaviors—and then moves to other treatment-interfering behaviors. As a result of this manualization of two years of TFP, this form of psychoanalytic psychotherapy is now uniquely capable of having its efficacy tested.

A major project in Stockholm is now under way that compares the bene-

TABLE 12–2. Hierarchy of targets for transference focused psychotherapy

1. Suicide or homicide
2. Overt threats to treatment continuity
   - Dishonesty or deliberate withholding
   - Contract breaches
   - In-session acting out
   - Between-session acting out
   - Nonaffective or trivial themes

Source. Adapted from Clarkin et al. 1999.

fits from 2 years of Kernberg's TFP (Clarkin et al. 1999) to the benefits of 2 years of DBT therapy. Both are manual guided, and thus far it has been established that training therapists to achieve satisfactory levels of adherence and competence represents a major problem (R. Weinryb, personal communication, April 1999; J. F. Clarkin, personal communication, November 1999). As with prior research in which different types of similarly intensive psychotherapy are compared, the outcomes seem likely to be similar. Still, as noted in Chapter 8, it would be validating for therapists with either dynamic or behavioral convictions to see some specificity in the relationship between outcome and goals: namely, that the DBT sample show added benefits in behavioral improvement and that the TFP sample show added benefits in interpersonal outcomes. Almost certainly this study will document the benefits of carefully delivered therapies by motivated and skilled therapists. Equally certain is that Swedish borderline patients will benefit from having these well-trained therapists as a nucleus who can teach others and thereby elevate the overall standards of psychotherapeutic care.

Psychoanalytic Contributions

In a scholarly review of the literature (by then already extensive) on psychoanalytic psychotherapies for BPD, Waldinger (1987) identified eight issues by which virtually all contributors distinguished effective therapies (see Table 12–3). Little has been learned that would revise that summary. Notably, the need for therapist activity is underscored; it is now clearly structured in case management activities (Chapter 5 of this book), in psychopharmacology (Chapter 6 of this book), and in the cognitive-behavioral therapies (Chapter 7 of this book)—all of which are important aspects of the early phases of treatment.

It would be misleading to conclude from the consensus features cited in Table 12–3 that major disagreements do not exist. In the 1970s and early 1980s, many conferences were held featuring expert psychoanalytic therapists who detailed competing theories and techniques that they felt were most effective. None was more widely attended than those featuring Kernberg and Adler (see Sidebar 12–1 and Table 12–4). During this period, the enthusiasm for the value of psychoanalytic therapies with borderline patients was at its peak. In a thoughtful commentary, Aronson (1985) pointed out that the authors responsible for this peak were all narrowly analytic and rarely focused on issues of diagnosis, attrition, treatment failure, or limitations of their model. Currently, although the existing research (Stevenson and Meares 1992 and the Menninger Psychotherapy Research Project [see above]) has lent support to the claims of the Adler/Kohut side of these debates, it is Kernberg's TFP that is the subject of by far the largest randomized controlled trial now under way.

TABLE 12–3. Distinguishing characteristics of effective intensive psychodynamic therapies

1. Stability of the framework of treatment
2. Increased activity of the therapist
3. Tolerance of the patient's hostility
4. Making self-destructive behaviors ungratifying
5. Establishing a connection between actions and feelings in the present
6. Blocking acting-out behaviors
7. Focusing early clarifications and interpretations in the here and now
8. Careful attention to countertransference feelings

Source. Adapted from Waldinger 1987.

TABLE 12–4. The debate

Kernberg	Adler/Kohut
(Transference analysis)	(Corrective relationships)
Confront	Validate
Limit	Avail yourself
Interpret	Empathize
Aggression intrinsic	Aggression reactive
Conflict model	Deficit model

Sidebar 12–1: The Debate of the 1970s

Kernberg's seminal papers on borderline patients (Kernberg 1967, 1968) bridged object relations theory (the concepts of introjection, self-representation, projective identification) and instinct theory (vicissitudes of basic aggressive drives). About the same time, Heinz Kohut's (1971) seminal contributions to self psychology (with its concepts of mirroring, selfobjects, and transmuting internalizations) became a counterpoint to Kernberg's theories about development and therapeutic technique. These theoretical contributions became part of a larger intellectual debate within psychoanalytic circles. Within the realm of psychopathology, Kohut's concepts became tied to pathological narcissism.

Yet Kernberg's construct of borderline personality organization subsumed what Kohut called pathological narcissism, and Kohut's concept of pathological narcissism offered different ways to explain borderline phenomena such as rage, feelings of entitlement, and intolerance of aloneness.

Gerald Adler, with Dan Buie (Adler and Buie 1979; Buie and Adler 1982) and in his own writing (Adler 1975, 1986), championed the application of Kohut's self psychology to the psychotherapeutic care of patients with BPD. As a result, the 1980s were marked by numerous, highly publicized, and widely discussed debates between those who stood by Kernberg's theoretical and clinical views and those who aligned themselves with Kohut and Adler. Table 12–4 characterizes the clinical differences.

Behind these debates was a fundamental difference: whether the inappropriate or excessive expressions of anger shown by borderline or narcissistic patients were understandable as reactive to insults to a fragile self (i.e., narcissistic injury) or as inadequately modulated expressions of an aggressive drive.

The theoretical and clinical controversy provided materials for a burgeoning number of books on psychoanalytic therapies. Among these, the books by Brandschaft and Stolorow (1987), Chessick (1977), and Volkan (1987) aligned themselves with self psychology, and those by Goldstein (1985), Grotstein (1988), Masterson (1972, 1976), Rinsley (1982), and Searles (1986) were more aligned with object relations theory.

Against the backdrop of the debate between the Kernbergian and Adlerian-Kohutian models, another approach to psychotherapies developed. A growing number of experts wrote accounts about psychodynamic psychotherapies that were more pragmatic and eschewed either theoretical pole (e.g.,

Benjamin 1993; Gabbard and Wilkinson 1994; Gunderson 1984, 1996; Kroll 1993; McGlashan 1993; Paris 1998; Stone 1990, 1993). My own experience indicated that there was often a distinction in the use of the various therapies: the supportive techniques advocated by Adler are needed early in therapy, are crucial for therapies done without support from other modalities, and are the techniques essential for making borderline patients feel cared for and become attached (in a relational alliance). It also seemed apparent that the interpretations advocated by Kernberg can be essential for managing early negative transferences, that they become increasingly valuable over time, and that, as noted by Kernberg, they are crucial to helping borderline patients recognize and own unacknowledged and misdirected aggression. But—as noted by Kernberg's many critics, and a point emphasized by Gabbard et al. (1994)—the acceptance of such interpretations depends on the presence (even though transitory) of a working alliance (to be discussed).

Overview of Change Processes

Table 12–5 offers a schematic survey of the processes of change that can be expected over the course of long-term successful therapies with borderline patients. It mirrors changes described in Chapter 3 of this book (Table 3–3) but elaborates on those changes by adding processes within the therapy.

The timeline may vary considerably, but the sequence in which changes occur is quite predictable. Above all, the table highlights the fact that when change ceases, it is wise for therapists to seek consultation rather than assume that further change is not possible.

Several studies have examined the alliance between borderline patients and their therapists. As noted, this topic has been central to many psychoanalytic discussions (see Sidebar 3–2). In the McLean prospective repeated-measures study of 35 BPD patients who were beginning individual psychotherapies, a rather steady improvement in the *relational* type of alliance was observed (see Figure 12–1) (Gunderson et al. 1997). Although in the Menninger Treatment Intervention Project, the long-term course of the *working* alliance demonstrated overall improvements with one patient (Gabbard et al. 1988, 1994), the level of alliance in three other patients was still found to fluctuate dramatically, even after they were in therapy for several years (Horwitz et al. 1996). Of note in both studies is that the initial alliance scores were higher than expected (Gunderson et al. 1997; Horwitz et al. 1996).

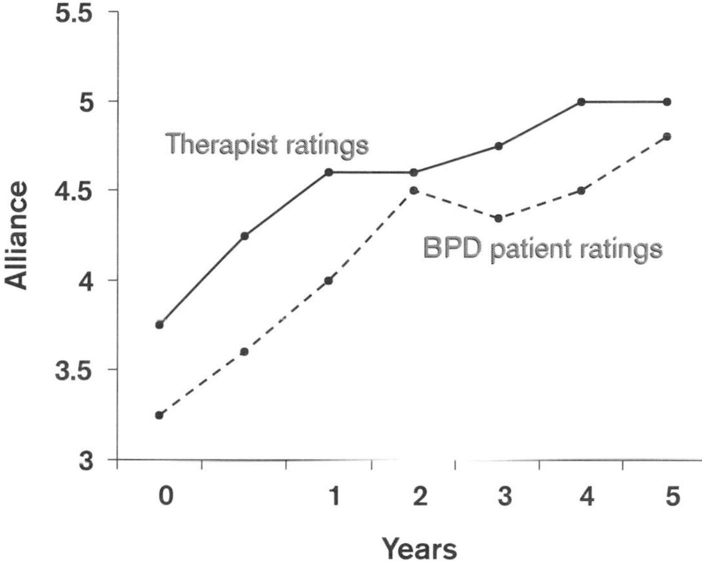

FIGURE 12–1. Change in therapist and patient ratings of their alliance during years of therapy.
Source. Adapted from Gunderson et al. 1997.

PHASE 2: A RELATIONAL ALLIANCE

After a patient has become engaged in therapy, the primary learning process involves behavioral control, and the primary relational process in the first year involves advancing from the contractual form of alliance, as discussed in Chapter 11 of this book, to establishing the second level of alliance, a relational alliance (see Table 12–5). With the borderline patient, a relational alliance involves likability, common goals, reliability, and hope for a better future (see Table 12–6). In effect the therapist becomes a selfobject (Stolorow 1995) or a transitional object (Giovacchini 1984; Modell 1963) with potential to offer corrective experiences.

The primary therapeutic techniques that make a relational alliance possible involve showing interest, conveying feasible expectations, possessing resilience in the face of opposition, and, above all, as emphasized by Adler (1986) and demonstrated by Stevenson and Meares (1992), deploying empathy and validation. Empathy involves acknowledgment of patients' dilemmas (e.g., "What a difficult situation," or "I can see why you were undecided")

TABLE 12–5. Indices of change in long-term psychotherapies

	Phase				
	Phase 1 (0–3 mo)	**Phase 2 (1 mo–1 yr)**	**Phase 3 (1 yr–2 or 3 yr)**	**Phase 4 (2 or 3 yr–?)**	**Result**
Change target	↓symptoms (moods)	↓self-destructiveness ↓impulsivity	↓maladaptive interpersonal problems ↓projection	↓splitting, leading to owning anger ↓Avoidance	↓emptiness ↑friends
Therapeutic relationship	Contractual alliance Agreed-upon goals and roles Counterdependent	Relational alliance Therapist valued Dependent/anxious	Relational alliance Therapy valued Dependent/positive	Working alliance Separation anxiety	Secure attachment
Major issues	Action, symptoms, fearfulness Anger and denial of anger Projection	Affect recognition and tolerance Accepting neediness Anger projected	Misattribution, assertiveness Fear of aggression Anger projected	Negative transference Reentering competition Developmental issues Trauma, self-image	Internal locus of control
Therapist activities	Interactive Responsive Educates and clarifies	Clarifies maladaptive responses to feelings (e.g., frustration) Validates and empathizes Develops formulation	Identifies conflicts and misattributions Supports functional capabilities Connects present to past	Interprets conflicts and transference Confronts avoidance	N/A
Outcome	Patient likes and is engaged by therapist	Capable of low-demand social role	Capable of low-demand relationships	Capable of competition, friendships	Patient does not have BPD

TABLE 12-6. Components of a relational alliance
Likability: responsive, real
Commonality: goals, interests, values
Reliability: conscientiousness, predictability
Hopefulness: change is possible; goals are attainable

and especially of their feeling states (e.g., "You must have been scared," or "You seem angry about that"). This is often complicated by a patient's fears that such feelings either are evidence of their "badness" or will be unacceptable to others. Fonagy and Target (1996) emphasized the corrective power of such interventions for those borderline patients whose feelings as children have been ignored, mislabeled, or rejected. They learn to observe themselves by being observed; to paraphrase Winnicott, they discover themselves in their mother's [or therapist's] eyes (Winnicott 1967). They also learn a useful new way to label and accept part of their experience.

Although patients' initial reaction to feedback about themselves is likely to be ambivalent, usually suspicious, and sometimes hostile, it helps to start by making observations at the surface. Uninvited observations by the clinician indicates that the clinician is attending to the task of helping patients learn about themselves. I often comment about facial expressions: "You look worried" or "You seemed sad when you talked about . . ." Actively identifying a patient's apparent feelings is most important when the patient looks either fearful or angry—feelings both of which may be hard to recognize or talk about and either of which, if not noted, can result in flight. Affirmation or disclosure by therapists about feelings, done with discretion, also asserts this process of *mentalization* (term developed by Fonagy [Fonagy 1991, 1995; Fonagy et al. 1995]): learning to represent feelings and affects in one's mind without action. It also presages a very important, recurrent thematic process in long-term therapies whereby borderline patients connect behaviors to events, to feelings, and to their thoughts.

Validation involves actively reinforcing the reality of borderline patients' perceptions and identifying the adaptive functions served by their defenses and behaviors. Of particular delicacy is the balance between listening sympathetically to disclosures of past mistreatment and, while validating the experience of unfairness, not assuming the validity of the realities as described (Gunderson and Chu 1994). This can be difficult, either because there is a natural impulse to convey support or because the borderline patient so clearly wants you to. It is usually sufficient to convey that the patient's life sounds as if it was awful, and that you can understand why, under such circumstances, they behave as they characteristically do.

Being liked occurs early (see Chapter 11 of this book) and is of value, but primarily because it helps create the engagement needed for a relational alliance. The valuation of *a therapist* is most directly a result of the therapist's empathy and validation. These activities make the therapist what is termed a good object. But valuing *therapy* derives from learning experiences. Interpretations or confrontations that bring to the patient's attention problems in themselves are activities that risk the therapist's becoming a bad object. Still, by 3–6 months, the value of the *tasks* in therapy should be evident in patients' reports that they've learned new things about themselves (Gunderson et al. 1997). Indeed, I like to underscore the therapy's task, understanding oneself, from the very first session by making observations about a patient and inquiring about whether he or she has learned anything new.

Empirical data that help identify key therapeutic processes are available from the Menninger Psychotherapy Research Project. As noted earlier, this study distinguished between two types of psychotherapy: expressive (meaning investigative, insight oriented, emotion generating) and supportive (meaning directive, defense reinforcing, emotion inhibiting). The original interpretation by Kernberg et al. (1972), buttressed by Guttman's formidable statistical techniques, was that the data indicated that expressive techniques and processes were effective. A reanalysis by Horwitz (1974) suggested that patients with borderline personality organization who had a strong therapeutic alliance with their therapists did improve significantly in supportive therapy. Wallerstein's (1986) further reanalysis of the data demonstrated that in actual practice almost all the therapies offered a less expressive—that is, less psychoanalytic and more supportive—approach than the study design called for. Moreover, patients frequently switched between treatment modes and between therapists. The study appears to yield quite different conclusions concerning the value of expressive therapy for borderline personality disorder. Kernberg has persisted in viewing expressive therapy as superior, whereas for Wallerstein and others the results pointed toward the critical role of supportive elements.

Of further note is the significance of relational factors emphasized in Stevenson and Meares' psychodynamic therapies. Stevenson and Meares (1992, 1999) defined their brand of therapy (and offered intensive supervision to assure adherence) as self psychological (Kohutian-Adlerian), with particular emphasis on empathic connection. The exploratory component focused on the identification of the inevitable triggers that disrupt that sense of connectedness. Thus the empirical evidence reinforces the clinical impression (Chapter 11 of this book) that supportive, attachment-generating interventions are critically important for successful psychotherapies. Notably, Linehan identified empathy and validation as critical components of DBT (Linehan 1993, 1997). The evidence offered from both Wallerstein (1986) and Stevenson and Meares that supportive, empathic interventions are critically important is consistent with the larger shifts in modern psychoanalytic thinking, which now, starting with Lang's "bipersonal field" (Lang 1976) and Gill's "dyadic relationship" (Gill 1979), have accepted the corrective power of relational processes (Lyons-Ruth 1998; Stern et al. 1998). For borderline patients this is a prototypical type of transitional object relatedness that can provide a "holding environment" (Modell 1976).

On reading Adler or Stevenson and Meares, there is a notable absence of concern about and focus on boundaries and behavioral control issues. This contrasts with the attention given to these issues by Kernberg, Linehan, and most others, including me. This first year in therapy is when the borderline patient's testing behaviors, or boundary violations (see Chapter 4 of this book) are most likely to occur. The primary benefits to be expected in this second phase of the first year of therapy are behavioral: fewer impulsive, desperate, and self-destructive behaviors. Although much attention has been given in the literature to the role of confrontations or limits in facilitating behavioral change, I believe that therapist activities in the area of learning or insight can also have a great deal to do with attaining the primary health and safety objectives of the first year.

The following vignette illustrates some of the processes that typify this phase of therapy, when the relational alliance is being built alongside a task orientation. This material illustrates my efforts to convert the meaning of depressive symptoms into maladaptive defensive phenomena—that is, convert the patient's depression into a meaningful communication of needs and fears. I use it also to introduce how a concept of mental deficits can link symptoms to meanings and how therapy can be transformative.

Vignette

Ms. K was 6 months into her thrice-weekly psychotherapy. She had started as an inpatient, moved through 3 months of partial hospital, and at this time was an outpatient. She appeared, looking pale and thin, walked slowly to her chair, seemed distracted, and didn't look at me.

Therapist: You look depressed. [a comment about a feeling]

Patient: I am.

Therapist: What's going on . . . how do you understand this? [a question]

Patient: I don't.

Therapist: I'm surprised you don't relate it to what we talked about last time, i.e., having started work . . . [a linking comment that creates a coherent narrative]

(Silence)

Therapist: Then, do you relate becoming depressed to starting work? [a question]

Patient: No.

Therapist [now I question her response to therapy, to me]: Does that mean that you think what I've been pointing out, interpreting, and even predicting about your depressions isn't correct? [I've been saying since we started that every time she takes a step toward more responsibility and less patient care, it represents a big threat to her and impels her to seek more supports.]

Patient (irritably interrupting): Yes, I know (rolls eyes disdainfully), every step forward will be followed by 10 backwards. I think that's just your theory.

Therapist: That theory helps explain why you're depressed: why taking a step—not a little one, by the way [here I provide validation]—like your new job, would predictably cause you to feel deprived and feel in need of more help. Unfortunately, to my mind, by becoming dysfunctional, you may evoke caring responses that you could otherwise attain more readily than you believe.

Patient: Fuck you.

Ms. K's depression can still be seen as an Axis I disorder: somatic symptoms (sleepless, lost appetite, anergic) with morbid preconceptions. Still, unlike earlier depressive episodes, at this time Ms. K is responsive to my efforts, even if she seems to disagree with the content of my remarks. My responses to her involve interpreting her depression as: 1) a regression in the face of abandonment and separation fears (including from the therapist) engendered by the job; 2) an angry attack on the meaning given to her depressive experiences in the therapy; 3) a communication of her need for added support.

I deploy a series of responses to Ms. K that are escalating in their intrusiveness and in their provocativeness—that is, in being difficult for her to ignore. First commenting, then questioning, and then a more affectively charged and interpersonally meaningful question: "Do you dismiss what we've talked about?" When I end up repeating the interpretation that put her depression into an interpersonal context—as fear of loss and an expression of need—the patient is affectively engaged with me. This aspect of the interaction highlights my readiness to get involved.

Let me add that though Ms. K seemed unable to see connections between her depression and recent events, and though she failed to validate my interpretative efforts, I believe these seemingly futile activities will make it increasingly difficult for her to ignore such connections in the future. This will change Ms. K's thinking from *teleological* to *intentional*. Whether the mechanism is conceptualized as education, transmuting internalization, or identification with the aggressor, or whether the effect is to subtly reconfigure the brain's neurophysiological response, the result is to introduce a disruptive new way of thinking. I believe that the prospect this offers—that her depressive experience can develop personal meaning—is an irresistibly hopeful and compelling message.

In this process, I am adding small increments to her capacity for thinking or introspection that will eventually allow her to be able to put words to her experience. A bridging conceptualization is offered by Fonagy's term *mentalization*, mentioned earlier in this chapter. Ms. K's childhood experience did not arm her with ways to label or identify her moods or her motivations. Either her feelings and motivations during childhood were mislabeled, or they were left unidentified, with the result that she is unable to conceptualize or communicate her inner experiences. From this perspective, the recurrence of her depression is a testimonial to the fact that she has not yet developed the ability to recognize the subtle precursory feelings or cognitions related to her depressed moods (e.g., her anxiety about the therapist's potential lack of interest or the early signals of her yearnings for supportive attention) that could foretell and forestall the emerging depressive state of mind.

The most central issue for helping borderline patients' insights to occur during the second phase involves helping patients understand how their wishes for caring attention prompt their interpersonal demands and evoke the rejections or anger that they fear (an issue repeatedly addressed with Ms. K). This issue is important for no one more than the therapist, who must help patients accept that their wish for caring attention is understandable and acceptable and that having those wishes frustrated prompts many of their behavioral problems. Although this issue sounds like transference analysis, it is usually first identified in situations outside the therapy: for example, "I knew that when your mother went on vacation you were likely to start drinking" or "When you leave the halfway house, as much as you hate it, it is going to represent a big loss for you." Such interpretations of meanings assigned to events by borderline patients underscore the therapist's role as an interested observer.

Other interpretations involve the defensive role of behaviors: for example, "You know when you yell that your husband will comply" or "Taking these drugs prevents you from feeling weak." Again, these are not transference interpretations; they are designed to increase self-awareness, and in the process they help patients to appreciate the therapist's ability to make their life more understandable. The primary use of transference interpretations involves the borderline patients' subtle or indirect expressions of hostility. This can become epidemic if not addressed, but hostility needs to be identified in a natural, instructive way, without implying that the patient has offended or scared the therapist—rather, the therapist can invite a more direct expression.

When interpretations are met by hostility, the patient's feelings need to be respected, but a therapist ought not to be apologetic; making observations is essential to a therapist's ability to be helpful. Indeed, I offer patients such observations in a psychoeducational way and buttress my observations by citing how well known and familiar such patterns of response are. In this way, the interpretation gets neutralized. (In much this same way, I believe Benjamin [1993] combines education with dynamic formulation.)

Obviously, the belief held by many borderline patients that "psychotherapy might help" after 6 months is enhanced by advances made both in the relational alliance and by any actual learning that has taken place. Though the former is essential, it should never be considered sufficient. By the end of 1 year, the patient should be involved in therapy and attached to the therapist (Table 12–5). This is another sign that the patient has fully achieved the goal of a relational (affective and empathic) alliance.

Continued involvement and investment by the therapist—as demonstrated by reliability, interest, and good judgment—evokes hope about the relationship that, in the first phase of treatment, is often experienced as dangerous vulnerability ("I'll get hurt, rejected," etc.). Still, most borderline patients consciously entertain the idea, some if not most of the time, that "this therapist cares." This idea only gradually becomes a conviction based on actual experience with the therapist, quite independently of whatever idealized or devalued attributions are professed about the therapist. (In response to requests for reassurance about caring, it is best to tell patients that the only way to know is through experience.) Unrealistic sexual or nurturant expectations (i.e., transferences) may fuel a borderline patient's attachment and will often endure well through the second year of a therapy. The quieter conviction about the therapist's caring for the patient is the bedrock for establishment of the relational alliance, and it develops slowly but inexorably from the largely nonverbal experience in the relationship.

PHASE 3: POSITIVE DEPENDENCY

Between 6 and 18 months of therapy, as has been shown in the previous examination of successful therapies (Waldinger and Gunderson 1989; Wallerstein 1986), positive dependency should have evolved. *Dependency* does not necessarily mean wanting to be told what to do; it primarily involves extreme sensitivity to the therapist's moods, attitudes, and absences. This is a type of relationship that can be established with nondynamic clinicians too, such as cognitive-behavioral therapists, case managers, or psychopharmacologists, although in these relationships the dependency is more apt to involve direction and reassurance. In essence, the therapist has become a transitional object (see Sidebar 12–2).

Sidebar 12-2: Transitional Objects–From Concept to Phenomenon

Winnicott (1953) identified the phenomenon in which children struggling with the recognition that their caregivers are separate from, not extensions of, themselves adopt inanimate transitional objects, whose presence can diminish their anxieties and whose absence causes great distress. This use has been confirmed (Roig et al. 1987). Although the use of transitional objects is not an uncommon phenomenon in normal development, it is particularly common (about 70%) for patients with borderline personality disorder, and it is significantly more common among them than among patients with other–most particularly antisocial–personality disorders (Arkema 1981; Cardasis et al. 1997; Horton et al. 1974; Morris et al. 1986). The sustained attachment to transitional objects in adults remains one of the simplest and most pathognomonic indicators for the diagnosis of BPD to nursing staffs, who bear witness to the importance placed on such objects (e.g., timeworn dolls, blankets, pandas) when borderline patients come to stay in hospital or residential settings.

Many borderline patients will deny being dependent on a therapist. Acknowledging their dependency is a cause of anxiety—particularly separation

("I'll be left") and paranoid ("I'll be mistreated") anxieties—that may evoke considerable defensive use of devaluation. Patients typically confess that "my therapist means too much"—thereby reflecting their dependency and their apprehension about it. Marking progress into phase 3, patients should no longer be denying a dependent attachment.

Under these circumstances—when dependency is acknowledged and the therapist is valued—patients are less resistant to self-disclosure and more responsive to learning from a therapist's observations. Many of the testing behaviors and boundary problems that characterized the first year are significantly diminished. The work of connecting feelings to situations and behaviors remains central. Similarly, the themes of needing caring attention and how their frustration can be managed without action recur. These themes can now be more easily addressed within the context of patients' responses to their therapist. This is the period in therapy when the exchanges can be quite intense, and a therapist's composure and containment can usually provide the needed holding without needing case management (parameters) or a second modality. Learning to think about the relationship of cause and effect, with respect to both feelings and interpersonal relationships, introduces delays of impulse discharge or avoidance behaviors. This learning to "think first" helps build affect tolerance. Mentalization, or being able to conceptualize, like any new habit, requires much repetition in order to be internalized (speaking psychologically) or to be embedded as new neural circuits (speaking biologically).

The Menninger study of alliance included a microanalysis of taped sessions from 39 BPD patients that documented multiple shifts in the level of collaboration (working alliance) within sessions (Allen et al. 1990). This work showed that advances apparent at one point in a session or even over longer periods of time will be dramatically reversed and then slowly regained. Nevertheless, I believe that the ontogeny of the alliance is a dialectic process, in which the more mature working form of the alliance progressively becomes more resilient and persistent over the course of therapy (see Figure 12–1) while the regressions from collaboration become less long lived and less dramatic. Within this iterative process, broad generalizations can be made about the time framework by which signs of a developing alliance should be noted. In phase 2, signs of a developing working alliance involve the ability to hear feedback without flight and with ability to think about the feedback. The absence of such signs once phase 1 ends is sufficiently troublesome that the viability and effectiveness of the therapy become questionable. For therapists, as Gabbard et al. (1994) pointed out, the rapid vicissitudes of the working alliance within sessions require therapists to be deft, resourceful, and adaptive in how they respond. In particular, he notes that interpretations are "high risk, high gain" interventions. This is especially true for the transference interpretations believed by Kernberg to be central.

Of value within the hurts and confusion due to projections, misunderstandings, and intense feelings is an ongoing review of what transpires in sessions in the interaction between patient and therapist. Not only does this mean a review within sessions of what was said, meant, etc.; this process is also greatly assisted by having sessions tape-recorded (Robbins 1988)—a technique introduced by Martin Orne to help Sylvia Plath (who probably had BPD; see Freed 1984). The encouragement to tape-record sessions is sometimes resisted, but once it is begun, borderline patients are usually quite responsive to what they can learn. Tape-recording makes possible a quite specific clarification of what "really" occurred (it's very nice to have a borderline patient volunteer that he or she understood what you said or why you said it). In addition, the tapes also serve (as can other office items) as concrete extensions of the therapist's involvement and attention between sessions—that is, as transitional objects (see Sidebar 12–2).

Therapists will allow themselves to be transitional objects and will want to make the silent functions that they serve as explicit as possible. Thus, for example, just as the therapist's task in the first year was helping the patient to understand that his or her actions stemmed from feelings and relational needs, in this second year (and third phase) it is valuable for the therapist to help the patient to identify what the patient depends on the therapist for. The essential component of this process will involve issues of not being alone and of feeling connected—in effect, issues involving object constancy. Being able to recognize this need to avoid aloneness will make such experiences more easily managed. Table 12–7 shows a hierarchy of ways in which prolonged separations from therapists can be managed. Although interpretations of intolerance of aloneness run the risk of imposing theory on a patient's experience, it is worth making these interpretations early and often, because awareness of this dilemma can so effectively diminish unnecessary regressive responses—and unnecessarily heroic acts of availability by therapists (see Gunderson 1996 and Sidebar 12–3).

Still, most interpretive or confrontational activity in the second year remains in the domain of connecting feelings and behaviors to interpersonal situations. Even though this activity occurs increasingly within the relationship to the therapist, it still does not quite conform to transference interpretations; it is learning to know oneself in new ways, not about oneself or why.

TABLE 12–7. Hierarchy of transitional options for use during therapist absences

1. Therapist accessible by phone
   As-needed call
   Prescheduled call
2. Therapist substitutes: coverage by colleagues
   Prescheduled meetings
   Meetings to be requested by the patient as needed
3. Therapist-associated transitional objects
   Tape-recorded sessions
   Notes from the therapist
   Cognitive-behavioral directives ("what to do")
   Items from the therapist's office
4. Self-initiated coverage options
   Increased contact with friends or relatives
   Increasing social networking (e.g., events, clubs)
   Distracting oneself (e.g., travel, movies)

Note. These options are generally needed only for absences of more than a week. Options are listed hierarchically from most soothing to least.
Source. Reprinted from Gunderson JG: "The Borderline Patient's Intolerance of Aloneness: Insecure Attachments and Therapist Availability." *Am J Psychiatry* 153(6):752–758, 1996. Used with permission.

Sidebar 12–3: Is Regression Therapeutic?–The Two Margarets

Although the capacity for borderline patients to regress in unstructured situations (from Rorschach tests to workplaces) was one of the first defining characteristics of borderline patients (Gunderson and Singer 1975), the clinical implications of this capacity have always teased therapists. There is the standard-issue warning: regressions are a danger in unstructured therapies. This danger was forcefully detailed by psychoanalysts who described the development of psychotic transferences in analyses (Hoch and Polatin 1949) or even psychotherapies (Frosch 1970; Zetzel 1971). Equally strong warnings were voiced against the danger of regression within unstructured milieu programs (Adler 1973; Knight 1953).

In contrast, in another tradition in psychoanalytic writing, regression is considered a necessary component of transference–necessary for a full transference to become convincingly evident to both patient and analyst. What is more difficult to trace is the idea that the therapist/analyst might then provide a corrective experience by fulfilling the patient's transference needs. Yet this is evident in Balint's (1992) book *The Basic Fault: Thera-*

peutic Aspects of Regression and is illustrated quite dramatically in practices deployed, with apparent success, by D. W. Winnicott in his treatment of Margaret Little (Little 1981).

Winnicott spoke openly with Dr. Margaret Little about the importance of completing a "full regression," even though she worked as a therapist more or less continuously during the 8 years of treatment. Winnicott responded to "the terrified child" that Little became "like" when she was in analysis. He was hesitant to note Little's strengths, because, in her "borderline" state (p. 24), she feared it meant losing him. He held her hands and extended the length of sessions when she was silent. He visited her daily at her home when she was ill. When she became terrified, he held her head and interpreted it as reliving her birth. He condemned her mother while explicitly providing the nurturance he felt Little's mother had failed to give, and to encourage Little's regression, he hospitalized her during one of his absences. Little reported that as a result of the therapy she went on to a more satisfying and stable interpersonal life and a successful career as a training analyst. She explicitly credited the power and learning of her "full regression" for enabling her to "find and free [her] true self" (p. 38).

Thirty-some years later, another female psychiatrist, Margaret Bean-Bayog, became infamous for efforts that were equally heroic, equally creative, and equally regressive. Bean-Bayog too did this to treat a very bright, promising, and tormented Harvard medical student with BPD. Here too, the therapist invited the patient's regression via addressing "the child within." She read children's books, inscribed gifts "for the baby," made herself available over vacations, arranged hospitalizations during her absences, and deliberately tried to provide Paul, her patient, with the nurturant attention he allegedly lacked from his mother. Paul did not improve. He had a series of hospitalizations that included a course of ECT, and after about 3 years this therapy eventually terminated. When Paul, unlike Margaret Little, ended up dead 6 months later (ostensibly by suicide but possibly from cocaine overuse), his family pursued legal action. As a result, the case became the featured topic of national news and two books (Chafetz and Chafetz 1994; McNamara 1994), and also as a result, Margaret Bean-Bayog regrettably lost her license to practice medicine.

Debates about the merits of regression are not related exclusively to borderline patients. The merits of regression were also actively debated in earlier literature about psychotherapy with schizophrenic patients (Gunderson and Mosher 1975). Underlying the claims for the effectiveness of long-term hospitalization were the claims of corrective action that the holding/parenting experiences given during such hospitalizations could provide for patients of many diagnostic types. Even now, reparenting is offered to some otherwise treatment-resistant anorexic patients.

In my view, what Margaret Bean-Bayog did was brave and potentially defensible—if all else had failed. The Margaret Little case offers a rationale that regressions might be powerfully helpful. It may be that Bean-Bayog just had the wrong patient, but I doubt it: regressive experiences can clearly be powerfully harmful for borderline patients.

I am skeptical about Margaret Little's conclusions. I suspect that an intensive schedule of sessions in which Little received the caring attention of an older, idealized man could have accomplished as much—maybe more quickly without the regressive transference enactments. At present, there may still be a role for deliberately regressive psychotherapy, but because of the dangers, regressions should be encouraged only when other therapies have failed and when the regressions are conducted with informed patient collaboration and ongoing professional consultations. At present, we have no guidelines regarding when regression is in the service of development.

A patient of mine once told me, "A need fulfilled will go away." I smiled skeptically, but sometimes I wonder.

The conclusion of phase 3 can occur as early as the end of the second year of therapy and usually occurs by year 3. At this point the borderline patient has acquired a capacity for stable, supportive relationships and a capacity for stable, low-demand work (see Table 12–5). At this point, many borderline patients can successfully leave therapy. They can get on with their lives if they have the good fortune of having established stable, supportive living or working situations. It is not unusual, for example, for borderline patients to find a romantic partner, or even a spouse, whose presence can greatly diminish the relational needs served by a therapist. Others find stable supports from extended families, self-help groups, or church communities that are sufficient. Borderline patients are still insecure about rejections, fearful about separations, and prone to cut themselves, drink, binge, rage, or withdraw in the face of conflicts. However, such reactions are less severe and less prolonged than before therapy or during phase 1. But patients are still unable to rely on a consistent inner locus of control; they remain too reactive (defiant or compliant) toward external pressures.

Phase 4: Secure Attachment, The Working Alliance, and Consolidation of Self

At this point, the psychotherapeutic techniques are no longer very specific to the borderline patient's psychopathology, except that the issues remain those unique to this diagnostic group. Although this phase is the least essential for mental rehabilitation, it is of the most indefinite duration (see Table 12–5).

A stable and increasingly secure relationship has formed, and a collaborative working alliance can generally be assumed. The capacity for a secure attachment to the therapist may at last become evident, meaning an attachment in which absences may cause anxiety or objections but do not require substitutes or any therapist-associated objects (see Table 12–7). The relationship is no longer contaminated by fears of rejection or abandonment, and criticisms, although unwanted, can be responded to effectively.

The direct expression of hatefulness toward the therapist that in Kernberg's theory is needed to remedy core psychopathology may occur during this phase. This behavior remains, in my experience, a critical process in rendering a borderline patient nonborderline. This process is not always possible: deeply ingrained moralistic prohibitions or deficient intellectual or organizational capabilities can prevent it. Nor does this process usually occur in the cathartic way that I had imagined. Rather, it is more likely to occur in the form of direct, cruel indictments over long periods of time, for which the therapist has become a safe container.

This is the phase of therapy when long-denied problems with early trauma can be revisited usefully or when the developmental regions of distortions in body image can be explored. Such issues may take years to open up and to have the needed desensitization or resolution occur. This process involves a patient's obtaining a coherent narrative of his or her life, without major gaps, thereby consolidating a sense of self.

Entering competition is always both desirable and conflictual for borderline patients insofar as it triggers fears of aggression and of rejection. In addition to clarifying such fears, therapists often need to actively urge borderline patients to compete. Competition requires that borderline patients take initiatives on their own behalf without guilt.

The acquisition of stable, nonsexual, intimate relationships is almost certainly a sign that someone is no longer borderline. The conclusion of this phase is marked by the patient's fullness of life—his or her investment in work and satisfaction from it and from relationships outside therapy.

IMPASSES

Usually, individual psychotherapies fail to achieve the initial and mutual goal of curative—or at least basic personality structure—changes. Table 12–8

TABLE 12–8. Major reasons for impasses ("can't leave, can't progress"): chronicity

Phase 2 (1 mo–1 yr)	Phase 3 (1 yr–2 or 3 yrs)	Phase 4 (2 or 3 yrs–?)
Too much frustration	Inadequate relational focus (transference)	Insufficient task (exploratory) orientation
Too little frustration	Insufficient vocational expectations	Insufficient support for non-therapy relationships (for life to replace therapy)
Insufficient attention to functioning	Overvaluation of the role of psychotherapy	Underestimation of the potential for normality

identifies the common reasons why impasses occur. The reasons vary within each phase of treatment.

Notably, whereas too much frustration in phase 2 causes dropout, too little causes regression. Because inexperienced therapists tend to worry too much about frustrating and thereby losing patients, they may become targets for devaluation and dismissal by borderline patients; or, more often, these therapists create a chronically dependent and potentially regressive relationship (see Sidebar 12–3). A major concern that all therapists need to be aware of is the capacity for borderline patients to regress in therapies that are too unstructured or seductive. This issue usually is not as obvious as that described in Sidebar 12–3, on the two Margarets. The issue more often takes the form of a patient's silent belief that his or her therapist is doing and will continue doing for the patient what he or she found lacking in their early parental relationships: listening kindly and empathically and offering an opportunity to be understood nonjudgmentally, spiced by some sound advice. Although this is not exactly a transference (insofar as the patient's attribution is exactly what the well-meaning therapist would say he or she is intentionally doing), the therapist is serving a parental role without examining its meaning and in the process may be perpetuating expectations for relationships that are unrealistic. Hence, the patient is grateful and dependent, but he or she is making no progress in the capacity for mature relationships outside the therapy. This type of therapeutic impasse, in my experience, is usually accompanied by a failure to address the patient's functional impairment. Such therapists may be too ready to sympathize with their patients' complaints about employers who are misunderstanding or their complaints about being assigned the same performance standards as other, less handicapped people.

On the other side of this dilemma is the reality that too much frustration will cause flight. "Too much frustration," with some borderline patients, may be very little. Some will perceive that any lack of reassurance, lack of indication of care, or sign of inattention is evidence of a therapist's cruelty or disinterest. The concept of a *negative therapeutic reaction* is appropriate here. These are the circumstances where readiness for psychotherapy needs to be evaluated. When "too much frustration" means an intolerance for confrontation or interpretation, then either less use of these techniques is required or the role of a second modality becomes critical. Early in the course of psychotherapies (phase 1 or phase 2), this second modality not only buffers transference distortions but also fulfills other and complementary goals (other modalities could be, e.g., sociotherapeutic or pharmacological; see Chapters 3 and 4 of this book).

As a further step-down refinement of the principle of split treatment, it is sometimes helpful to introduce a second individual clinician during the course of an intensive individual psychotherapy that is already under way. Stiver (1988) discussed how the introduction of an ongoing consultant (for 2 to 6 months) can mitigate the regressive (or, I would add, rageful) transferences that can develop. A further variation on this that I've seen successfully employed is the introduction of an intermittent cotherapist. The primary problem with such arrangements is not the danger of splitting but the potential that such use of a cotherapist may, if unexamined, verify the patient's belief in the destructiveness of his or her hostilities.

SUMMARY

Much of the clinical literature about psychoanalytic therapies has wrestled with the relative merits of supportive, attachment-enhancing interventions and those that are more explicitly insight-enhancing ones. In this chapter I have clarified the necessity of both the relational and the learning components if therapies are to be successful. Both empirical work and clinical experience document the overriding importance of supportive forms of intervention (e.g., empathy, validation, reassurance, clarification) during the second phase of therapy if the therapy is conducted within the agreed-upon usual framework. Nonetheless, it is of critical importance, even early in therapies, to underscore the tasks of therapy: to learn about oneself and to change as a result of what is learned. When this task orientation is combined with the development of a trusting and dependent relationship, the borderline patient will be able to function and the therapy will move into a third phase. During this period, the focus in sessions is often on the borderline patient's learning to identify his or her feelings and how they relate to the therapist's behaviors or words. The gradually improved ability to understand feelings correctly and to accept *unsupportive* feedback (e.g., interpretations, confrontations, impatience, criticisms) enables the patient to form stable relationships. The fourth phase of therapy will be more fully insight oriented, and the patient's ownership of hostilities and resolution of developmental failures allow the previously borderline patient to compete and to take independent, self-serving initiatives.

The hope that borderline patients can undergo curative change is justified, but such change rarely occurs. It is critically important that therapists appreciate the sequence of changes and their approximate timetable so as not to foreshorten unwittingly this long-term process.

References

Adler G: Hospital treatment of borderline patients. Am J Psychiatry 130:32–35, 1973

Adler G: Transference, real relationship and alliance. Int J Psychoanal 61(pt 4):547–558, 1980

Adler G: Borderline Psychopathology and Its Treatment. New York, Jason Aronson, 1986

Allen JG, Gabbard GO, Newsom GE, et al: Detecting patterns of change in patients' collaboration within individual psychotherapy sessions. Psychotherapy 27(4):522–530, 1990

Arkema PH: The borderline personality and transitional relatedness. Am J Psychiatry 138(2):172–177, 1981

Aronson TA: A historical perspective on the borderline concept: a review and critique. Psychiatry 48(3):209–222, 1985

Balint M: The Basic Fault: Therapeutic Aspects of Regression, Evanston, IL, Northwestern University Press, 1992

Benjamin LS: Interpersonal Diagnosis and Treatment of Personality Disorders. New York, Guilford, 1993

Brandschaft B, Stolorow RD: The borderline concept: an intersubjective viewpoint, in The Borderline Patient, Vol 2. Edited by Grotstein JS, Solomon MF, Lang JA. Hillsdale, NJ, Analytic Press, 1987, pp 103–126

Buie DH, Adler G: Definitive treatment of the borderline personality. International Journal of Psychoanalytic Psychotherapy 9:51–87, 1982

Cardasis W, Hochman JA, Silk KR: Transitional objects and borderline personality disorder. Am J Psychiatry 154(2):250–255, 1997

Chafetz GS, Chafetz ME: Obsession: The Bizarre Relationship Between a Prominent Harvard Psychiatrist and Her Suicidal Patient. New York, Crown, 1994

Chessick R: Intensive Psychotherapy of the Borderline Patient. New York, Jason Aronson, 1977

Clarkin JF, Yeomans FE, Kernberg OF: Psychotherapy for Borderline Personality. New York, Wiley, 1999

Fonagy P: Thinking about thinking: some clinical and theoretical considerations in the treatment of a borderline patient. Int J Psychoanal 72(Pt 4):639–656, 1991

Fonagy P: Playing with reality: the development of psychic reality and its malfunction in borderline personalities. Int J Psychoanal 76(Pt 1):39–44, 1995

Fonagy P, Target M: Playing with reality: theory of mind and the normal development of psychic reality. Int J Psychoanal 77(Pt 2):217–234, 1996

Fonagy P, Leigh T, Kennedy R, et al: Attachment, borderline states and the representation of emotions and cognitions in self and other, in Emotion, Cognition, and Representation (Rochester Symposium on Developmental Psychopathology, Vol 6). Edited by Cicchetti D, Toth SL. Rochester, NY, University of Rochester Press, 1995, pp 371–414

Freed AO: Differentiating between borderline and narcissistic personalities. Social Casework 65(7): 395–404, 1984

Frosch J: Psychoanalytic considerations of the psychotic character. J Am Psychoanal Assoc 18:24–50,1970

Gabbard GO, Wilkinson SM: Management of Countertransference with Borderline Patients. Washington, DC, American Psychiatric Press, 1994

Gabbard GO, Horwitz L, Frieswyk S, et al: The effect of therapist interventions on the therapeutic alliance with borderline patients. J Am Psychoanal Assoc 36(3):697–727, 1988

Gabbard GO, Horwitz L, Allen JG, et al: Transference interpretation in the psychotherapy of borderline patients: a high-risk, high-gain phenomenon. Harv Rev Psychiatry 2(2):59–69, 1994

Gill MM: The analysis of the transference. J Am Psychoanal Assoc 27(suppl):263–288, 1979

Giovacchini PL: The psychoanalytic paradox: the self as a transitional object. Psychoanal Rev 71(1):81–104, 1984

Goldstein WN: Introduction to Borderline Conditions. New York, Jason Aronson, 1985

Grotstein JS: Transitional phenomena and the dilemma of the me/not-me interface, in The Solace Paradigm: An Eclectic Search for Psychological Immunity. Edited by Horton PC, Gewirtz H, Kreutter KJ. Madison, CT, International Universities Press, 1988, pp 59–74

Gunderson JG: Borderline Personality Disorder. Washington DC, American Psychiatric Press, 1984

Gunderson JG: The borderline patient's intolerance of aloneness: insecure attachments and therapist availability. Am J Psychiatry 153(6):752–758, 1996

Gunderson JG, Chu JA: Treatment implications of past trauma in borderline personality disorder. Harv Rev Psychiatry 1(2):75–81, 1994

Gunderson JG, Mosher LR (eds): Psychotherapy of Schizophrenia. New York, Jason Aronson, 1975

Gunderson JG, Singer M: Defining borderline patients: an overview. Am J Psychiatry 132:1–10, 1975

Gunderson JG, Frank AF, Katz HM, et al: Effects of psychotherapy in schizophrenia, II: comparative outcome of two forms of treatment. Schizophr Bull 10:564–598, 1984

Gunderson JG, Frank AF, Ronningstam EF, et al: Early discontinuance of borderline patients from psychotherapy. J Nerv Ment Dis 177(1):38–42, 1989

Gunderson JG, Zanarini MC, Kisiel C: Borderline personality disorder, in DSM-IV Sourcebook, Vol 2. Washington, DC, American Psychiatric Press, 1996, pp 717–733

Gunderson JG, Najavits LM, Leonhard C, et al: Ontogeny of the therapeutic alliance in borderline patients. J Psychotherapy Research 7(3):301–309, 1997

Hoch P, Polatin P: Pseudoneurotic forms of schizophrenia. Psychiatr Q 23:248–276, 1949

Horton PC, Louy J, Coppolillo HP: Personality disorder and transitional relatedness. Arch Gen Psychiatry 30:618–622, 1974

Horwitz L: Clinical Prediction in Psychotherapy. New York, Jason Aronson, 1974

Horwitz L: Clinical and projective assessments of borderline patients. Paper presented at a symposium, The Borderline Patient: A Multiaxial View, Department of Psychiatry, University of Miami School of Medicine, Key Biscayne, FL, 1982

Horwitz L, Gabbard GO, Allen JG, et al: Borderline Personality Disorder: Tailoring the Psychotherapy to the Patient. Washington, DC, American Psychiatric Press, 1996

Howard KI, Kopta SM, Krause MS, et al: The dose-response relationship in psychotherapy. Am Psychol 41:159–164, 1986

Kernberg O: Borderline personality organization. J Am Psychoanal Assoc 15:641–685, 1967

Kernberg O: The treatment of patients with borderline personality organization. Int J Psychoanal 49:600–619, 1968

Kernberg O: Final report of the Menninger Foundation's psychotherapy research project: summary and conclusions. Bull Menninger Clin 38:181–195, 1972

Kernberg OF, Burstein ED, Coyne L, et al: Psychotherapy and psychoanalysis (final report of the Menninger Foundation's Psychotherapy Research Project). Bull Menninger Clin 36:1–275, 1972

Kernberg O, Selzer M, Koenigsberg HW, et al: Psychodynamic Psychotherapy of Borderline Patients. New York, Basic Books, 1989

Knight R: Borderline states. Bull Menninger Clin 17:1–12, 1953

Kohut H: The Analysis of the Self. New York, International Universities Press, 1971

Kroll J: The Challenge of the Borderline Patinet: Competency in Diagnosis and Treatment. New York, WW Norton, 1988

Linehan MM: Cognitive-Behavioral Treatment of Borderline Personality Disorder. New York, Guilford Press, 1993

Linehan MM: Theory and treatment development and evaluation: reflections on Benjamin's "models" for treatment. J Personal Disord 11(4):325–335, 1997

Little MI: Transference Neurosis and Transference Psychosis. New York, Jason Aronson, 1981

Lyons-Ruth K: Implicit relational knowing: its role in development and psychoanalytic treatment. Infant Mental Health Journal 19:282–289, 1998

Masterson J: Treatment of the adolescent with borderline syndrome (a problem in separation-individuation). Bull Menninger Clin 35:5–18, 1971

Masterson J: Treatment of the Borderline Adolescent: A Developmental Approach. New York, Wiley, 1972

Masterson J: Psychotherapy of the Borderline Adult. New York, Brunner/Mazel, 1976

McGlashan TH: Implications of outcome research for the treatment of borderline personality disorder, in Borderline Personality Disorder: Etiology and Treatment. Edited by Paris J. Washington, DC, American Psychiatric Press. 1993, pp 235–260

McNamara E: Breakdown: Sex, Suicide, and the Harvard Psychiatrist. New York, Pocket Books, 1994

Meares R, Stevenson J, Comerford A: Psychotherapy with borderline patients, I: a comparison between treated and untreated cohorts. Aust N Z J Psychiatry 33:467–472, 1999

Modell A: Primitive object relationships and the predisposition to schizophrenia. Int J Psychoanal 44:282–291, 1963

Morris H, Gunderson JG, Zanarini MC: Transitional object use and borderline psychopathology. Am J Psychiatry 143(12):1534–1538, 1986

Najavits LM, Gunderson JG: Better than expected: improvements in borderline personality disorder in a 3-year prospective outcome study. Compr Psychiatry 36(4): 296–302, 1995

Paris J: Working with Traits: Psychotherapy of Personality Disorders. Northvale, NJ, Jason Aronson, 1998

Rinsley D: Borderline and other Self Disorders. New York, Jason Aronson, 1982

Robbins M: Use of audiotape recording in impasses with severely disturbed patients. J Am Psychoanal Assoc 36(1):61–75, 1988

Roig E, Roig C, Soth N: The use of transitional objects in emotionally-disturbed adolescent inpatients. International Journal of Adolescence and Youth 1(1):45–58, 1987

Sabo AN, Gunderson JG, Najavits LM, et al: Changes in self-destructiveness of borderline patients in psychotherapy: a prospective follow-up. J Nerv Ment Dis 183(6):370–376, 1995

Searles HF: My Work with Borderline Patients. Northvale, NJ, Jason Aronson, 1986

Stanton AH, Gunderson JG, Knapp PH, et al: Effects of psychotherapy in schizophrenia, II: design and implementation of a controlled study. Schizophr Bull 10:520–563, 1984

Stern D, Sanders L, Nahum J, et al: Noninterpretive mechanisms in psychoanalytic therapy: the "something more" than interpretation. Int J Psychoanal 79:903–921, 1998

Stevenson J, Meares R: An outcome study of psychotherapy for patients with borderline personality disorder. Am J Psychiatry 149(3):358–362, 1992

Stevenson J, Meares R: Psychotherapy with borderline patients, II: a preliminary cost benefit study. Aust N Z J Psychiatry 33:473–477, 1999

Stiver IP: Developmental dimensions of regression: introducing a consultant in the treatment of borderline patients. McLean Hospital Journal 13:89–107, 1988

Stolorow RD: An intersubjective view of self-psychology. Psychoanalytic Dialogues 53:393–399, 1995

Stone MH: Treatment of borderline patients: a pragmatic approach. Psychiatr Clin North Am 13(2):265–285, 1990

Stone MH: Abnormalities of Personality: Within and Beyond the Realm of Treatment. New York, WW Norton, 1993

Volkan VD: Six Steps in the Treatment of Borderline Personality Organization. New York, Jason Aronson, 1987

Waldinger RJ: Intensive psychodynamic therapy with borderline patients: an overview. Am J Psychiatry 144(3):267–274, 1987

Waldinger RJ, Gunderson JG: Completed psychotherapies with borderline patients. Am J Psychother 38(2):190–202, 1984

Waldinger RJ, Gunderson JG: Effective Psychotherapy with Borderline Patients: Case Studies. Washington, DC, American Psychiatric Press, 1989

Wallerstein R: Forty-Two Lives in Treatment. New York, Guilford, 1986

Winnicott DW: Transitional objects and transitional phenomena. Int J Psychoanal 34:89–97, 1953

Winnicott DW: The Mirror-role of mother and family in child development, in The Predicament of the Family: A Psychoanalytic Symposium. Edited by Lomas P. London, Hogarth Press, 1967, pp 26–33

Zetzel ER: A developmental approach to the borderline patient. Am J Psychiatry 127:867–871, 1971

13

Future Considerations

PATIENTS WITH BORDERLINE PERSONALITY DISORDER are an imposing presence within clinical populations. The validity of the diagnosis is now widely accepted by clinicians (B. Pfohl, K. Silk, C. Robins, M. Zimmerman, and J. Gunderson, "Attitudes Towards Borderline PD: A Survey of 752 Clinicians," unpublished data, May 1999). Moreover, the disorder has attained the forms of validation traditionally given by academic psychiatry in specificity about its familial transmission, developmental risk factors, course, and treatment (Gunderson 1994; Paris 1994). This is a remarkable achievement, since recognition of this diagnosis has only emerged within a 30-year time span. There is, however, a glaring need for good epidemiological data to document the incidence, prevalence, and natural comorbidities of this disorder. There remains also a glaring need to document the enormous social and public health significance of this disorder. The diagnosis is still new, and, within the present historical context of radical changes in health care and the neurosciences, the diagnostic construct and the treatments recommended for these patients will undoubtedly undergo further change in the years ahead. In this chapter I anticipate what these changes are likely to involve.

The Diagnosis: Self-Disorder and Relationship to DSM-IV Axes I and II

The recognition and usage of this diagnosis arose because of the particularly troublesome and specific problems these patients create for unsuspecting health care providers: regressive responses to usual supports, intense transferences, splitting the treaters, nonresponsiveness to treatments for comorbid

DSM-IV (American Psychiatric Association 1994) Axis I diagnoses, noncompliance with or overdosing on medications, and intense, hateful countertransference responses. The value of the borderline diagnosis in helping clinicians anticipate and explain this set of troubling and specific problems will not disappear.

Still, the borderline diagnosis itself faces challenges. One challenge involves its name. Even those who strongly endorse the construct argue that "borderline" is an adjective that belies the disorder's categorical integrity and that the name carries psychoanalytic baggage that can mislead treatment and can turn off families, pharmaceutical companies, and many mental health professionals. Despite these unfortunate reactions, I believe that to change this name would mistakenly underestimate the clinical traditions that sustain interest in these patients; I also believe that any of the alternative names (e.g., emotional dysregulation personality disorder or mood/impulse personality disorder) could unwisely prejudice the ongoing search for identification of the core aspects of borderline psychopathology (discussed below).

A second challenge relates to BPD's place in the nosological system. Some of the current personality disorders may be better conceptualized as extreme variants of normal personality, others as spectrum variants of Axis I disorders (see Figure 13–1). As discussed in Chapter 2 of this book, the high rates of comorbidity with selected Axis I disorders and with other personality disorders leaves BPD still vulnerable to being considered a "wastebasket diagnosis" (Hudziak et al. 1996). Despite these concerns, I believe that BPD should survive as a self-disorder, given priority akin to Axis I disorders (Gunderson 1994, 1999). BPD's extensive validation, its severity of impairment, and its specificity of treatment needs should, I believe, withstand the otherwise valuable pruning of the present Axis II classification system.

The Search for the Core Psychopathology of Borderline Personality Disorder

Table 13–1 identifies major theories about the core (i.e., basic, underlying, requisite) psychopathology of borderline personality disorder that has derived from clinical observations. Some of these theories have attributed core psychopathology to constitutional (i.e., temperamental) variables with predominantly genetic origins. Others have emphasized environmentally induced character failures. These theories have all emphasized failures in early preborderline children's experience with their primary caregivers. Advocates for any

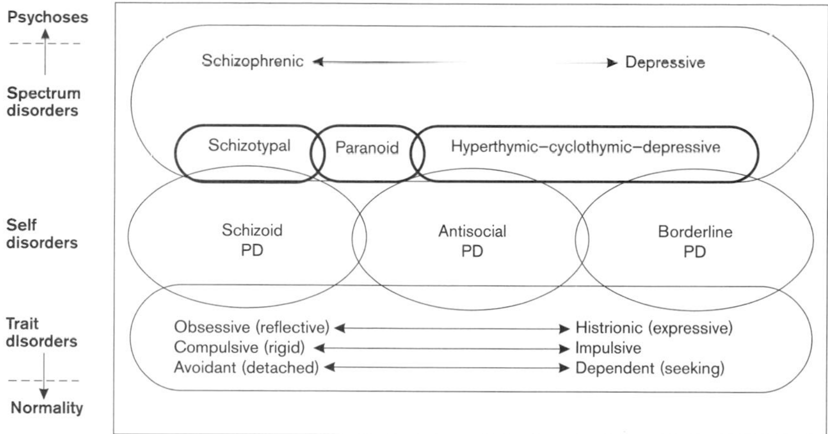

FIGURE 13–1. Relationship of BPD with other personality disorders.
Source. Adapted from Gunderson and Phillips 1995.

of these theories, as noted throughout this book, use them to organize their clinical practices. Increasingly, these theories are becoming subjects for research. Mahler and Kaplan (1977), for example, showed that rapprochement failures, assigned a central role by Masterson, are neither necessary nor sufficient cause for BPD. The theory of affective dysregulation was disconfirmed by testing emotional responses to excitatory photographs and finding that borderline subjects' responses were similar to those of normal control subjects (Herpetz et al. 1999). On a more positive note, work on attachment failures by Fonagy et al. (1999) and others (Lyons-Ruth 1998) seems to confirm their potential explanatory power.

TABLE 13–1. The core psychopathology of BPD: seminal clinical theories

Excessive aggression: Kernberg (1967)	T or E[a]
Abandonment anxieties secondary to rapprochement failures: Masterson (1972)	E
Affective dysregulation: Klein (1975); Akiskal (1981); Stone (1979); Linehan (1993)	T
Intolerance of aloneness secondary to attachment failures: Gunderson and Singer (1975); Adler and Buie (1979); Fonagy (1991)	E
Complex posttraumatic stress disorder: Herman (1992)	E

[a] T = primarily a temperamental disposition; E = primarily an environmentally caused disposition.

A significant recent development is the effort to identify the core dimensions of psychopathology from the scientifically based perspectives of neurobiology or academic psychology. Table 13–2 indicates that almost all the scientifically based hypotheses about BPD's core psychopathology involve formulations of a core temperament—that is, the heavily genetically determined way in which a child perceives and reacts to the environment. Yet very few medical illnesses are purely genetic—none within psychiatry. Even a disorder such as schizophrenia almost certainly involves multiple genes, whose penetrance (i.e., whether the gene is manifestly, meaning phenotypically, expressed) depends on environmental conditions or stimulation. Thus an interaction between temperament (genetic disposition or tendency) and environmental conditions determines whether an illness occurs.

TABLE 13–2. BPD's core psychopathology: scientific perspectives from biology and psychology

Affective/impulsive psychobiological disposition (T)[a]	Siever and Davis (1991)
High reward dependence (T) Low harm avoidance (T) Low self-transcendence (E)	Cloninger (1987)
Emotional dysregulation (T)	Livesley et al. (1993)
High nurturance needs (E) Angry response to frustrations (E)	Benjamin (1993)
High neuroticism (T) Low agreeableness (E)	Costa and Widiger (1994)

[a] T = primarily a temperamental disposition; E = primarily an environmentally caused disposition.

BPD reflects this interactional complexity. Until recently, the only twin study was too small to be persuasive, but, by showing no concordance in three monozygotic twin pairs and in only two of seven dizygotic pairs, it suggested that BPD has a low level of heritability (Torgersen 1984). This is congruent with the overwhelming evidence indicating severe environmental failures and/or stressors during childhood for borderline patients (Gunderson and Zanarini 1989; Paris 1992; Zanarini et al. 2000). Still, the usual level of heritability operating for normal personality types is about 50% (Tellegen et al. 1988) and in subsequent analyses with a larger sample, Torgersen has demonstrated a similar level of heritability for BPD (Torgerson et al., in press).

As research sorts out the relative strengths of these scientifically based theories, the theories can be expected to gain more importance for practicing clinicians. For example, with respect to Costa and McCrae's (1990) widely acclaimed "Big Five" factors of normal personality, the theory suggests that individuals with high neuroticism *and* low agreeableness (a combination that would occur in only a minority of the population) will possess a temperament predisposing them to the development of BPD (Widiger 1994; Widiger et al. 1991). Such high-risk individuals could then be targets for preventive interventions (e.g., education of their parents, school counseling). From another perspective, these dimensions of personality can be used as outcome variables. Neuroticism could, for example, prove responsive to SSRIs, whereas low agreeableness might improve only after individual psychotherapy based on self psychology. It can be expected that the other variables contending for the core role (Table 13–2) would, once verified, similarly be targets for intervention.

BRAIN MEETS MIND: FRONTIERS FOR BPD IN THE NEUROSCIENCES

Advances in the neurosciences are forcing a conceptual and clinical revolution in which the traditionally distinct conceptions of the brain and the mind are being ever more closely linked. The concepts and language by which to communicate these changes are still in a primitive state. Reflecting this already outdated division is the identification by the National Alliance for the Mentally Ill (NAMI) of only a few psychiatric disorders as "brain diseases" to distinguish them from other disorders that are "mental illnesses." As Sidebar 13–1 describes, for a disorder like BPD, which has clear, strong environmental causes, this distinction of brain and mind has had unfortunate political consequences.

Sidebar 13–1: Is BPD a Brain Disease or Not?

The problem with the question is that it presumes distinctions that don't exist. The primary brain diseases, according to the National Alliance for the Mentally Ill (NAMI), are schizophrenia, manic-depressive disorder, and depressive disorder. Still, it is easy to find scientific evidence demonstrating that psychosocial factors are important in causing or treating these alleged brain diseases. They are not diseases that are the inevitable, or probably even the usual, expressions of some heritable dispositions. People with these diseases vary enormously in the degree to which the etiology is genetic and in what types of environmental problems contribute to their pathogenesis.

On another level of scientific evidence, the traditional dichotomy of body and mind is increasingly debatable. Environmental events affect gene expression; trauma can have the same effect on brain neurophysiology as genetic disposition; psychotherapy affects brain anatomy; placebos can mimic antidepressants in their effect on brain functioning; and all mental learning is recorded neurologically and then affects the brain's aptitude for processing and the ways in which it processes subsequent stimuli (Kandel 1998).

So what about BPD? Since all etiological and therapeutic schemes with respect to BPD include psychosocial factors, is it therefore not a brain disorder? No. If *brain disease* means that BPD psychopathology must be located in the brain, of course it is. If *brain disease* means including heritable dispositions, of course BPD does. (Whether what's inherited involves affect dysregulation, impulsivity, neuroticism, or excessive hostility is controversial. Yet 50% of "normal" personality is also heritable.) If *brain disease* means including neurobiological abnormalities, of course BPD does. Lowered intersynaptic serotonin levels and the like have all been found in patients with BPD (Coccaro et al. 1989). If *brain disease* is meant only to designate chronic, severely dysfunctional public health disorders, BPD surely qualifies. Therefore, if these definitions are included when some severe mental illnesses are identified as brain diseases, then BPD is a brain disease.

A powerful coalition of NAMI and academic psychiatrists have pushed the hope that major, severe ("real") mental illnesses should be set apart as brain diseases. This campaign is designed to link these designated mental illnesses conceptually to other organ-specific medical illnesses like heart or lung disease. The purpose of removing the mind from these mental illnesses is to focus attention on genetic and neurobiological etiological forces. When this concept is used to exclude psychosocial components from considerations of etiology or treatment, the concept is a shortsighted one.

It is now evident that environmental events have great influence on gene expression and that psychotherapies can influence neural capacities in just the way medications do (Kandel 1998). Advances made in the study of anxiety disorders (Gorman 1996) will almost certainly be a template for what can be expected for BPD. With respect to anxiety disorders, a spectrum of neural activities is associated with the spectrum of clinical anxiety: terror is heavily encased by the amygdala, responding to stimuli before conscious perception.

Panic attacks involve the limbic regions of the brain, and, although panic is linked to perceptions, the connection isn't rational (e.g., as in panic triggered by a mouse). Being worried occurs in the frontal cortex and almost always has rationalization in its associated mental content—although, of course, some individuals worry more or less than others because of a temperamental disposition, such as neuroticism.

How can these ideas apply to BPD? When a father wrote to his alienated borderline daughter that, if she remained unemployed, they would need to discuss rearranging her budget, she anxiously told her therapist that her father was planning to "cut off" her funding. Her dialectical behavior therapy (DBT) therapist thought that her reaction was due to emotional dysregulation—that an emotion of inappropriate intensity had erupted, to which she attached inappropriate ideas. Her psychoanalytic therapist thought that her reaction was due to her father's message having evoked a withdrawing, punitive part-object. Her cognitive therapist believed this was all-or-nothing thinking due to her inability to manage uncertainties, that is, not knowing. Her interpersonal therapist believed she altered (consciously or unconsciously) her father's message to evoke a sympathetic and protective response from her therapist. Teasing apart these competing theoretical possibilities can be assisted by having a better map of where and how her father's message was processed in the brain. The use of cognitive, emotional, or pharmacological activation to look at functional brain imaging is a frontier where investigations are just beginning (Teicher et al. 1994).

It is possible that early abuse or other traumatic experiences lead to neuropsychological difficulties in processing information and in memory (Post 1992; Teicher et al. 1994). But it remains unclear whether affect drives cognitive and memory problems, or vice versa—that is, whether cognitive and memory problems render someone vulnerable to intense, inappropriate emotional responses (O'Leary and Cowdry 1994). The science of learning, memory, and perceptions has still rarely been applied to the perceptual and mental processes of borderline patients. An illustrative application is found in a study by Bohus et al. (1999). These researchers are studying the ability of borderline patients to use a psychophysiological monitor of emotional arousal as a signal to improve their self-awareness and then invoke appropriate self-soothing strategies.

Of equal promise are studies examining the neurobiological effects of early separation experiences. Those conducted with primates have already shown a clinical picture similar to abandonment depression when rhesus monkeys were separated from their mothers; the degree to which this syndrome was ameliorated by imipramine was related to the state of the brain's development when the separation occurred (Suomi 1985). The recent surge of interest in studying human infant attachment behaviors offers wonderful opportunities to test theories about the centrality of insecure attachments to later development of BPD (Hazan and Shaver 1994). Here too it can be expected that the impact of failed attachment will be detectable in brain imaging or neurophysiological measures that may become markers for risk of later BPD.

Development of Specialists and Special Services

This book's recurrent messages have implications for the care of borderline patients. First, a range of services is usually needed. It is and always has been rare for any individual with BPD to make major gains from any one therapy. The hope that one person or one modality might effect such gains has most frequently been attributed to individual psychotherapy delivered by experts. Yet accounts of successful individual therapy show that it has almost always used other modalities (considered adjunctive), such as long-term hospitalization, medications, or family meetings. Even with an optimal, skilled individual therapist (primary a clinician), treatment with other modalities will facilitate change and address some problems better than individual therapy could.

A less explicit but even more compelling message in this book is that standards of clinical care need to be defined because, in their absence, bad things often happen: regressions, psychotic transferences, noncompliance, increasing self-destructiveness, and lawsuits. Borderline patients have achieved a bad reputation, because when treated wrongly, they become worse, and their hostilities and behavioral problems become unmanageable. Because of this the American Psychiatric Association is writing practice guidelines for BPD treatment.

An implication of these basic messages is that specialists and specialized clinical services are needed. A proposal was outlined by the European branch of the International Society for the Study of Personality Disorders (ISSPD) in 1998 to develop identifiable centers in each European country for specialized training, research, and treatment services for personality disorders, with obvious reference to borderline patients (ISSPD Newsletter 1998). Such centers are clearly justifiable; borderline patients are known to be a significant (15%–20%) clinical presence everywhere that they've been systematically looked for (Gunderson 1999). Table 13–3 identifies components that a BPD specialty

TABLE 13–3. Components of BPD specialty centers

Special services at all levels of care primarily designed for BPD patients
Clinicians primarily dedicated to the care of BPD
Expertise (as measured by recognized leadership, e.g., invited talks, publications)
All modalities available (minimally including psychopharmacology, individual, and group therapies)
Research on BPD
Special training programs for treating BPD
Family support services
Public advocacy/education

center might optimally include. At present, if such specialty services were to require being able to provide all levels of care and to have skilled, enthusiastic, collaborative practitioners in multiple modalities, only a very few such centers would be available.

From this perspective, knowledgeable and comprehensive treatment for BPD patients is rarely available. In the United States, most major departments of psychiatry or major psychiatric hospitals have staff who are identified as experts on borderline personality disorder, but only a small number have a BPD-related specialty service. Most of the time, borderline patients have the components of their treatment administered by people or services without skill, experience, or enthusiasm. This deplorable situation is even worse in most countries outside the United States.

Economic, scientific, and clinical forces all push for the development of specialized services and clinical specialists to treat borderline patients. The economic forces will be further pushed by documentation of the enormous public health costs of this diagnostic group, from the perspectives of both health care utilization (see Bender et al., in press; Walker et al. 1999) and vocational disability (for example, A. E. Skodol, T. H. McGlashan, C. M. Grilo, R. L. Stout, and J. G. Gunderson, unpublished manuscript, July 2000). The economic incentive will become further magnified by the current cost-benefit consciousness. Even managed-care organizations, who dread long-term care, recognize that the revolving door in hospitalizations and emergency rooms signifies the failure and cost ineffectiveness of nonspecialized and short-term treatments. Insofar as the first year of treatment can make serious changes in self-destructive and/or suicidal behaviors, it can greatly reduce health care costs. The costs to society of unemployment and interpersonal conflicts far exceed health care costs. To address these problems requires longer-term treatments with both rehabilitative and interpersonal goals.

The scientific forces that encourage specialization for BPD are propelled by the increasing body of evidence that diagnosis-specific, manual-guided therapies for BPD invariably exceed generic types in their efficacy (and cost effectiveness).

The clinical forces are described throughout this book: many clinicians don't like working with these patients; poorly conceived and executed therapies easily and frequently result in patients' getting worse, with subsequent liability issues for the treaters. Above all, the proper care of these patients at every level of the health care system, and with every modality, involves very distinctive features customized to the particular needs of this patient group.

Credentialing Therapists

A very important lesson that has emerged from the recent efforts to study the efficacy of therapies with borderline patients is the difficulties that investigators discover in training motivated trainees to achieve competence. Much was made of this in Chapter 11 of this book, and its implications are quite profound.

First of all, although this problem may be true for many therapies, I am convinced that it is more true for borderline patients than for any other patient group. The most obvious implication is that one cannot easily generalize from efficacy studies to one's own clinical practice or clinical setting. Also obvious is that excellence in one modality, such as psychoanalytic therapy, does not translate easily into expertise in another modality, such as DBT or family psychoeducation. More worrisome is that, although it seems that standards need to be established for clinicians who undertake therapies with borderline patients, it is not clear how this is feasible. A natural-selection system has always existed, but this system is a good one only if clinicians who are not capable with borderline patients choose (or are selected out by colleagues) to see fewer of them, and that clinicians who do well with borderline patients will choose to work with them or will get more referrals. The experience of both Linehan and Kernberg is that self-selected would-be practitioners of their quite different treatments often are not well suited to borderline patients. In the ongoing study at the Karolinska Institute in Sweden (J. F. Clarkin, personal communication, November 1999; also discussed in Chapter 12 of this book), it is clear that training therapists to become adherent to either a DBT or a psychoanalytic therapy model is very time consuming and fraught with difficulties. Some reasons for this are obvious. To do well, one must be empathic and flexible, and both modalities require composure in the face of predictably intense feelings and demands. As noted in Chapter 11 of this book, to attain such composure, in my experience, therapists usually need to have had several years' exposure within residential or hospital settings where structures, supports, and collaboration are built in.

In 1998, the European Branch of the ISSPD approved a plan to develop quality assurance guidelines for personality disorder assessment and interventions that require that they be audited and monitored to ensure high standards. The introduction of quality assurance considerations is difficult. (Table 13–4 outlines the sort of rigorous credentialing requirements that a new therapist might expect.) On an informal basis, quality assurance is conducted by clinicians' having supervision and being required to present cases to others for feedback. Supervision provides both support and continuing education and is sufficient for most purposes. Certainly, the development of the specialty centers discussed previously in this chapter will be extremely useful to those who work there in this way. Auditing and monitoring outside such settings would require unforeseeable pressures from professional organizations—pressures that seem very unlikely.

TABLE 13–4. Proposed credentialing requirements for primary clinicians/therapists treating borderline patients

Experience
___ [to be identified] years of exposure to borderline patients within residential/inpatient units
___ [to be identified] hours of 1-to-1 contact in either psychopharmacological or nonintensive psychotherapies
Training
___ [to be identified] hours of supervision by a qualified (credentialed) professional in the modality to be practiced
Didactic training in the theory and technique of the modality
Working knowledge of the relevant BPD-specific literature for the modality
Mental health
Good affect tolerance, empathic ability, self-sufficiency

STANDARDS OF CARE

In 1997, the development of BPD practice guidelines was authorized by the American Psychiatric Association, and in fall 1998, the committee, chaired by John Oldham, began the task of reviewing literature. The committee's initial draft was completed in spring 2000, and the ensuing process of review and revision is continuing as this book is published. Although much of what these guidelines will include can be expected to overlap with this book's content, this book is not constrained by the same consensus-building processes or by the inherent reservations about clinical theory or experience.

What I would propose as standards of care (see Table 13–5) contains little that is empirically based. Readers will recognize that the rationale for these guidelines has been anchored in the experiences and literature included in this book. Adoption of these standards would require radical changes in the present health service system. It is probably feasible to expect these standards to be met only in specialty centers (as described above). At present the types and quality of care available to these patients are highly variable. Without standards of care, a natural selection process will continue, with the risk that cost containment will be more valued than cost benefit.

TABLE 13–5. Standards of care for borderline personality disorder in the year 2000

BPD patients and their significant others should receive psychoeducation about this diagnosis and its treatment.
Treatments should be tailored to meet goals for change agreed to by the BPD patient.
BPD patients should have a primary clinician (Chapter 4) who is experienced with borderline patients or is under skilled supervision.
Impulsive BPD patients should have two or more collaborating components in their treatment (Chapters 3–6, 9, 10) until they are stabilized in the community.
The least restrictive level of care consistent with safety and social rehabilitation should be used (Chapter 5).
BPD patients should be offered medications with the explicit expectation of partial relief and with plans to test the effects of tapered dosage every few months thereafter (Chapters 6 and 7).
Self-injurious patients should be offered cognitive-behavioral skills training (Chapter 8).
Therapists who offer psychotherapy should be trained to give BPD-specific therapies or be under skilled supervision (Chapter 11).
Psychodynamic psychotherapy should be reserved for BPD patients without disabling social and vocational impairments (Chapter 11).

Note. All chapters cited are in this book.

Public Awareness and Advocacy

The dramatic expansion of communications via the Internet is making information available about private concerns, like psychiatric disorders, that were otherwise uninvestigated because of fear or shame. On one level, the privacy and distance that communication via the Internet allows has provided isolated borderline individuals with a means of finding support from peers (Ginther 1997; Silk 1997). On another level, it encourages families and others to learn about this condition safely. As shown in Sidebar 13–2, many types of information are available for consumers.

Sidebar 13–2: Borderline Personality Disorder on the Internet—Proceed Enthusiastically...With Caution

by Jason Fogler, M.A.

Much of the growth in self-help and consumer empowerment that has taken place in this decade can be attributed to the accessibility to information offered by the Internet, specifically the World Wide Web. The Internet allows users to gather a tremendous amount of information in a vastly shorter period of time than it would take to gather the same information from a library, for instance. In addition, the Internet allows users to gather (and publish) information at a protective, anonymous distance. For these reasons, many people with BPD, their relatives, and clinicians use the Internet as a preferred outlet for support networks and for gathering and disseminating information about the illness.

Since the Internet is in constant flux and transformation, it would be impossible to accurately survey the BPD-relevant Web sites that are available when this is being read. However, I would recommend beginning any Internet search about BPD with these two sites:

- BPD Central (http://www.bpdcentral.com/)
- Mental Help Net (http://www.mentalhelp.net)

Unlike other Web sites about BPD, both are overseen by professionals (Paul Mason, M.S., C.P.C., and Randi Kreger, BPD Central; and Mark Dombeck, Ph.D., Mental Help Net), and both sites provide regularly updated, comprehensive links to, and evaluations of, the available BPD Internet resources, including Web sites and e-mail or live-chat support groups.

In addition, a comprehensive database of professional journal articles—has become available on the Net at

- Medline (http://www2.ncbi.nlm.nih.gov/PubMed/)

This comprehensive database of articles from journals in every field of medicine is a superb psychoeducational resource; articles cited on Medline are all from journals that have publication criteria.

- Rating Criteria for Mental Health Sites (http://www.mentalhelp.net/help/ratings.htm

This rating criteria site, by John Grohol, is a fine example of critical reviews of Web sites. Caution needs to be exercised with many Web sites, which may not have publication criteria or check Webmasters' credentials. Anyone can publish on many Web sites, and at present, Webmasters are not required to publish such disclaimers as "This site is not a substitute for professional advice and counseling" (although, thankfully, many do). As with any service, I strongly encourage consumers to consider the source of a Web site's information carefully and to check that information against professional advice and research.

Bridging the gap between clinicians and families has far-reaching consequences. The fact, cited earlier, that family members usually do not define themselves as patients means that they can easily convert their parental hopes for better treatment and their alliance with the treating clinicians into advocacy. This has been dramatically evident in the success of national organizations like NAMI and the National Depressive and Manic-Depressive Association (National DMDA), who have relentlessly worked to decrease stigma and increase research into mental illnesses. The same need is evident for borderline patients. They have a chronic disease, of great public health significance, that enormously burdens families who too often are deeply shamed by it.

In 1993, Valerie Porr founded an organization in New York City, Treatment And Research Advancements: Association for Personality Disorder (TARA APD), dedicated to advocacy. In 1995, a small group of graduates ("veterans") of the PE/MFGs described in Chapter 9 of this book formed a similar organization, the New England Personality Disorders Association (NEPDA). Both organizations are struggling to increase membership, develop avenues for funding, and draw attention to the little-recognized plight of this population.

These goals have received support from two publicized events. In the best-selling book, *Diana in Search of Herself: Portrait of a Troubled Princess,* her biographer, Sally Bedell Smith (1999), identified the famous princess as having BPD. Shortly thereafter, Susanna Kaysen's (1993) book *Girl, Interrupted* became an acclaimed movie, in which the borderline diagnosis, though viewed skeptically by Kaysen, was much discussed. An even better route to public recognition would be a living celebrity who has or did have BPD becoming a spokesperson who would work to educate the public about this disorder and destigmatize it (see Sidebar 13–3).

Sidebar 13-3: Were a Famous Borderline to Go Public...

It would be a major step forward for someone with fame to identify himself or herself publicly as having BPD. Of course, most people with this disorder are either too dysfunctional to achieve fame or, if able to achieve it, too ashamed of or insecure about their inner devils to want to go public. The most famous person until Princess Diana to have been alleged to have this disorder was Marilyn Monroe. Her life has been the subject of many biographies, all of which capture her desperation, her impulsivity, and her series of clinging, demanding, ultimately failed relationships, culminating in suicide. There have been others whose borderline personality has been inferred, such as Sylvia Plath and Judy Garland.

Should such a famous person go public with the illness, he or she could at best evoke a public outcry for better recognition, less stigma, more research, and better clinical services. Princess Diana's desperate life evoked sympathy. It was only after her death that her biographer identified her as having BPD and chronicled how her public persona reflected her inner emptiness and her lack of access to good treatment (in spite of wealth and position).

As welcome as the coming out of a much-beloved spokesperson would be, it seems more likely that a famous person with BPD would surface because of venting the negative side of this personality–for example, through unreasonable demands or violence. This behavior might of course evoke a counterproductive public attitude toward the community of borderline patients that the celebrity could come to represent.

The ability of famous individuals to go public effectively as an advocate for both more compassionate attitudes and better clinical services probably requires that they have already benefited significantly from treatment. There is increasing reason to believe that better-quality care will yield a new generation of borderline patients who privately, if not publicly, will become advocates for themselves. One of them may also become famous.

Both NEPDA and TARA APD hope to convert the despair of BPD patients into protests and public action. These efforts will be buttressed by recent and improved research documenting that comorbidity with BPD accounts for much of the resistance to treatment of anxiety and mood disorders—disorders that have far more extensive recognition, research, and insurance support—and by documentation of the enormous costs to society of BPD, both in disability and in liability.

Among the early initiatives of both NEPDA and TARA APD are these:

- Petitioning NIMH to create a well-informed brochure—long overdue for a population that constitutes 15% of clinical populations
- Sponsoring talks that are open to the public
- Publicizing newsletters and Web sites to disseminate information—including research findings and events whereby parents and interested others may learn more and, more importantly, take action on behalf of the mentally ill

A by-product of advocacy groups is the development of social support networks for families and for patients. In the past, I've often been grateful if a borderline patient had a substance abuse problem sufficient to warrant their taking advantage of the round-the-clock, no-cost support network offered by Alcoholics Anonymous (AA). Now the mental health community should encourage the development of self-help support groups for borderline patients, modeled on AA and the National DMDA. Such groups have the potential to help reduce the aloneness and isolation that borderline patients experience after they've given up their acting out or other attention-getting behaviors. Such groups also offer a semicontrolled opportunity to care and be cared for, support self-esteem, and provide ongoing self-financed psychoeducational services (Brightman 1992). Here too the self-help groups will be particularly valuable for patients who have given up the "bad habit" of demanding exclusivity (begetting rejections that typify prototypical borderline relationships) but who still have unfulfilled wishes for relationships and often have modest social skills.

Everyone in the mental health disciplines should applaud the efforts of NEPDA and TARA APD. It has taken strength for families to become spokespersons for the very offspring who often condemn them. Without doubt, the goals of these organizations are the same as those of clinicians who labor in different ways to be helpful.

The Swiss Foundation

As this book was written, a remarkable gift has been given by an anonymous Swiss donor. A foundation has been established to support research on borderline personality disorder. The foundation has funded four sites that are using multidisciplinary, highly sophisticated methods to examine the neurobiology, genetics, and psychotherapeutics of BPD. As a side effect, this initiative has engaged world-class scientists who otherwise know little about BPD, both in the research effort and in consultative and administrative roles. An immediate dividend of the financial and intellectual strength of this initiative has been the heightened awareness by NIMH, pharmaceutical companies, and other foundations of the need for more research attention to this extremely needy and underrepresented patient population. The possibilities are breathtaking.

SUMMARY

In the past 30 years an industrious and diverse group of clinicians and scientists have created a space for borderline personality disorder in the collective minds of the mental health community. The results of these efforts are evident in the greatly expanded body of knowledge about this disorder. This book has reviewed the advances in treatment of persons with BPD, and it makes clear, I hope, that we already know enough to significantly improve the prognosis of these patients. Knowledge will continue to grow. The more immediate task is to implement and disseminate what is already apparent. For those tasks, this book is intended to provide a template.

The space created for the borderline diagnosis exists on another, more abstract level. For the mental health field it provides a needed asylum for creative theory building and research. This disorder has thus far warded off conceptual reductionism or the constraints of entrenched standards of care. BPD is not the intellectual or clinical property of psychoanalysts, of psychologists or psychiatrists, of researchers or clinicians, of theoreticians or practitioners. All are part "owners" who remain vitally necessary contributors. I hope that the book communicates the excitement and challenge of being a part of this community.

In the years ahead, a different task awaits. It is of critical importance to the welfare of these patients that their tragedies—and their potential for change enter the collective mind of the larger society of which the mental health community is only a small part. Successfully attaining this much higher level of collective consciousness will be assisted by initiatives from those who are prepared to become public advocates. However, this attainment will ultimately rest upon the appeal for rescue that, to their credit, these patients continue to evoke.

REFERENCES

Adler G, Buie DH Jr: Aloneness and borderline psychopathology: the possible relevance of child development issues. Int J Psychoanal 60:83–96, 1979

Akiskal HS: Subaffective disorders: dysthymic, cyclothymic and bipolar II disorders in the "borderline" realm. Psychiatr Clin North Am 4(1):25–46, 1981

American Psychiatric Association: Diagnostic and Statistical Manual of Mental Disorders, 4th Edition. Washington, DC, American Psychiatric Association, 1994

Bender DS, Dolan RT, Skodol AE, et al: Treatment utilization by patients with personality disorders. Am J Psychiatry (in press)

Benjamin LS: Interpersonal Diagnosis and Treatment of Personality Disorders. New York, Guilford, 1993

Bohus M, Ebener U, Stiglmayr C, et al: On the development of interactive, outpatient monitoring of psychophysiological and endocrinological parameters among patients with a borderline personality disorder. Paper presented at the Sixth International Congress of the International Society for the Study of Personality Disorders, Geneva, Switzerland, September 1999

Brightman BK: Peer support and education in the comprehensive care of patients with borderline personality disorder. Psychiatric Hospital 23(2):55–59, 1992

Cloninger CR: a systematic method for clinical description and classification of personality variance. Arch Gen Psychiatry 44:573–588, 1987

Coccaro E, Siever L, Klar H et al: Serotonergic studies in patients with affective and personality disorders: correlates with suicidal and impulsive aggressive behavior. Arch Gen Psychiatry 46:587–599, 1989

Costa PT Jr, McCrae RR: Personality disorders and the five-factor model of personality. J Personal Disord 4(4):362–371, 1990

Costa PT Jr, Widiger TA (eds): Personality Disorders and the Five-factor Model of Personality. Washington, DC, American Psychological Association, 1994

Fonagy P: Thinking about thinking: some clinical and theoretical considerations in the treatment of a borderline patient. Int J Psychoanal 72(pt 4):639–656, 1991

Fonagy P, Target M, Gergely G: Attachment and borderline personality disorder: a theory and some psychiatric evidence. Psychiatr Clin North Am 23(1):103–122, 1999

Ginther C: The Web as resource for patient advocacy groups. Psychiatric Times, November 1997

Gorman JM: The New Psychiatry: The Essential Guide to State-of-the-Art Therapy, Medication and Emotional health. New York, St Martin's Press, 1996, p 388

Gunderson JG: Building structure for the borderline construct. Acta Psychiatr Scand (suppl) 379:12–18, 1994

Gunderson JG: Personality disorders, in The New Harvard Guide to Psychiatry. Edited by Nicholi AM. Cambridge, MA, Harvard University Press, 1999

Gunderson JG, Phillips KA: Personality disorders, in Comprehensive Textbook of Psychiatry, 6th Edition. Edited by Kaplan HI, Sadock BJ. Baltimore, MD, Williams & Wilkins, 1995, p 1450

Gunderson JG, Singer M: Defining borderline patients: an overview. Am J Psychiatry 132:1–10, 1975

Gunderson JG, Zanarini MC: Pathogenesis of borderline personality, in American Psychiatric Press Review of Psychiatry, Vol 8. Edited by Tasman A, Hales RE, Frances AJ. Washington, DC, American Psychiatric Press, 1989, pp 25–48

Hazan C, Shaver PR: Attachment as an organizational framework for research on close relationships. Psychological Inquiry 5(1):1–22, 1994

Herman J: Trauma and Recovery. New York, Basic Books, 1992

Herpetz SC, Kunert HJ, Schwenger UB, et al: Affective responsiveness in borderline personality disorder: a psychophysiological approach. Am J Psychiatry 156:1550–1556, 1999

Hudziak JJ, Boffeli TJ, Kreisman JJ, et al: Clinical study of the relation of borderline personality disorder to Briquet's syndrome (hysteria), somatization disorder, antisocial personality disorder, and substance abuse disorders. Am J Psychiatry 153(12):1598–1606, 1996

ISSPD Newsletter, Vol 3, no 1, December 1998

Kandel ER: A new intellectual framework for psychiatry. Am J Psychiatry 155:457–469, 1998

Kaysen S: Girl, Interrupted. New York, Random House, 1993

Kernberg O: Borderline personality organization. J Am Psychoanal Assoc 15:641–685, 1967

Klein D: Psychopharmacology and the borderline patient, in Borderline States in Psychiatry. Edited by Mack I. New York, Grune & Stratton, 1975, pp 75–92

Linehan MM: Cognitive-Behavioral Treatment of Borderline Personality Disorder. New York, Guilford, 1993

Livesley WJ, Jang KL, Jackson DN, et al: Genetic and environmental contributions to dimensions of personality disorder. Am J Psychiatry 150:1826–1831, 1993

Lyons-Ruth K: Implicit relational knowing: its role in development and psychoanalytic treatment. Infant Mental Health Journal 19:282–289, 1998

Mahler M, Kaplan L: Developmental aspects in the assessment of narcissistic and so-called borderline personalities, in Borderline Personality Disorders: The Concept, the Syndrome, the Patient. Edited by Hartocollis P. New York, International Universities Press, 1977, pp 71–86

Masterson J: Treatment of the Borderline Adolescent: A Developmental Approach. New York, Wiley, 1972

O'Leary KM, Cowdry RW: Neuropsychological testing results in borderline personality disorder, in Biological and Neurobehavioral Studies of Borderline Personality Disorder. Edited by Silk KR. Washington, DC, American Psychiatric Press, 1994, pp 127–157

Paris J: Social risk factors for borderline personality disorder: a review and hypothesis. Can J Psychiatry 37(7):510–515, 1992

Paris J: Borderline Personality Disorder: A Multidimensional Approach. Washington, DC, American Psychiatric Press, 1994

Post RM: Transduction of social stress into the neurobiology of recurrent affective disorder. am J Psychiatry 149:999–1010, 1992

Siever LJ, Davis KL: A psychobiologic perspective on the personality disorders. Am J Psychiatry 148:1647–1658, 1991

Silk K: Email, transitional relatedness, and borderline patients. Paper presented at the 5th International Congress on the Disorders of Personality, Vancouver, BC, Canada, June 1997

Smith SB: Diana in Search of Herself: Portrait of a Troubled Princess. New York, Times Books/Crown Publishing, 1999

Stone M: Contemporary shift of the borderline concept from a sub-schizophrenic disorder to a subaffective disorder. Psychiatr Clin North Am 2:577–594, 1979

Suomi SJ: Response styles in monkeys: experiential effects, in Biologic Responses Styles: Clinical Implications. Edited by Klar H, Siever LJ. Washington, DC, American Psychiatric Press, 1985, pp 1–17

Teicher MH, Ito Y, Glod CA, et al: Early abuse, limbic system dysfunction, and borderline personality disorder, in Biological and Neurobehavioral Studies of Borderline Personality Disorders. Edited by Silk R. Washington, DC, American Psychiatric Press, 1994, pp 177–207

Tellegen A, Lykken DT, Bouchard TJ, et al: Personality similarity in twins reared apart and together. J Pers Soc Psychol 54:1031–1039, 1988

Walker EA, Unutzer J, Rutter C, et al: Costs of health care use by women HMO members with a history of childhood abuse and neglect. Arch Gen Psychiatry 56:609–613, 1999

Widiger TA: Conceptualizing a disorder of personality from the five-factor model, in Personality Disorders and the Five-Factor Model of Personality. Edited by Costa PT, Widiger TA. Washington, DC, American Psychological Association, 1994

Widiger TA, Frances AJ, Harris M, et al: Comorbidity among Axis II disorders, in Personality Disorders: New Perspectives on Diagnostic Validity. Edited by Oldham JM. Washington, DC, American Psychiatric Press, 1991, pp 165–194

Widiger TA, Trull TJ, Clarkin JF, et al: A description of the DSM-III-R and DSM-IV personality disorders with the five-factor model of personality, in Personality Disorders and the Five-Factor Model of Personality. Edited by Costa PT, Widiger TA. Washington, DC, American Psychological Association, 1994, pp 41–58

Zanarini MC, Frankenburg FR, Reich DB, et al: Biparental failure in the childhood experiences of borderline patients. J Personal Disord 14(3):264–273, 2000

Index

*Page numbers printed in **boldface** type refer to tables or figures.*
Page numbers followed by an s refer to sidebars.

B

D

E

F

G

J

K

N

O

P

R

S

T

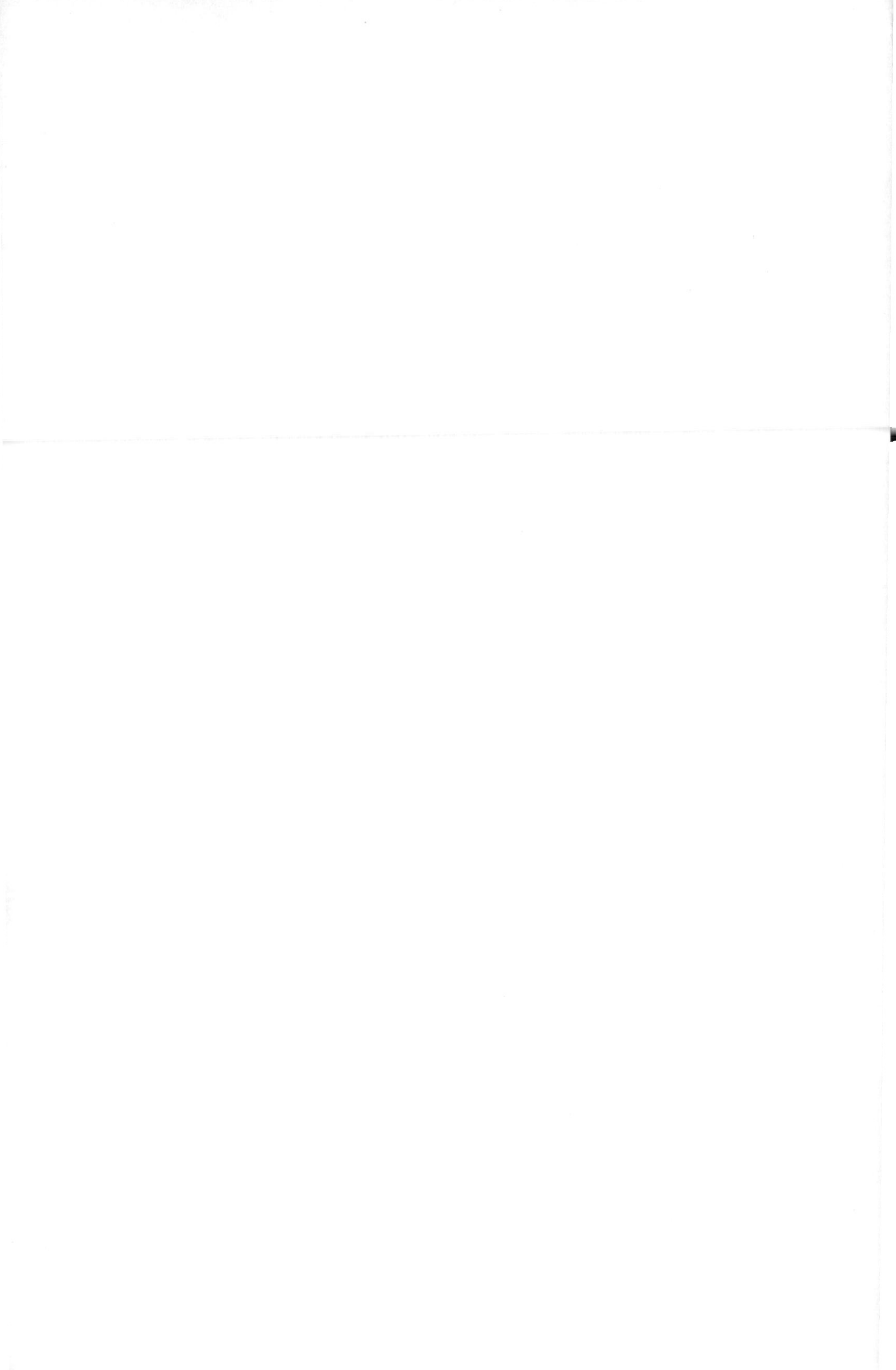